D1759123

Surgical

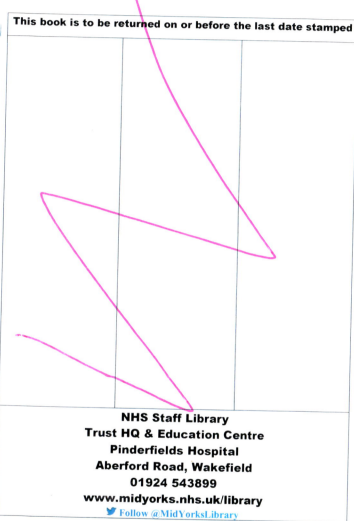

013622

Surgical pathology of the mouth and jaws

R.A. Cawson MD, FRCPath, FDS, RCS and RCPS (Glasgow)
Emeritus Professor of Oral Medicine and Pathology
Department of Surgery
Guy's Hospital
London

J.D. Langdon MB, BS, FDS, MDS, FRCS
Professor of Oral and Maxillofacial Surgery
King's College School of Medicine and Dentistry
London

J.W. Eveson BDS, PhD, FRCPath, FDS, RCS and RCPS (Glasgow)
Reader in Oral Pathology
Bristol Dental School
University of Bristol

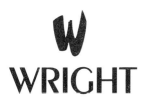

WRIGHT

Wright
An imprint of Butterworth-Heinemann
Linacre House, Jordan Hill, Oxford OX2 8DP
225 Wildwood Avenue, Woburn, MA 01801-2041
Reed Educational and Professional Publishing Ltd

A member of the Reed Elsevier plc group

OXFORD AUCKLAND BOSTON
JOHANNESBURG MELBOURNE NEW DELHI

First published 1996
Paperback edition 2000

British Library Cataloguing in Publication Data
A catalogue record for this book is available from
the British Library

ISBN 0 7236 1083 5

Typeset by BC Typesetting, Bristol
Printed in Scotland by Cambus Litho Ltd, Glasgow

Contents

Preface x

1 Investigational methods 1
Clinical investigation 1
Surgical biopsy 1
Frozen sections 4
Limitations of histopathological diagnosis 5
Immunocytochemistry 7
Fine-needle aspiration cytology 8
Simple aspiration 10
Exfoliative cytology 10
Aspiration and other ancillary methods –
conclusions 11
DNA hybridization and the polymerase chain
reaction 11
Radiography and other imaging
techniques 11
Salivary flow measurement 14
Laboratory investigations 14
Medical assessment of the patient 14
References 15

**2 Major infections of the mouth, jaws and
perioral tissues 16**
Acute osteomyelitis 16
Osteoradionecrosis and radiation-associated
osteomyelitis 19
Chronic osteomyelitis 20
Chronic osteomyelitis in childhood 21
Chronic specific osteomyelitis 21
Chronic focal sclerosing osteomyelitis 21
Chronic osteomyelitis with productive
periostitis (non-suppurative osteomyelitis,
Garrés osteomyelitis) 22
Diffuse sclerosing osteomyelitis 22
Pulse granuloma (chronic periostitis) of the
jaw 23
Sclerotic (dense) bone islands (idiopathic
osteosclerosis) 23

Fascial space infections (cervicofacial
cellulitis) 23
Cavernous sinus thrombosis 26
Necrotizing fasciitis 27
Cancrum oris (noma) 27
Soft tissue abscesses 28
Actinomycosis 29
The deep mycoses 30
Systemic infections by oral bacteria 35
References 37

**3 Cysts and cyst-like lesions of the
jaws 38**
Apical periodontal (radicular) cysts 40
Paradental cysts 44
Dentigerous (follicular) cysts 44
Eruption cysts 45
Gingival cysts 45
Lateral periodontal cysts 46
Botryoid and sialo-odontogenic cysts 46
Odontogenic keratocysts 47
Primordial cysts 51
Calcifying odontogenic cyst 51
Nasopalatine, incisive canal and related
cysts 52
Globulomaxillary cyst 53
Nasolabial cyst 53
Median mandibular cyst 53
Cyst-like lesions without epithelial lining 54
Cystic neoplasms 56
Benign mucosal cysts of the antrum 57
Sublingual dermoids 57
References 58

**4 Odontogenic tumours and tumour-like
lesions 59**
Ameloblastoma 59
Odontoameloblastoma 63

Malignant ameloblastoma and ameloblastic carcinoma   63
Primary intra-alveolar carcinoma   64
Adenomatoid odontogenic tumour   64
Calcifying epithelial odontogenic tumour   65
Clear cell odontogenic carcinoma   66
Odontogenic ghost cell tumour (calcifying odontogenic cyst, Gorlin cyst)   67
Odontogenic ghost cell carcinoma   67
Squamous odontogenic tumour   67
Ameloblastic fibroma   68
Ameloblastic sarcoma (ameloblastic fibrosarcoma)   69
Odontogenic myxoma   70
Odontogenic fibroma   71
Cemental tumours and dysplasias   71
Odontomas   76
References   78

5   Non-odontogenic tumours of the jaws   79
Ossifying (cemento-ossifying) fibroma   79
Osteoma and other bony overgrowths   79
Osteochondroma   80
Osteoid osteoma and osteoblastoma   81
Giant cell granuloma of the jaw   82
Osteosarcoma   84
Chondroma and chondrosarcoma   86
Chondrosarcoma   86
Chondromyxoid fibroma (fibromyxoid chondroma)   88
Chondroblastoma   89
Ewing's sarcoma   90
Desmoplastic fibroma   91
Fibrosarcoma of bone   92
Malignant fibrous histiocytoma   92
Haemangioma of bone   93
Angiosarcoma of bone   94
Leiomyosarcoma of bone   94
Melanotic neuroectodermal tumour of infancy   94
Primary lymphoma of bone   95
Multiple myeloma and solitary plasmacytoma   96
Amyloidosis   97
Langerhans cell histiocytosis   98
Eosinophilic ulcer (atypical or traumatic eosinophilic granuloma)   100
Metastatic tumours   100
References   101

6   Genetic, metabolic and other non-neoplastic bone diseases   103

Craniofacial defects – surgical considerations   103
Facial clefts and associated anomalies   103
Hemifacial microsomia (Goldenhar syndrome, oculo-auriculovertebral dysplasia, first and second branchial arch syndrome)   105
Down's syndrome (mongolism; trisomy 21)   106
Osteogenesis imperfecta (brittle bone syndrome)   107
Osteopetrosis (marble bone disease)   108
Hypophosphatasia   109
Cleidocranial dysplasia   109
Marfan's syndrome   110
Sickle cell disease and the thalassaemias   110
Fibro-osseous lesions   112
Fibrous dysplasia   112
Cherubism   114
Paget's disease of bone   116
Hyperparathyroidism   118
Idiopathic osteosclerosis (solitary bone islands)   119
Massive osteolysis (phantom bone disease)   120
References   120

7   Disorders of the temporomandibular joints and periarticular tissues   122
Limitation of movement (trismus)   122
Permanent limitation of movement (ankylosis)   123
Pseudoankylosis   123
Extracapsular ankylosis   123
Intracapsular ankylosis   126
Arthritis and other causes of pain in or around the joint   126
Cranial arteritis   129
Pain dysfunction syndrome   130
Condylar hyperplasia   132
Neoplasms   132
Loose bodies in the temporomandibular joints   133
Dislocation   133
References   134

8   Diseases of the oral mucous membranes   136
INFECTIONS   136
Primary herpetic stomatitis   136
Herpes labialis   138
Herpes zoster of the trigeminal area   138

Hand-foot-and-mouth disease   139
Cytomegalovirus infection   140
The acute specific fevers   140
Kawasaki's disease (mucocutaneous lymph node syndrome)   140
Tuberculosis   140
Syphilis   140
Candidosis   142
NON-INFECTIVE ULCERATION   142
Traumatic ulcers   142
Aphthous stomatitis (recurrent aphthae)   143
Behçet's syndrome   145
Lichen planus   146
Lupus erythematosus   149
Pemphigus vulgaris   150
Darier's disease (keratosis follicularis)   152
Epidermolysis bullosa   152
Mucous membrane pemphigoid   153
Linear IgA disease   154
Dermatitis herpetiformis   155
'Desquamative gingivitis'   155
Bullous erythema multiforme (Stevens–Johnson syndrome)   155
Reiter's disease   156
Acanthosis nigricans   156
Pyostomatitis vegetans   157
'Allergic stomatitis'   158
Oral mucosal reactions to drugs   159
Tongue complaints   160
References   164

9   White, red and pigmented lesions of the oral mucosa   166
ORAL WHITE LESIONS   166
White sponge naevus   166
Pachyonychia congenita   167
Fordyce's spots   167
Dyskeratosis congenita   168
Frictional keratosis and cheek biting   168
Smoker's keratosis ('nicotinic stomatitis')   169
Snuff dipper's keratosis and other smokeless tobacco lesions   169
Syphilitic leucoplakia   170
Candidosis   170
Lichen planus   173
Lupus erythematosus   173
Sublingual keratosis   173
Psoriasis   174
HIV-associated hairy leucoplakia   175
Oral keratosis of renal failure   175
Verruciform xanthoma   176

Oral submucous fibrosis   177
Idiopathic (including dysplastic) leucoplakia   177
Carcinoma-in-situ   178
Speckled leucoplakia   179
Erythroplasia ('erythroplakia')   180
Early squamous cell carcinoma   180
RED, PURPLE AND PIGMENTED LESIONS   180
Melanomas and pigmented naevi   181
Malignant melanoma   184
Melanotic neuroectodermal tumour of infancy (progonoma)   185
Miscellaneous oral pigmentations   185
References   188

10   Epithelial tumours and cancer of the mouth   190
Papilloma   190
Florid oral papillomatosis   190
Papillary hyperplasia of the palate   191
Cowden's (multiple hamartoma) syndrome   191
Verruca vulgaris   191
Condyloma acuminatum   191
Molluscum contagiosum   192
Verruciform xanthoma   192
Focal epithelial hyperplasia (Heck's disease)   192
Adenomas and adenocarcinomas   193
Cancer and precancerous lesions   193
Verrucous carcinoma   211
Keratoacanthoma   212
Other variants of oral carcinoma   213
Merkel cell carcinoma   213
Carcinoma of the maxillary antrum   214
References   214

11   Non-neoplastic diseases of salivary glands   217
Developmental disorders   217
Infections and other inflammatory diseases   217
Post-irradiation sialadenitis   222
Sialadenitis of minor glands   222
Necrotizing sialometaplasia   222
Allergic sialadenitis   223
Obstruction and trauma   224
Calculi (sialolithiasis)   224
Mucoceles   226
Sjögren's syndrome   227
Functional xerostomia   230
HIV-associated salivary gland disease   231

Irradiation damage   232
Mikulicz's disease and Mikulicz's
syndrome   232
Sialosis   233
References   233

12   Tumours of salivary glands   234
BENIGN EPITHELIAL TUMOURS   238
Pleomorphic adenoma   238
Myoepithelioma   240
Warthin's tumour (adenolymphoma,
cystadenolymphoma)   241
Oncocytoma (oxyphilic adenoma)   242
Duct adenomas   243
Clear cell adenoma   244
Papillary cystadenoma   244
Sebaceous lymphadenoma and sebaceous
adenoma   244
Duct papillomas   244
CARCINOMAS OF SALIVARY GLANDS   245
Mucoepidermoid carcinoma   245
Acinic cell carcinoma   246
Adenoid cystic carcinoma (cylindroma)   247
Adenocarcinomas   248
Polymorphous low-grade adenocarcinoma
(terminal duct carcinoma)   249
Salivary duct carcinoma   250
Clear cell tumours   250
Basal cell adenocarcinoma   252
Squamous cell (epidermoid) carcinoma   252
Undifferentiated carcinomas   253
Carcinoma in pleomorphic adenoma   254
Metastasizing mixed tumour   254
Other rare carcinomas of salivary
glands   255
NON-EPITHELIAL TUMOURS AND TUMOUR-LIKE
LESIONS OF SALIVARY GLANDS   255
Benign lymphoepithelial lesion   255
Lymphoma   255
Hodgkin's disease   256
Salivary gland tumours in infancy and
childhood   257
Other mesenchymal tumours of salivary
glands   258
Metastatic tumours in salivary glands   258
Juxtaglandular tumours   258
Intraosseous salivary gland tumours   259
References   259

**13   Tumours and tumour-like lesions of
mesenchymal tissues   260**
FIBROMAS AND FIBROUS NODULES   260

Fibrous epulis, denture-induced hyperplasia
and other fibrous nodules   260
Giant cell fibroma   261
Pyogenic granuloma and pregnancy
epulis   261
Giant cell epulis   262
Neoplastic epulides   263
Nasopharyngeal (juvenile) angiofibroma   263
Spindle cell and pseudo-mesenchymal
tumours of salivary glands   264
Fibromatoses   264
Myofibromatosis   265
Gingival fibromatosis   266
Fasciites   266
Fibrosarcoma   268
Fibriohistiocytic tumours and fibrous
histiocytoma   269
TUMOURS OF NEURAL TISSUE   270
Traumatic neuroma   270
Neurolemmomas (schwannomas)   270
Neurofibroma   271
Plexiform neurofibroma   271
Neurofibromatosis (von Recklinghausen's
disease)   272
Mucosal neuromas in endocrine adenoma
syndromes   273
Malignant schwannomas and
neurofibrosarcomas   273
Cervical paragangliomas (chemodectomas,
'glomus tumours')   274
TUMOURS OF FATTY TISSUE   275
Lipoma   275
Liposarcoma   275
DISEASES OF MUSCLE   276
Proliferative myositis   276
Myositis ossificans   277
Extraskeletal osteosarcoma and
chondrosarcoma   277
Granular cell tumour ('myoblastoma')   277
Congenital granular cell epulis   278
Rhabdomyoma   278
Rhabdomyosarcoma   279
TUMOURS AND HAMARTOMAS OF BLOOD AND
LYMPHATIC VESSELS   281
Leiomyoma and angioleiomyoma   281
Leiomyosarcomas   281
Haemangiomas   282
Glomus tumours (glomangiomas)   283
Lymphangiomas   283
Haemangiopericytoma   284
Haemangioendothelioma   285
Kaposi's sarcoma   285

Bacillary epithelioid angiomatosis   286
Synovial sarcoma   286
References   287

14   Lymphoreticular and granulomatous diseases   289
LYMPHORETICULAR TUMOURS – LYMPHOMAS   289
Burkitt's lymphoma   291
Hodgkin's disease   292
Causes and management of enlarged cervical lymph nodes   293
Indications for lymph node biopsy   293
Tuberculous cervical lymphadenopathy   296
Syphilis   296
Cat scratch disease   296
Lyme disease   297
Infectious mononucleosis   297
Acquired immune deficiency syndrome   297
Toxoplasmosis   298
Mucocutaneous lymph node syndrome (Kawasaki's disease)   298
Sinus histiocytosis   299
Giant (angiofollicular) lymph node hyperplasia (Castleman's disease)   299
Angiolymphoid hyperplasia with eosinophils (epithelioid haemangioma, Kimura's disease and related diseases)   300
Phenytoin and other drug-associated lymphadenopathies   300

IMMUNODEFICIENCY DISEASES   301
Acquired immune deficiency syndrome (AIDS)   301
Primary IgA deficiency   308
Hereditary angio-oedema   308
Allergic angio-oedema   308
granulomatous diseases   308
Midline granuloma syndrome (lethal midline granuloma, midfacial destructive disease, etc.)   308
Wegener's granulomatosis   309
Peripheral T cell lymphomas   310
Tuberculosis   311
Deep mycoses   311
Sarcoidosis   311
Crohn's disease   312
Melkersson–Rosenthal syndrome and cheilitis granulomatosa   313
Foreign body reactions   313
Granulomatous reactions secondary to radiotherapy or chemotherapy   313
Granulomatous reactions of unknown cause   314
Differential diagnosis of oral granulomatous lesions   314
References   315

Index   316

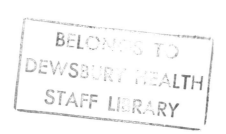

Preface

Surgeons have a natural interest in pathology, or if they haven't, they should. Only by understanding pathological processes involved in the diseases with which they have to deal can they manage them rationally and effectively.

Surgeons also have to understand the vocabulary of pathology and the full implications of a pathology report. Moreover, they need to appreciate some of the limitations of histopathological diagnosis. To provide helpful diagnoses, pathologists frequently need to know what the clinical findings are. Only by mutual understanding of their different tasks can surgeon and pathologist acquire that happy degree of cooperation that is ultimately in the best interest of the patient.

Vast numbers of publications on all aspects of oral and maxillofacial pathology continue to appear. To help the busy surgeon cope with this flood of material, this book aims to provide as much information as possible in concise, accessible and readily digestible form. Also, to serve the needs of the oral surgeon as well as possible, this book has been written jointly by a surgeon and two pathologists. Unusually great emphasis has therefore been placed on the principles of treatment of the conditions that have been discussed.

Non-surgical conditions, particularly mucosal diseases, have been included as these so frequently come under the wing of the oral surgeon. We earnestly hope therefore that this book will help to ease the many difficult problems that the oral surgeon often has to face.

We are anxious to express our gratitude to our publishers for their patience in waiting for this text to be put together and their generous allowance of colour illustrations. Inevitably, however, to provide an adequate coverage of the histopathology, the constraints of cost have forced on us some restriction on the number of illustrations. We therefore made it a matter of policy to omit clinical pictures. While one kind of lump may look much the same as another, we accept that the lack of clinical illustrations of mucosal diseases may be regarded as regrettable.

We would also like to thank Mr Bob Pearson for the unenviable task he has had in editing this text, and Mr Sidney Luck for his untiring efforts in tracing publications.

R.A.C.
J.D.L.
J.W.E.

1

Investigational methods

Malignant disease is inevitably one of the most important conditions that must be confirmed or excluded. Many biopsies of the mouth are taken primarily for this purpose and, in most cases, early recognition leads to better treatment results. The approach to the diagnosis of oral tumours is straightforward and can be used to illustrate the path to the diagnosis of all types of oral disease. The oral cavity is accessible and requires no special facilities for its examination. Moreover, unlike those in many other sites, early, even minute, oral lesions can cause symptoms. Biopsy is usually an essential adjunct to clinical and other investigations and is readily carried out under local analgesia. Nevertheless, between 25% and 50% of patients with oral cancer have late disease when referred for treatment and this may be, in part, due to failure to biopsy the lesion when first seen.

Provided that the biopsy is adequate, the microscopic diagnosis of most malignant tumours rarely presents major problems. Difficulties mainly arise in such conditions as dysplastic lesions, undifferentiated tumours and rare tumours, particularly if mesenchymal or lymphoreticular. In some cases, immunocytochemistry, as discussed later, can be decisive, but it must be appreciated that, on rare occasions, it may be difficult to reach a diagnosis with absolute certainty.

essential for all those attending patients with oral symptoms. It should be needless to add that a detailed history, with special care to record the dates of onset of particular signs and symptoms, should precede clinical examination.

All areas of the oral mucosa should be closely inspected in sequence and any suspicious area palpated for texture, tethering to adjacent structures and deep induration. The World Health Organisation's *Mucosa Manual* suggests a technique for sequential examination of each site within the mouth. If a systematic approach such as this is used, there is little chance of overlooking even a minute abnormality.

Accurate clinical records are essential for the care of any patient, and are valuable for any prospective or retrospective analyses of treatment methods and results. These notes must provide a detailed description of the lesion including site, precise measurements, appearance, extent, texture, fixation and induration. A photographic record is particularly valuable.

It is important to emphasize that this initial record is the basis upon which treatment is planned and progress assessed. Even a biopsy irrevocably changes the presenting lesion in some degree. Precise records are also essential should there be any medico-legal complications.

Clinical investigation

The provisional diagnosis of all disease must initially be clinical and a high index of suspicion is

Surgical biopsy

Biopsy of any suspicious area in the mouth should be undertaken, not as a substitute for sound clinical diagnosis, but for objective confirmation of its nature and, in some cases, efficacy of excision (see later). If the clinician suspects a particular disease, but the pathology report is at variance, there should be no hesitation in repeating the biopsy to obtain a more adequate or representative specimen.

It is sometimes claimed that malignant tumours should not be biopsied before definitive treatment, on the grounds that surgical manipulation increases the risk of bloodstream or lymphatic spread or of seeding tumour cells into previously healthy tissue planes. However, there is little evidence to support such arguments for most tumours and, in any case, there is rarely any practical alternative to biopsy for establishing a definitive diagnosis. Nevertheless, the biopsy should always be planned in such a way that, should surgical excision be necessary, then the resection can include the track of the previous biopsy.

Salivary gland tumours are an important exception to this rule, as pleomorphic adenomas are among the few that have a strong tendency to seed and recur if cells are released at biopsy or attempts at enucleation. This is a serious hazard in the parotid glands, and incisional biopsy should not therefore be carried out in this site.

It is often tempting to remove small lesions *in toto* by an excisional biopsy. However, this may be dangerous. Without histological confirmation of the malignant nature of the disease it is difficult to be certain of adequate margins. Moreover if the lesion is excised locally, subsequent management is compromised. It may also be difficult to persuade the patient to undergo further treatment for a lesion which appears to have been eliminated. Further, once the primary lesion has been excised, the surgeon no longer has a guide to the necessary extent of further excision and the radiotherapist cannot be certain of the field that needs to be treated.

For these reasons an incisional biopsy is recommended whenever cancer is suspected. For obviously benign lesions, such as most fibrous nodules, excisional biopsy is often curative as well as diagnostic.

When malignant disease is suspected, it is useful to tattoo the margins with Indian ink at the time of the initial biopsy. Any surgical resection must be planned according to the original dimensions of the tumour and the latter should be accurately delineated.

Biopsy technique

Biopsies in the mouth can usually be carried out under local analgesia. Infiltration of local anaesthetic solution should be made well away from the biopsy site. Distending the tissues with anaesthetic solution distorts them, with subsequent difficulties with diagnosis. It is also important not to crush the specimen with dissecting forceps or artery clips (Figure 1.1). This can be avoided by passing a suture through the specimen to immobilize it. Whenever possible, a representative piece of the lesion should be taken in continuity with adjacent normal tissue, as the changes at or near the junction may be important diagnostically. Specimens of lymphoid tissue need to be particularly gently handled. Lymphocytes are fragile and readily damaged to produce streaking artefacts (Figures 1.2 and 1.3).

Soft tissue biopsies should usually be taken using a double semilunar incision (Figures 1.4 and 1.5). This is not merely simple but also leaves a wound that is readily sutured. The triangular biopsy that has been advocated in the past not only leaves a good deal of waste tissue after the main slice has been taken for processing, but also leaves an awkwardly shaped wound.

The incision should include an adequate depth of underlying connective tissue. It is not possible to lay down hard-and-fast rules as to how deeply the incision should extend, as the requirements for diagnosis vary from one condition to another.

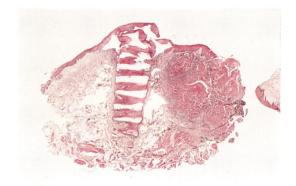

Figure 1.1 Forceps artefact in a biopsy specimen adjacent to a focus of squamous cell carcinoma which could readily have been missed if the damage had been in that area or if the specimen had been orientated in a different plane

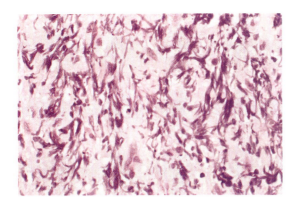

Figure 1.2 Streaking artefact in a lymphoma due to stretching of the tissue, making a definitive diagnosis impossible

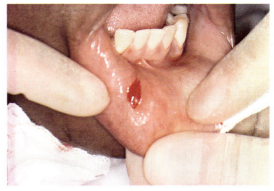

Figure 1.4 Labial salivary gland biopsy showing the incision

In many mucosal diseases no great depth of connective tissue is necessary, but in Crohn's disease, for example, granulomas may only be found deeply (Figure 1.6). Biopsies should also be extended more deeply when there is superficial necrosis, in order to reach living lesional tissue.

Thin biopsy specimens tend to curl up in the fixative and it may then be impossible to orientate the specimen for microscopy. Curling can be prevented by placing the specimen, deep surface downwards, on a square of blotting paper.

The specimen should be put in fixative as soon as possible. Delay can lead to autolysis and any drying distorts the tissues. Formal saline (10%) is generally acceptable unless electron microscopy is to be undertaken.

As important as any other aspect of biopsy procedure is completion of the pathology request form. Essential information includes:

- Name, age and sex of the patient. The sex may not be apparent from the given (first) name, especially in the case of immigrants.
- The provisional diagnosis and as much clinical information as possible (including, where relevant, details of any previous treatment, medical and drug history), but particularly the precise biopsy site and some indication of the rate of growth of the lesion and symptoms.
- The name of the clinician, the date of the biopsy and the hospital number.

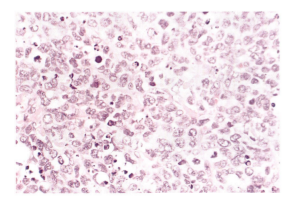

Figure 1.3 The same specimen as in Figure 1.2 showing how the cells should appear with more careful handling of the specimen

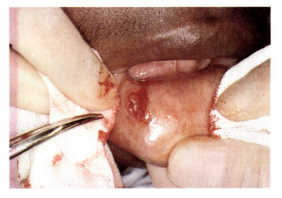

Figure 1.5 Labial salivary gland biopsy showing a lobule of salivary gland tissue bulging through the incision

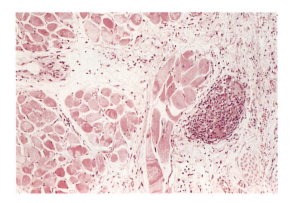

Figure 1.6   Crohn's disease. A granuloma is present well within the buccal musculature. This shows the depth of incision sometimes required to find diagnostic features

Though all this seems obvious enough, essential information of this sort is depressingly frequently left out.

A laboratory with automatic processing should usually be able to provide diagnoses within about 48 hours after submission of the specimen. With purely manual processing, the answer may not be available for up to a week. With difficult material, immunostaining may also delay diagnosis. If decalcification is necessary, there may be a delay of anything up to a month according to the type and size of the specimen and the kind of information required. However, this sort of delay can often be avoided by removing some of the tumour tissue from the bone. Genuine urgency in getting a diagnosis should also be mentioned if a frozen section is not possible or feasible. In the case of fibro-osseous and intra-bony cystic lesions, the pathologist frequently needs to know radiographic or other findings and joint discussion in the light of such information may sometimes be decisive.

Toluidine blue marking   Vital staining for delineating malignant and dysplastic lesions depends on the binding of toluidine blue to DNA in the superficial cells. Binding should therefore be proportional to the amount of DNA present and the number and size of superficial nuclei in the tissues. Though this test has been widely advocated

in the past, false negatives are so frequent as to make it unreliable.

Frozen sections

Frozen sections are indicated under such circumstances as the following:

● to establish, at operation, whether or not the tumour is malignant and to determine the extent of the excision
● to confirm that excision margins are free of tumour at the time of operation
● on rare occasions such as in an infant when it has not been feasible to take a biopsy under local anaesthesia preoperatively
● for immunofluorescence microscopy or for immunocytochemistry when reagents are ineffective in paraffin sections
● if the patient is from abroad and needs an immediate diagnosis to decide whether to return or stay.

Frozen sections are only justifiable if the definitive operation will follow immediately. Fixed, paraffin blocked sections are always to be preferred for light microscopy if the elective operation is going to be carried out some days later.

With reasonable precautions and facilities, frozen sections for tumour diagnosis usually provide a rapid and highly reliable answer and the only problem may be that of conveying the specimen, from theatre to laboratory, simply, rapidly and without deterioration. The usual methods include the following:

● With a cryostat in a side room of the theatre, the specimen can be prepared for sectioning within minutes of having been taken.
● If theatre and laboratory are close, then the wet specimen can be taken direct to and frozen in the laboratory. It is not possible to generalize about the maximum permissible delay when this is done, since lymphoma cells (for example) deteriorate faster than carcinoma cells. For most oral tumours, up to 20 minutes between excision and freezing is unlikely to cause serious deterioration, though it is clearly better to lose as little time as possible. The specimen can first

be put in frozen section embedding material such as OCT, if the pathologist wishes, and then taken immediately to the laboratory.

● The specimen can be dropped into liquid nitrogen, kept in the theatre in a vacuum flask, or into isopentane chilled with liquid nitrogen. If the specimen is very small it should be put in a capsule.

● If liquid nitrogen is not available, the specimen can be put on dry ice in an insulated container or snap-frozen in the theatre using a CO_2 jet spray freezer and then transported on dry ice.

● Instant freezing aerosol sprays (using, for example, dichlorodifluoromethane) will produce temperatures of $-50°C$ and are suitable and convenient for small specimens apart from muscle.

Rapid freezing is important to prevent autolysis and to reduce freezing artefacts. It is far better to take a wet unfrozen specimen immediately to the laboratory where it can be snap-frozen at $-50°C$, rather than to put it in an ordinary deep freeze (about $-40°C$) where serious freezing artefacts will develop, and take it later.

Under normal circumstances, using a cryostat, a stained section is obtainable in about 5 minutes from receipt of the specimen.

Limitations and contraindications Frozen section diagnosis is susceptible to error as a result of

● poor or inadequate sampling of the mass
● technical defects (freezing artefacts)
● difficulties of interpretation.

Sampling errors can result from sheer inadequacy of the specimen or from the fact that it may not be representative of the whole of the tumour. An obvious example is the case of a small area of malignant change in a salivary gland tumour. In other cases, the difficulties of diagnosis of some rare tumours may be such that immediate diagnosis cannot be made on a frozen section alone. Obvious examples are lymphoreticular diseases, including some of the midfacial granulomas (Chapter 14).

Finally, the initial verbal report on a frozen section must always be confirmed in writing and further confirmed by examination of paraffin sections which provide a permanent record. Misunderstandings can arise, especially if the message is relayed by a third party, and have unfortunate

effects on the patient. This in turn can lead to medico-legal complications.

Limitations of histopathological diagnosis

In many cases, such as cysts, the diagnosis is made largely on the clinical and radiographic features together with the findings at operation and is usually confirmed by the histological findings. Nevertheless, the pathological findings are occasionally unexpected and if, for example, a mural ameloblastoma or other cystic neoplasm is found, the management and prognosis are affected accordingly.

Histological examination of as much excised material as possible is therefore essential and there can be important medico-legal implications if this is neglected.

On the other hand, the surgeon should be aware of the limitations of histopathology and should not expect the pathologist always to be able to give a definitive answer as to the prognosis or what may be the optimal line of management for all possible diseases.

The apparent failures of histopathology stem from several factors, namely:

● Limitations imposed by the specimen. In this connection the following problems can arise if
  (a) the specimen fails to include a border with normal tissue and hence may fail to show (for example) peripheral invasion; in other cases, submission of no more than part of a cyst wall may prevent the identification of ameloblastoma in another area
  (b) the specimen is too large to examine completely; in the case of parotid gland tumours in particular, even multiple blocks might fail to find a focus of carcinomatous change
  (c) the specimen has been damaged by diathermy, crushing with forceps, injection of local anaesthetic solution or other means
  (d) the specimen is too thin and has been allowed to curl so that correct orientation is impossible

(e) poor fixation or autolysis; the specimen may have been put in *normal* rather than *formal* saline or put into fixative after too long a delay.

● Microscopy provides only a two-dimensional view and strictly speaking may never give an answer as to whether excision of a tumour is complete. Though the tumour may have a wide border of normal tissue in the plane of section, it could extend beyond the excision margins in another plane. Pathologists may therefore report that 'the margins of the specimen are clear of tumour *in the planes of section*', and try to take sections in as many planes as possible. This problem is perhaps greater in the mouth than in many other sites because of the lack of space for wide excisions.

● In a few cases, there are no absolute criteria for malignancy, particularly when the material shows no invasion. Some salivary gland tumours in particular can be cytologically benign, yet prove by their behaviour to be malignant.

● In some uncommon tumours, especially chondromas and neurofibromas, the borderline between being benign and malignant is indefinable.

● Some tumours are so uncommon that knowledge of behaviour is deficient. Prognostication is therefore impossible and there may be no consensus as to the optimal management.

● In the case of dysplastic leucoplakias, grading is no more than a subjective visual assessment of the degree of epithelial atypia. Though the diagnosis of severe dysplasia is frequently equated with inevitable development of frankly invasive carcinoma, this is no more than a probability as a significant number regress spontaneously.

● Occasionally, previously unrecognized tumours or other diseases still appear. These may have such unusual microscopic features as to fail to fall into any of the recognizable categories, and a group of even the most experienced pathologists will be unable to reach a consensus. Despite the fact that the current WHO typing of salivary gland tumours (Seifert, 1991) includes no fewer than 32 categories of epithelial tumours alone, it can be difficult to fit a particular tumour into one of these categories as van der Wal *et al.* (1992) have pointed out.

Table 1.1 lists a variety of problems which may affect in histological diagnosis and prognosis.

Table 1.1   Some problems in histological diagnosis and prognosis

Keratocysts	Inflammation can destroy the characteristic appearances to simulate a simple cyst
Ameloblastoma	Cystic expansion can flatten the epithelium to mimic a simple cyst over a large area
Salivary gland tumours	
Pleomorphic adenomas	Rarely, an area of carcinomatous change can be missed in a large specimen. Even more rarely, a cytologically benign tumour can behave as a carcinoma
Mucoepidermoid carcinomas	Behaviour not reliably related to histological features
Acinic cell carcinomas	Histologically benign specimens can be invasive
Papillary cystic adenomas/adenocarcinomas	Cytologically benign tumours can metastasize widely many years after apparently adequate excision
Clear cell tumours	Several different entities. Most are undoubtedly malignant
Neurofibromas	Hazy borderline between benign and malignant
Chondromas	Can prove to be sarcomas despite benign microscopic appearances
Fibro-osseous lesions	A grey area where differentiation between dysplasias and tumours may only ultimately be confirmed by behaviour
Fibrous histiocytomas, fasciites and fibromatoses	Differentiation from sarcomas or prediction of behaviour from the microscopic features may be difficult
Dysplastic leucoplakias and erythroplasias	Degree of dysplasia cannot be objectively assessed and behaviour not entirely related to microscopic features
Deep mycoses	Often no entirely specific features, and fungi or spores may be impossible to find

Immunocytochemistry

Antigenic substances can be identified in cells or tissues by the use of specific antibodies. Binding of the antibody to the antigen is made visible by conjugating the antibody with a stain or a stainable substance and using fluorescence microscopy.

Fluorescence immunocytochemistry has long been helpful in the diagnosis of immunologically-mediated diseases, by identifying deposits of immunoglobulins or complement in the tissue and thus to provide presumptive evidence of immunologically-mediated damage. A well-established application has been in the diagnosis of pemphigus vulgaris (Chapter 8) where, using frozen sections of fresh unfixed material, local-ization of pemphigus autoantibodies along the intercellular junctions can be demonstrated by fluorescence of conjugated anti-human immuno-globulin. This technique is relatively non-specific in that it does not identify pemphigus autoantibodies specifically, but merely takes advantage of the fact that these autoantibodies are immunoglobulins, but are antigenic.

Immunocytochemical techniques have been extended by the introduction of monoclonal anti-bodies. In essence, the identification of cyto-chemical markers depends on the antigen being insoluble and on a suitably sensitive detection system; the most widely used at present is peroxidase–antiperoxidase, but there are increasing numbers of alternatives such as avidin–biotin, each with its attendant advantages and limitations. Horseradish peroxidase labelling, conjugated with a suitable antibody, enables many antigenic sub-stances to be identified in fixed paraffin-blocked material, though some antibodies can only be used on frozen sections. The hope underlying the use of monoclonal antibodies is that each type of cell or structural component has sufficiently well-defined antigenic characteristics to differentiate it from every other. In tumours particularly, the cells of origin, however poorly differentiated, may there-fore be identifiable by such means.

An early application was the identification of monoclonal immunoglobulin production by lym-phoreticular tumours (Figure 1.7). Nevertheless, despite the availability of commercial monoclonal antibodies to an enormous number of tissue components, it can still happen that they fail to provide a definitive diagnosis. An important

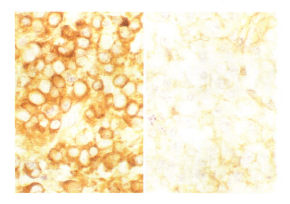

Figure 1.7 Plasmacytoma showing, by the brown staining in the cells, monoclonal production of light chains (kappa left; lambda right)

limitation is that, in addition to any difficulties of technique, tissue components from different types of cell may share antigenic determinants (epitopes). Thus some sarcomas, for example, stain positively for epithelial markers (keratins).

Frequently, a panel of monoclonal antibodies has to be applied. The panel chosen depends on general and personal experience. It is not feasible simply to apply all the monoclonal antibodies available, partly because of time and cost, but also because of the fact that the specificity of some of them is questionable and positive staining by one of these may only cause confusion.

The limitations of these techniques have become widely appreciated, but the continued stream of publications on unexpected findings testifies to the problems. Moreover, overconfidence in their value may lead to lack of care in assessment by light microscopy. Important difficulties are as follows:

- effects of fixation and other aspects of processing
- false-positive or false-negative results
- problems of specificity
- lack of adequate controls
- distinguishing between tissue (tumour) or infil-trating cells which mark positively
- loss of specific epitopes by tumour cells
- inability to distinguish malignant from benign cells by immunostaining alone.

Immunocytochemistry has become a speciality in itself, sufficient to fill substantial textbooks, and it is not feasible to discuss it in detail here but only to point out that the techniques demand considerable experience in their performance and in the interpretation of the results.

Nevertheless, among tumours of the mouth or jaws, several points can be clarified (Figures 1.8 and 1.9). At the least, what used sometimes to be called small dark cell tumours, which might be anaplastic carcinomas or lymphomas, can now be distinguished with certainty by positive staining of carcinomas for epithelial antigens and lymphomas for leucocyte common antigen (CD45). B cell lymphomas can also be confidently differentiated from T cell lymphomas. Some of the latter are so pleomorphic as not to have been recognized as lymphomas in the past (Chapter 14).

Surgeons, naturally enough, usually want answers in a hurry. Unfortunately immunostaining is slow and labour-intensive unless it can be reliably automated.

Relatively recently, the possibility of differentiating benign from malignant lesion has been studied by identifying markers of cell proliferation, oncogenes and mutations of the p53 oncogene-suppressor gene (Birch, 1992). Changes in the p53 gene lead to nuclear accumulation of p53 protein and this has been found in many different types of malignant neoplasms. Nevertheless, Dei Tos *et al.* (1993) have shown that p53 protein can also be expressed in many benign neoplasms or non-neoplastic lesions.

Antibodies used to recognize cell proliferation of potential value in the diagnosis or prognosis of cancer include KiSi (Sampson *et al.* 1992), Ki67 (Sawhney and Hall, 1992) and JC1 (Garrido *et al.*,

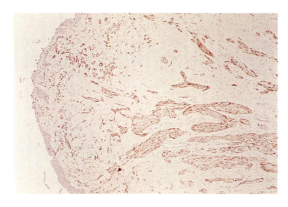

Figure 1.9 Amputation neuroma. The same specimen as in Figure 1.8 but the neural elements have been made clearly visible by positive staining for S-100 protein

1992). However, immunocytochemistry will not reliably distinguish between all tumours of similar origin, such as the many varieties of salivary gland tumour.

Flow cytometry measures the DNA content of 10 000 or more nuclei in suspension. The presence of diploidy, haploidy or aneuploidy has been correlated with behaviour for some salivary gland neoplasms (Chapter 11). However, the results are mainly of statistical value and as yet of little use in predicting the behaviour of a particular tumour. The method itself also has limitations, as discussed by Robinson (1992).

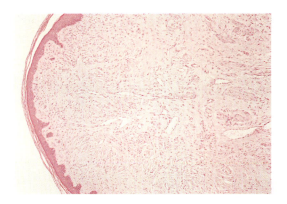

Figure 1.8 Amputation neuroma, haematoxylin and eosin stained section shows predominantly fibrous tissue. Neural elements are present but inconspicuous

Fine-needle aspiration cytology

This technique is applicable mainly to lumps in the neck, especially suspect lymph nodes in a patient with a known primary carcinoma, and to parotid gland tumours. It is valuable when open biopsy is inadvisable or contraindicated. It consists of percutaneous puncture of the mass with a fine needle and aspiration of material for microscopic examination. This technique needs no elaborate equipment and is quick, almost painless and without complications.

Nevertheless, the technique is often incorrectly performed and too little tissue obtained. Two aspects are critical, namely successful puncture of the mass and the transfer of material from the needle to a microscope slide. The mass is immobilized between finger and thumb and then punctured with a 21- or 23-gauge needle (depending on the size of the mass) on a 10 ml syringe. Important points to note are that

- the needle is tightly fitted on to the syringe to prevent air leaking in when the plunger is withdrawn, and
- about 2 ml of air is already in the syringe before puncturing the node in order to expel all the aspirate from the needle on to the slide.

Aspiration should be forceful and, at the same time, the needle should be moved around different parts of the mass. Having aspirated for 10–30 s, the plunger is released and the needle withdrawn through the skin. The needle contents are then expelled on to a glass slide using the 2 ml of air drawn into the syringe beforehand. To do this, the tip of the needle must touch the slide to prevent splashing the material, which can be gelatinous or sticky, over a wide area. Blobs of material can be deposited on several slides and then smeared with a second slide to provide a thin film for staining and microscopy. Some pathologists prefer wet-fixed material which must be sprayed with an alcoholic spray fixative immediately. Others prefer thinner films which can be left to dry.

After aspirating the tissue, instead of making a smear directly on to the microscope slide, 2 ml of 95% ethanol can be aspirated as fixative into the syringe to avoid losing material. The syringe containing fixative and cells is then sent to the laboratory where the contents are centrifuged and a smear prepared from the deposit.

Fine-needle aspiration has become widely used to obviate the need for open biopsy and the risk of spreading malignant cells into the surrounding tissues where they cannot be detected at the time of radical surgical excision. Further, any displaced cells having lost their blood supply and rendered anoxic may be more resistant to radiotherapy. Schelkun and Grundy (1991) have reported the results of 213 fine-needle aspiration biopsies of head and neck lesions and found a false-positive rate of 0.5% and a false-negative rate of 2.3%. Sensitivity was 81.1% and specificity was 99% for malignant tumours.

Tumour implantation into the needle track has been reported when large (Vim–Silverman) biopsy needles have been used. It is widely believed that there is no risk of needle track dissemination of cancer after aspiration using 21- or 23-gauge needles. However, this hazard cannot be dismissed, as discussed by Hix and Aaron (1990) and Nankhonya and Zakhour (1991). Increasing experience with other tumours, particularly of the lung, shows that the risk of seeding of tumour cells along the needle track is real (though small) rather than theoretical. This complication has not as yet been shown in the case of salivary gland tumours, and Frable (1983) did not consider that there was any significant risk. However, the slow growth of pleomorphic adenomas in particular may mean that such recurrences may eventually appear.

Fine-needle aspiration cytology offers great potential advantages for the diagnosis of parotid gland tumours, since benign and malignant tumours are frequently not clinically distinguishable and open biopsy is contraindicated (Figure 1.10). However, the diagnosis of salivary gland tumours is by no means always straightforward even when the gross specimen is available. For example, malignant change in a salivary pleomorphic adenoma may occupy only a minute part of the mass and could be missed during needling. In other cases, dysplasia within a pleomorphic adenoma, in the absence of invasion of surrounding tissues, might be mistaken for carcinoma in a fine-needle aspiration biopsy. In any case, from the practical viewpoint, parotidectomy is the treatment required for pleomorphic adenomas, as for malignant tumours. In practice, the chief factor limiting

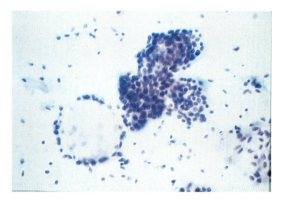

Figure 1.10 Fine-needle aspiration cytology of an adenoid cystic carcinoma. A pseudocyst is surrounded by darkly staining cells and there is an adjacent dense clump of small darkly staining cells (Papanicolaou stain) (By courtesy of Dr E. Malberger)

the usefulness of cytological diagnosis of salivary gland tumours is that it may be difficult for the cytologist to build up sufficient experience in the appearances of the aspirates of the many different types of neoplasms, unless working in a specialist centre.

Punch/drill/Trucut needle biopsy

Several techniques are available for obtaining samples of deep-seated solid lesions. These may be obtained using a small punch, a rotating trephine or a special wide-bore needle. Each of these techniques results in a solid core of material and may be useful for solid intra-osseous lesions. However, there is a high risk of seeding malignant cells along the track of the instrument.

Simple aspiration

Simple aspiration of radiolucent areas to confirm whether or not they are cysts and if possible to make a precise diagnosis has been extensively used in the past.

This technique can be performed at the chairside using a wide-bore hypodermic needle and syringe. Infiltration with a local anaesthetic makes the procedure pain free.

If it is impossible to aspirate anything (assuming that the needle has entered the lesion), the lesion is probably either solid or the uncommon variant of keratocyst, filled with semi-solid keratin. If the lesion is in the maxilla and air is aspirated, the needle is in the antrum. This may be confirmed by injecting a little sterile saline, when the patient will complain of a salty taste at the back of the throat as the saline passes into the nose via the antral ostium. Gas obtained from a mandibular lesion indicates a solitary bone cyst. These cysts sometimes contain serosanguineous fluid resulting from breakdown of red cells, and biochemical analysis may show a high bilirubin content.

Uninfected dentigerous or radicular cysts typically contain clear straw-coloured aspirates containing cholesterol crystals. The characteristic shimmering of these crystals may be seen by running some of the aspirate on to a dry swab

and examining it in a strong oblique light. Alternatively, a smear on a slide enables cholesterol crystals to be identified by their characteristic notched rhomboid shape by microscopy. However cholesterol crystals are not pathognomonic of cysts.

If blood is aspirated, this suggests either a vascular tumour (haemangioma) or an aneurysmal bone cyst. This finding is probably the most valuable application of simple aspiration and may prevent torrential bleeding when an intraosseous haemangioma is unknowingly opened surgically.

Any infected lesion may yield pus on aspiration and occasionally yeast forms of a deep mycosis may be identifiable in the smear. An odontogenic keratocyst may contain cheesy material unlike the clear fluid from other odontogenic cysts. If this material can be aspirated, a smear can be made and stained (haematoxylin and eosin) to show keratin squames. Alternatively, the aspirate can be sent to the laboratory for protein analysis. Less than 4 g per 100 ml of total protein in the aspirate indicates a keratocyst, whereas a protein content of more than 5 g per 100 ml excludes the diagnosis.

In practice, however, competent clinicians are rarely mistaken in their diagnosis of jaw cysts on the basis of the clinical and radiographic findings. On rare occasions, a monolocular cystic ameloblastoma can be mistaken for a simple cyst, but even then aspiration is unlikely to provide useful information. Aspiration of cystic lesions is, therefore, increasingly rarely performed.

Exfoliative cytology

Cervical smears are a valuable mass screening method for detecting early cervical cancer, where Papanicolaou staining helps to differentiate the varied appearances of epithelium during the oestrous cycle from malignant cells. Exfoliative cytology has also been used for suspected oral carcinomas, but for this purpose haematoxylin and eosin staining is simpler and satisfactory. The specimen is obtained by scraping the moist oral mucosa with a blunt-edged instrument such as a spatula. The scrapings are transferred to a clean microscope slide. A smear is made, allowed to dry briefly, then fixed and stained. Skill is required in interpreting the results, and a specialist cytologist should be consulted. A positive result is an indication for surgical biopsy.

However, the technique is unreliable and there can be a false-negative rate of over 30%. Since the mouth is so readily accessible for biopsy, it should always be used in preference to exfoliative cytology and a biopsy should also be taken for confirmation. As cytology can produce false-negative findings, and positive findings need to be confirmed by biopsy, there is virtually no justification for the use of this technique in the mouth for the diagnosis of tumours.

One possible exception is the appearance of ulceration following radiotherapy, when there is doubt as to whether this is due to recurrence of the tumour. In such cases, a biopsy wound can be very slow to heal or can precipitate serious infection. If cancer cells are found by cytological examination, an immediate answer is thus obtained and biopsy may be avoided. However, only positive findings are informative.

Another use for exfoliative cytology in the mouth is for the diagnosis of infections, particularly herpetic or candidal and for the preliminary diagnosis of pemphigus vulgaris. Haematoxylin and eosin stains are also satisfactory for smears of herpetic or candidal lesions. Virally damaged cells with ballooning degeneration and syncytial multinucleate cells are seen in both herpes simplex and zoster infections. A refinement of this technique is to use antibodies to these viruses to confirm the nature of the infection. The diagnosis of thrush is readily confirmed by the finding of many strongly Gram-positive hyphae in and among epithelial and inflammatory cells.

Aspiration and other ancillary methods – conclusions

Fine-needle aspiration cytology is a valuable technique for examining equivocal masses in the submental and submandibular areas, and the neck in patients whose primary tumour has been treated but who develop palpable nodes later. Metastases should always be suspected, but the lymph nodes sometimes show only reactive changes. Alternatively, it is sometimes difficult to distinguish such a mass from a chronically inflamed submandibular

salivary gland. If aspiration biopsy confirms either the presence of tumour or salivary tissue, the nature of the mass is certain. Failure to find tumour or salivary tissue leaves the same doubts as a negative biopsy and in particular whether the aspiration needle missed the mass. Fine-needle aspiration under computer tomography (CT) guidance may be helpful under such circumstances.

Exfoliative cytology and toluidine blue tests cannot be recommended. They are only applicable to surface lesions accessible to surgical biopsy which avoids the risk of false-negative results.

DNA hybridization and the polymerase chain reaction

The diagnostic applications of recombinant DNA technology are as yet limited to (a) the diagnosis of genetic disorders, (b) identification of some micro-organisms in tissues or body fluids, and (c) phenotyping of some lymphomas and leukaemias (Arends and Bird, 1992). Of these, identification of microorganisms is most likely to be useful in the present context, because of the great sensitivity and rapidity. *In situ* DNA hybridization has the advantage that it is more readily applied to formalin-fixed tissues and can be used, for example, for identification of human papilloma virus (HPV) in papillomas, carcinomas and other oral lesions.

Radiography and other imaging techniques

Conventional radiography is essential for investigating any lesion of the mouth and jaws other than superficial soft tissue lesions. The facial bone structure is so complex that confusion with overlying structures sometimes makes X-ray diagnosis difficult. However, rotational pantomography of the jaws can be helpful in assessing alveolar and antral involvement, provided that the limitations are understood (Whaites, 1992).

Conventional tomography can be useful for assessing bony involvement by antral lesions where posterior extension beyond the pterygoids may render a lesion inoperable. However, CT scanning has largely replaced conventional radiographs for the pterygoid and orbital regions.

Chest radiographs are essential if metastases, sarcoidosis, tuberculosis or Wegener's granulomatosis are suspected. Skull radiographs or skeletal surveys will help to confirm the diagnosis of multiple myeloma and are occasionally required in cases of hyperparathyroidism.

Sialography

Sialography depends on instillation of contrast medium into the salivary tree to demonstrate such changes as obstruction or tumours obliterating or displacing the duct system. Sialography is discussed in more detail in Chapter 11.

Computed tomography (CT) and magnetic resonance imaging (MRI)

The increasing availability of CT scanning and MRI has been of enormous benefit in the investigation of head and neck lesions (Figure 1.11a,b) and particularly for salivary gland tumours where they have displaced and are considerably more informative than sialography.

However, for intraoral tumours the value of CT scanning is more limited. For the evaluation of antral tumours, particularly assessment of the pterygoid regions, CT has largely displaced plain radiography and conventional tomography. CT is also of value in the investigation of metastatic disease in the lungs, liver and skeleton.

The principles of magnetic resonance imaging have been described by Komoroski *et al.* (1992). The patient is placed in the structured magnetic field of the MRI apparatus and the field subjected to a radiofrequency pulse, to generate an MRI signal. The signal reflects the status and environment of hydrogen molecules within the body. Diseased tissue produces different signals from healthy tissue. These signals are computer processed to produce an image on a visual display unit. However, hard tissues produce no image.

The sensitivity of MRI to differentiate diseased from healthy tissues sometimes enables it to detect metastatic oral cancer in clinically negative necks and the absence of disease in suspicious necks. However, Kabala *et al.* (1992) remain sceptical of the ability of MRI to detect micrometastases. Until this question has been satisfactorily answered by the use of gadolinium enhancement, use of STIR sequences or other means, the management of patients with oral cancer but clinically normal neck nodes (Chapter 10) remains controversial.

Ultrasonography

Ultrasonography provides a quick, safe and cheap method of imaging which provides the expert with remarkably detailed and informative pictures. For example, the valvular vegetations of infective endocarditis can be visualized in this way.

However, CT and/or MRI scanning are even more informative and provide readily interpreted images. Their value is limited mainly by their availability and cost.

Radionuclide scanning

Technetium pertechnetate bone scans of the facial skeleton are of little value in the diagnosis of primary oral cancers. Obvious clinical disease long precedes bone changes visible on a technetium scan and the procedure is not without risk to the patient.

Radionuclide scans for liver metastases have been used but have been displaced by CT scanning or ultrasound scans which are both non-invasive and more sensitive techniques.

Technetium scanning of the salivary glands has been advocated in the past, but is rarely diagnostic. Many tumours and functional disorders show up unpredictably as either hot or cold spots and the only lesion showing a consistent appearance in technetium scans is Warthin's tumour (adenolymphoma) which appears as a hot spot. Technetium scanning may be useful in the investigation of functional activity of salivary glands, although emptying films on sialography are more informative and do not require special apparatus.

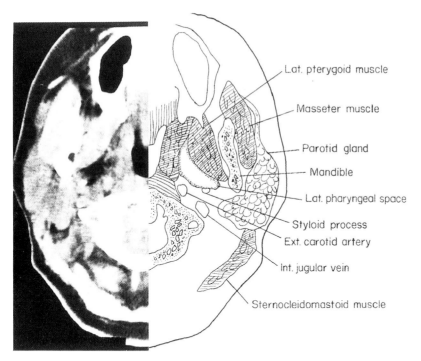

Lat. pterygoid muscle

Masseter muscle

Parotid gland

Mandible

Lat. pharyngeal space

Styloid process
Ext. carotid artery

Int. jugular vein

Sternocleidomastoid muscle

(a)

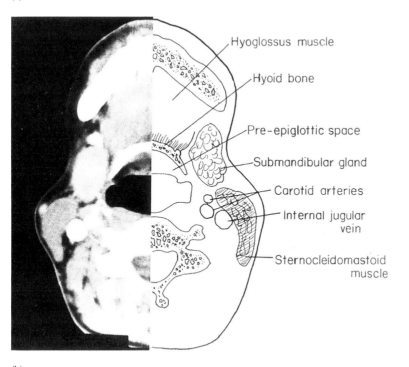

Hyoglossus muscle

Hyoid bone

Pre-epiglottic space

Submandibular gland

Carotid arteries

Internal jugular
vein

Sternocleidomastoid
muscle

(b)

Figure 1.11(a,b) CT scans with accompanying orientation diagrams to identify structures shown in the radiographic image

Gallium-67 is taken up by leucocytes and may be useful in staging lymphomas. However, it is also taken up by leucocytes in inflammatory lesions and those passing through vascular tumours. It has therefore been used as an alternative to angiography.

Salivary flow measurement

Impairment of salivary flow, unless of extreme degree, is not usually detectable clinically and patients frequently make no direct complaint of it even when it is present. By contrast, other patients with normal salivary flow may complain of a dry mouth. Objective confirmation of complaints of dry mouth is frequently therefore necessary, particularly in the diagnosis of Sjögren's syndrome. Techniques are discussed in Chapter 11.

Laboratory investigations

Innumerable investigations can be asked for, but unless the clinician is clear about their relevance to the disease in question and the likely yield in terms of diagnostically useful information, the findings are unlikely to be helpful. Further, the habit of asking for unnecessarily many investigations is likely eventually to antagonize laboratory staff and may result in lessened cooperation.

Important examples of investigations relevant to and often crucial in the diagnosis of oral lesions are shown in Table 1.2.

It should be emphasized that there are no tests which will provide a direct, positive diagnosis of immunologically-mediated disease, and autoantibody studies must be interpreted in relation to the clinical and other findings. In a few cases such as Sjögren's syndrome the autoantibody findings (associated with objective confirmation of a reduced salivary flow rate) may obviate the need for biopsy. However, even in this case a labial salivary gland biopsy may be just as informative.

With regard to bone diseases, newer methods for assessment of bone formation such as osteocalcin, procollagen, bone specific alkaline phosphatase have been developed but are not yet widely

Table 1.2   Examples of clinically useful laboratory investigations for oral diseases

Haematology
Lymphomas, leukaemias, myelomas, sore tongues, HIV infection (lymphopenia), recurrent aphthae (particularly in older patients)

Microbiology
Osteomyelitis, cellulitis, acute parotitis, deep mycoses (frequently mistaken for tumours)

Serology
Confirmation of some infections, particularly syphilis and theoretically for others such as herpes or mumps, HIV infection (rarely), infectious mononucleosis (Paul–Bunnell test)

Erythrocyte sedimentation rate
Raised in all inflammatory diseases, but especially important in cranial (giant cell) arteritis

Blood chemistry (calcium or phosphatases)
Giant cell lesions of bone to exclude hyperparathyroidism, Paget's disease of bone, prostatic metastases

Autoantibodies
Sjögren's syndrome, rheumatoid arthritis, lupus erythematosus, pemphigus vulgaris and mucous membrane pemphigoid (immunofluorescence of tissue specimen)

Urine
Bence-Jones protein in amyloid disease (myeloma or other paraproteinaemia)

available. Similarly, markers of bone resorption, such as pyridinoline and deoxypyridinoline, are likely to improve accuracy of diagnosis. Lytic metastatic bone lesions may be associated with production of parathyroid hormone-related peptide, while secondaries from prostatic cancer may be identifiable by raised (up to 100 u/l) levels of prostate specific antigen (PSA).

Medical assessment of the patient

However certain the surgeon is of the diagnosis and his ability to eliminate the disease, these advantages will be of little value to a patient who fails to survive the operation. In general, the anaesthetist is responsible for the preoperative assessment, but it is advisable also for the surgeon to take a careful medical and drug history. This may be initiated by use of a proforma questionnaire, but needs to have any areas of doubt confirmed by clinical examination and further investigation.

The latter may include haemoglobin estimation, blood picture, sickling test in Afro-Caribbeans and blood pressure estimation. The taking of an electrocardiogram (ECG), particularly for patients over 60, and a chest radiograph may seem to be desirable precautions, but rarely yield more information than can be obtained clinically or from the history. Similarly, the history is the most important guide to defective haemostasis. Wagner and Moore (1991) reviewed an extensive literature on the value of many screening procedures and found that 60% of oral surgery patients were overinvestigated without benefit, and that some tests could even be hazardous to the patient.

References

Arends, M.J. and Bird, C.C. (1992) Recombinant DNA technology and its diagnostic applications. *Histopathology*, **21**, 303–313

Birch, J.M. (1992) Germline mutations in the p53 tumour suppressor gene: scientific clinical and ethical challenges (editorial). *British Journal of Cancer*, **66**, 424–426

Dei Tos, A.P.T., Doglioni, C., Laurino, L. *et al.* (1993) p53 protein expression in non-neoplastic lesions and benign and malignant neoplasms of soft tissue. *Histopathology*, **22**, 45–50

Frable, W.J. (1983) *Fine-needle Aspiration Biopsy*, W.B. Saunders, Philadelphia

Garrido, M.C., Cordell, J.L., Becker, M.H.G. *et al.* (1992) Monoclonal antibody JC1. New reagent for studying cell proliferation. *Journal of Clinical Pathology*, **45**, 860–865

Hix, W.R. and Aaron, B.L. (1990) Needle aspiration in lung cancer. Risk of tumor implantation is not negligible (editorial). *Chest*, **97**, 516–517

Kabala, J., Goddard, P. and Cook, P. (1992) Magnetic resonance imaging of extracranial head and neck tumours. *British Journal of Radiology*, **65**, 375–383

Komoroski, R.A., Pappas, A. and Hough, A. (1992) Nuclear magnetic resonance in pathology: 1. Principles and general aspects. *Human Pathology*, **22**, 1077–1084

Nankhonya, J.M. and Zakhour, H.D. (1991) Malignant seeding of needle aspiration tract: a rare complication. *British Journal of Dermatology*, **124**, 285–286

Robinson, R.A. (1992) Defining the limits of DNA cytometry. *American Journal of Surgical and Pathology*, **16**, 275–277

Sampson, S.A., Kriepe, H., Gillet, C.E. *et al.* (1992) KiS1 – a novel monoclonal antibody which recognizes proliferating cells: evaluation of its relationship to prognosis in mammary carcinoma. *Journal of Pathology*, **168**, 179–185

Sawhney, N. and Hall, P.A. (1992) Ki67 – structure, function and new antibodies (editorial). *Journal of Pathology*, **168**, 161–162

Schelkun, P.M. and Grundy, W.G. (1991) Fine-needle aspiration biopsy of head and neck lesions. *Journal of Oral and Maxillofacial Surgery*, **49**, 262–267

Seifert, G. (in collaboration with pathologists in 6 countries) (1991) *Histological Typing of Salivary Gland Tumours*, World Health Organisation/Springer-Verlag, Berlin

Van der Wal, J.E., Snow, G.B., van der Waal, I. (1992) Histological reclassification of 101 intraoral salivary gland tumours (new WHO classification). *Journal of Clinical Pathology*, **45**, 834–835

Wagner, J.D. and Moore, D.L. (1991) Preoperative laboratory testing for the oral and maxillofacial surgery patient. *Journal of Oral and Maxillofacial Surgery*, **49**, 177–182

Whaites, E. (1992) *Essentials of Dental Radiography and Radiology*, Churchill Livingstone, Edinburgh

2

Major infections of the mouth, jaws and perioral tissues

Severe oral and perioral infections are uncommon, but may take any of the forms discussed in the text. Oral bacteria can also cause dangerous metastatic infections or septicaemias and these are sometimes a significant hazard, particularly in immunodeficient patients, as discussed later.

Acute osteomyelitis

Acute osteomyelitis of the jaw has a different aetiology and microbial causes from long bone infections. The latter are largely a disease of childhood as a result of haematogenous spread of bacteria. By contrast, osteomyelitis of the jaws is a disease of adults and the infection typically originates from the mouth. The source of infection can be any of the following:

● periapical infection
● a periodontal pocket when the jaw is fractured
● acute gingivitis or pericoronitis (even more rarely)
● the skin or other external sources (open fractures or gunshot wounds).

Predisposing causes
Now that apparently spontaneous severe infections in or around the jaws have become rare in the general population, predisposing conditions have become relatively more important. The main examples include:

1. Local damage to or disease of the jaws:
   (a) open fractures including gunshot wounds

(b) radiation damage
   (c) Paget's disease or osteopetrosis (Chapter 6).
2. Impaired immune defences. Examples include acute leukaemia, immunosuppressive treatment, poorly controlled diabetes mellitus, sickle cell anaemia, chronic alcoholism or malnutrition. In such cases, and particularly in alcoholics, serious infection of the bone is typically precipitated by injury, sometimes of a minor nature. Acute osteomyelitis of the jaw has been described in HIV infection but appears to be uncommon in this group; indeed it has been shown by Robinson *et al.* (1992), that in such patients healing is normal after extractions and the incidence of localized osteitis is no more frequent than in a control group.

In a review of 35 cases, Koorbusch *et al.* (1992) found that odontogenic infections and trauma each accounted for 36% of osteomyelitis of the jaws. Immunosuppressive treatment was associated in only 9% of cases. None of the patients was diabetic, but this may reflect better control of the disease. Alcohol and tobacco use were recorded in 46% and 51%, respectively, but their contribution to the infection is unclear.

Clinical features
The great majority of patients are adult males and the mandible is usually affected. Acute osteomyelitis of the maxilla is usually a disease of neonates or infants and follows either birth injuries (due to forceps, for example) or uncontrolled middle ear infection. It is also therefore rare now in developed countries. In adults it is also a rare complication of trigeminal herpes zoster.

Early complaints are severe, throbbing, deep-seated pain, and swelling. The external swelling is initially due to inflammatory oedema. Later distension of the periosteum with pus, and finally subperiosteal bone formation, cause the swelling to become progressively firmer. The overlying gingiva is red, swollen and tender.

Associated teeth are tender to percussion. In severe cases they may become loose and pus may exude from an open socket or from round the necks of the teeth. Muscle oedema causes difficulty in opening the mouth and swallowing. Regional lymph nodes are enlarged and tender, and anaesthesia or paraesthesia of the lower lip is characteristic.

During the acute phase there may be fever, malaise and leucocytosis, but frequently the patient remains surprisingly well. A severely ill or very pale patient suggests underlying disease which should be investigated.

Radiography

Bony changes do not appear until after at least 10 days. The sharp trabecular pattern of the bone is lost where bone has been resorbed and areas of radiolucency indicate bone destruction. These areas have ill-defined margins and have a fluffy or moth-eaten appearance. Areas of dead bone appear relatively dense. These become more sharply defined as they are progressively separated as sequestra (Figures 2.1–2.3). Later, there is subperiosteal new bone formation which is most often seen in young patients. It typically appears as a

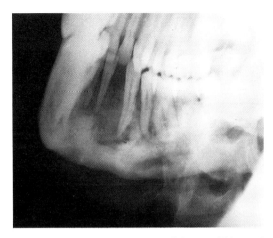

Figure 2.2 Acute osteomyelitis of the mandible. In the same patient as in Figure 2.1, sequestrum formation has produced typical, irregular areas of relative radiolucency and radiopacity

thin, curved strip of new bone below the lower border of the jaw.

Microbiology

Unlike osteomyelitis of long bones, which is usually a haematogenous infection, staphylococci are only likely to cause osteomyelitis of the jaw when they come from an external source, such as the skin, as a result of an open fracture. In such cases *S. epidermidis* is more frequently the cause than *S. aureus*. In most cases, oral bacteria, particularly anaerobes such as Bacteroides, Porphyromonas or Prevotella species, are the main cause and it is often a mixed

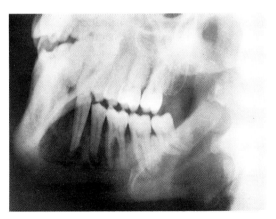

Figure 2.1 Acute osteomyelitis of the mandible. Bone destruction in the early stages has produced irregular areas of radiolucency

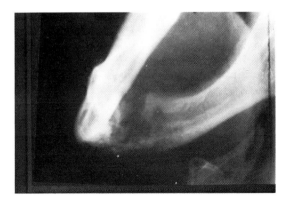

Figure 2.3 Acute osteomyelitis. The radiolucent area has the typical irregular moth-eaten appearance

Table 2.1   Important bacteria implicated in osteomyelitis of the mandible

Eikenella corrodens	Klebsiella
Staphylococcus aureus	Actinomyces
Staphylococcus epidermidis	Bacteroides (various)
Pseudomonas aeruginosa	*Fusobacterium nucleatum*
Viridans streptococci	Anaerobic or aerophilic
Salmonellae	streptococci
Streptococcus pyogenes	*Serratia marcescens*

infection (Table 2.1). Strict care in sampling is necessary to isolate anaerobes which may not be found unless the isolation technique is adequate. Gram-negative infections have also been reported, particularly in sickle cell disease and in alcoholics.

Pathology

The mandible has a relatively limited blood supply, dense bone with thick cortical plates and coarse trabeculae. Osteomyelitis is likely only to follow a straightforward extraction if the patient is immunocompromised and has a neutrophil defect as in acute leukaemia.

Fractures of the tooth-bearing regions of the jaw are usually open to the oral cavity through torn mucoperiosteum, but there is little risk of infection from the saliva. However, periodontal pockets form a reservoir of virulent bacteria and if the fracture line involves a periodontal ligament, infection can spread from this source, unless controlled by prophylactic antibiotics. In the case of gunshot wounds there may be the combined effects of gross trauma and implantation of foreign material together with staphylococci or other bacteria from the skin.

Once infection involves the medullary soft tissue it provokes an acute inflammatory response. Outpouring of inflammatory exudate carries infection through the marrow spaces. However, the rigid boundaries of the vascular canals cause exudate to compress the blood vessels; thrombosis and obstruction then lead to further bone necrosis. Bacteria can proliferate in this dead tissue and are then relatively inaccessible to some antibiotics such as the penicillins. Dead bone is readily recognizable microscopically by the lacunae empty of osteocytes but filled with neutrophils.

Pus formed by liquefaction of necrotic soft tissue and inflammatory cells is forced along the medulla, but is eventually able to reach the subperiosteal region by resorption of bone. Distension of the periosteum by pus stimulates subperiosteal bone formation, but perforation of the periosteum by pus and formation of sinuses on the skin or oral mucosa is rarely seen now.

At the boundary between the infected and healthy tissue, osteoclasts resorb the periphery of the dead bone which eventually becomes separated as a sequestrum (Figure 2.4). Once the infection starts to localize, new bone forms around it, particularly subperiosteally. In the past this could lead to involucrum formation and enclosure of sequestra; however, no more than a rim of new bone below the lower border of the mandible is usually seen now.

Where bone has died and been removed, healing is by granulation with formation of coarse fibrous bone in the proliferating connective tissue. Gradually fibrous bone is replaced by compact bone and remodelled to restore normal morphology.

Management

The following are main requirements:

1. *Bacteriological diagnosis.* A specimen of pus or, failing that, a swab from the depths of the lesion should first be obtained for culture and sensitivity testing.
2. *Antimicrobial treatment.* Once a specimen has been obtained, vigorous antibiotic treatment should be started. Initially, penicillin, 600–1200 mg daily can be given by injection, provided that the patient is not allergic, with metronidazole 200–400 mg 8-hourly.

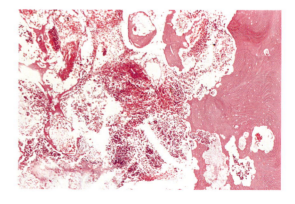

Figure 2.4   Acute osteomyelitis showing necrotic bone with empty osteocyte lacunae and pus cells in the marrow spaces

Clindamycin has unusually good penetration of poorly vascular tissue and has been effective for the treatment of osteomyelitis of the mandible as well as of long bones. The precise regimen will be determined a few days later by the bacteriological findings.

3. *Debridement*. If there has been a gunshot wound or other penetrating injury, careful debridement, removal of foreign material and immobilization of any fracture is necessary.

4. *Drainage*. Pressure within the bone must be relieved by tooth extraction, burr holes or decortication, as necessary, and exudate drained into the mouth or externally.

5. *Removal of sequestra*. This should be delayed until the acute phase has been controlled. Dead bone should not forcibly be separated and vigorous curetting is inadvisable, but in the later stages a loosened sequestrum may have to be removed. Teeth should be extracted only if loosened by tissue destruction.

Complications
- Involvement of the inferior dental nerve may cause anaesthesia of the lower lip, but sensation should recover with elimination of the infection.
- Pathological fracture may be caused by extensive bone destruction and requires immobilization, but is unusual.
- Chronic osteomyelitis may rarely follow inadequate treatment.
- Cellulitis due to spread of exceptionally virulent organisms is also rare.
- Septicaemia is only likely to be seen in an immunodeficient patient.

Osteoradionecrosis and radiation-associated osteomyelitis

Osteoradionecrosis is death of irradiated bone which is highly susceptible to infection. Watson and Scarborough (1938) reported an incidence of 13% in a series of 1819 patients with oral cancer treated by irradiation. With modern techniques and antimicrobials, the incidence is considerably lower.

The mandible is usually affected. It has a far more dense cortical plate and trabeculae than the maxilla and its blood supply in the elderly is poor, being predominantly via the periosteum. Infection can enter, particularly via injuries such as tooth extractions, and can spread to cause widespread necrosis of bone, periosteum and mucosa. However, radiation-associated osteomyelitis is highly unpredictable and can occasionally develop even in the absence of obvious infection or trauma.

The role of dental disease in the aetiology of bone infection after irradiation is uncertain. Clinically significant radiation necrosis of the mandible is usually associated with open mucosal wounds. Dental disease is the usual cause of disruption of these tissues and allows the ingress of microorganisms. There is a clear relationship between the dental state before radiation and subsequent infection. All dental disease should be treated thoroughly before radiotherapy, but removing teeth before radiotherapy is a subject of some controversy. One unsettled point is the interval between the time of extractions and the initiation of radiotherapy, and many authors have indicated the risks of irradiating a mandible shortly after extractions. Others have just as strongly advocated that all teeth in the beam should be extracted before starting radiotherapy. In practice, with modern high-energy beams it is safe to leave healthy teeth, but any non-vital or periodontally involved teeth in the radiation field should be removed before radiotherapy.

Jansma *et al.* (1992), in their protocol for prevention of oral complications after radiotherapy, consider that a delay of 3 weeks is necessary after extractions.

Management
The approach should be conservative. Any intraoral wounds should be regularly irrigated and the patient must maintain meticulous oral hygiene. Dilute eusol, hydrogen peroxide or chlorhexidine solutions are suitable, but the nature of the irrigation fluid is less important than the mechanical dislodgement of food debris and necrotic tissue. The patient should be shown how to irrigate the cavity and at the very least should rinse the mouth thoroughly with a chlorhexidine mouthwash, after any food.

Sequestra should be allowed to separate spontaneously. Active curettage only encourages extension of the infection. Only loose bony sequestra should be removed. Any sharp edges or spicules of bone should be smoothed off with rongeurs to prevent irritation of the tongue. Spontaneous healing is accomplished in approximately 50% of cases by natural sequestration and granulation. Because of its avascular nature, resorption of non-vital bone may take many months or even years, and great patience is required to resist the temptation to intervene surgically even after pathological fracture.

Osteoradionecrosis is usually relatively painless and any discomfort may be controlled with anti-inflammatory analgesics. Persistent severe pain is an indication for surgical intervention.

The avascularity of the tissues makes antibiotic therapy unlikely to help, though clindamycin diffuses well into poorly vascular areas and is the drug of choice for some anaerobic infections such as *Bacteroides fragilis*. However, in long-term treatment, the risk of pseudomembranous colitis becomes significant. Long-term low-dose tetracycline therapy (oxytetracycline 250 mg b.d.) or long-term sodium fusidate (500 mg q.d.s.) may, therefore, be more appropriate. It also seems logical to include metronidazole (200 mg t.d.s.) to help combat anaerobes. Healing takes many months, even when antibiotics are given, so that their value is difficult to assess.

Hyperbaric oxygen therapy has been shown to encourage healing by accelerating revascularization and increasing both osteoblastic and osteoclastic activity. Hart and Mainous (1976) reported on 46 patients with osteoradionecrosis of the mandible who had been treated at 2 atm for 2 h each session. A course of treatment consisted of a total of 120 h of hyperbaric therapy. Daily irrigation and long-term tetracycline were also employed. After such treatment, 37 of the 46 patients were symptom free, with complete intraoral soft tissue healing. Nine of the patients had dental extractions and trimming of the alveolar bone without complications. A further 4 patients required bone grafts to restore mandibular continuity – all were successful. Marx (1983) reported successful treatment of 27 cases of osteoradionecrosis with hyperbaric oxygen, combined with surgery in 5 of them. By contrast, van Merkesteyn *et al.* (1984) had limited success with it for chronic osteomyelitis. The procedure is generally safe, but Foster (1992) has described the contraindications and a formidable range of possible complications.

If pain or infection persists despite conservative measures, surgical intervention is required. Failure of conservative measures to bring about healing should prompt investigation for residual or recurrent tumour. Often when the necrotic bone is removed, active tumour becomes apparent. When surgery is undertaken, all heavily irradiated bone must be removed and the line of resection must be within healthy bleeding bone. Failure to achieve this will result in further necrosis. In patients who have been treated for large tumours or even small anterior tumours, both sides of the mandible may have received high-dose irradiation. Bilateral mandibular resection may then be necessary and considerable subsequent deformity can result.

Long-term management No reconstructive surgery should be attempted until the lesion has undergone fibrosis and contraction for at least a year. Often this will result in extra-articular ankylosis which makes subsequent intubation for general anaesthesia hazardous. Ankylosis must be released before soft tissue reconstruction (using local and distant flaps) can be attempted. Ankylosis often recurs due to the strong tendency to fibrosis and osteogenesis in the affected tissues. Active jaw movement exercise postoperatively for an indefinite period is therefore essential.

Chronic osteomyelitis

Inadequately treated osteomyelitis may become chronic. Rarely, chronic osteomyelitis may develop without any apparent acute episode. The infection is localized, but persistent because of the inaccessibility to host defences of bacteria growing in dead bone. There is intermittent discharge of pus and new bone formation. Pain tends to be mild and intermittent. Sequestra are slowly shed, but may often be felt by probing along a sinus. They give a characteristic rough, grating sensation, and may be felt to be loose. Radiologically a small area of bone destruction may be seen and there may be sclerosis of surrounding bone, together with subperiosteal new bone formation.

Treatment
Chronic osteomyelitis is best treated by decortication of the affected area and insertion of

gentamicin-impregnated acrylic beads in the adjacent tissues.

Chronic osteomyelitis in childhood

This entity has been recognized only in recent years. It typically begins at 8–10 years, with intermittent dull aching pain in the posterior mandible. Painful episodes are sometimes accompanied by diffuse swelling in the cheek, but usually respond to antibiotics.

Serial radiographs show migrating areas of moth-eaten destruction of the cancellous and cortical bone throughout the ramus and body of the mandible, eventually followed by complete regeneration with no residual changes.

Despite attempts to establish a bacterial cause, pathogenic bacteria have not been found, but the rapid response to fusidic acid suggests that *Staphylococcus aureus* may be responsible. There is some evidence that many of these patients may have a leucocyte defect which allows the infection to persist. Ord and El-Attar (1987) described three cases of chronic osteomyelitis in children, one of whom responded to extraction of the causative tooth and the others to clindamycin.

Management

Fusidic acid, clindamycin or erythromycin are most likely to be effective, but recurrent symptoms may persist for several years and only resolve in late adolescence. If pain is frequent or persistent, it may be necessary to maintain continuous antibiotic therapy for months or even years, but surgery seems to offer little benefit.

Chronic specific osteomyelitis

Syphilitic, actinomycotic and tuberculous osteomyelitis of the jaws are recognized entities and show the histological features typical of these diseases, but are unlikely to be seen now.

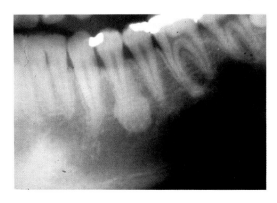

Figure 2.5 Chronic focal sclerosing osteomyelitis related to the apex of a lower premolar

Chronic focal sclerosing osteomyelitis (condensing osteitis)

This is an uncommon bony reaction to exceptionally low-grade periapical inflammation or, alternatively, to an unusually high degree of local tissue resistance to infection.

Patients are typically under 20 and the focus is most commonly related to a mandibular first permanent molar which, though grossly carious and non-vital, is either asymptomatic or causes only mild pain.

Radiographs show a well-circumscribed radiopaque area up to 2–3 cm in diameter below the apex of one or both roots, which typically retain an intact lamina dura (Figure 2.5). The margins of the lesion can be sharply defined or merge with the surrounding normal bone.

Microscopy shows a dense mass of compact bone with few lacunae, many of which are empty of osteocytes, but prominent resting and reversal lines give it a pagetoid appearance. There are only small amounts of fibrous interstitial tissue infiltrated by small numbers of lymphocytes.

Removal of the infected tooth is followed by slow resolution of the lesion, but an area of sclerotic bone may remain indefinitely.

Chronic osteomyelitis with productive periostitis (non-suppurative osteomyelitis, Garrés osteomyelitis)

This uncommon reaction to periapical or peri-follicular infection is characterized by subperiosteal new bone formation.

Only young patients are affected and the lesion is a response to low-grade chronic infection, usually in the mandible and, particularly, the lower first permanent molar. There may be mild pain before the formation of a non-tender, bony hard swelling, usually on the lower border or lateral aspect of the jaw.

Radiographs show a carious tooth with a periapical area of radiolucency or, less commonly, folliculitis round an unerupted tooth. On the cortical surface there is a smooth convex over-growth of bone. The new bone may show parallel, concentric (onion skin) laminations. The rest of the jaw may appear normal or show radiolucent or osteosclerotic areas due to osteomyelitis.

Microscopy shows the newly formed bone to consist of primitive bone (osteoid) in fibrous connective tissue, patchily infiltrated by lympho-cytes and plasma cells.

Other diseases which resemble proliferative periostitis radiographically include Ewing's sar-coma, osteosarcoma, infantile cortical hyperostosis, fracture callus, ossifying subperiosteal haematoma and peripheral osteoma.

Removal of the infection should lead to gradual remodelling of the jaw.

Diffuse sclerosing osteomyelitis

So-called diffuse sclerosing osteomyelitis was described by Shafer *et al.* (1983) as an unusual proliferative response to low-grade infection, par-ticularly widespread periodontal disease. How-ever, it has the same microscopic appearance as florid osseous dysplasia (gigantiform cementoma) and they are probably not distinct entities (see Chapter 4), though the term may possibly be

justified if infection has become superimposed. However, Schneider and Mesa (1990) dispute this view and give reasons for regarding florid osseous dysplasia and chronic sclerosing osteomyelitis as separate entities.

This disease is most frequently seen in middle-aged or elderly Blacks. The mandible, which may be dentate or edentulous, is usually affected and the main symptoms are episodes of mild suppuration with fistula formation and vague pain or an unpleasant taste.

Radiographs show areas of diffuse or nodular sclerosis, resembling the cottonwool radiopacities of Paget's disease, often bilaterally, and sometimes involving both the mandible and the maxilla (Figure 2.6).

Microscopy shows dense, irregular bone with a pagetoid ('mosaic') pattern of reversal lines. Fibro-blastic connective tissue fills the marrow spaces and is patchily infiltrated by variable numbers of chronic inflammatory cells. During acute exacerbations, neutrophils become numerous.

Management
Chronic diffuse sclerosing osteomyelitis needs to be distinguished from Paget's disease, osteopetrosis and late-stage fibrous dysplasia. Removal of any offending teeth and antibiotic therapy are the initial treatment. Often the dense 'cemental' masses form sequestra and when this happens the affected area should be guttered and the dense masses removed. Healing then follows.

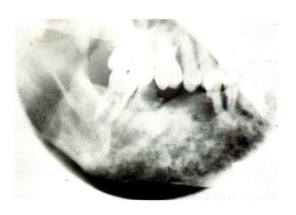

Figure 2.6 Chronic diffuse sclerosing osteomyelitis

Pulse granuloma (chronic periostitis) of the jaw

Pulse (hyaline ring) granuloma is an uncommon lesion which usually affects the edentulous posterior mandible. It can cause recurrent swelling and tenderness. Radiographically, there is typically a radiolucent area with an irregular outline, or erosion of the crest of the alveolar bone, but there is sometimes subperiosteal bony thickening.

Microscopy
Eosinophilic hyaline rings are surrounded by granulation tissue with chronic inflammatory and multinucleated giant cells. The rings may be incomplete but may enclose giant cells, connective tissue and blood vessels. They resemble residues from leguminous vegetable matter by light and electron microscopy. Somewhat similar changes have been produced experimentally by implantation of homogenized cooked pulses: the starch component was gradually digested and the residual cellulose formed rings. These were less grossly thickened than those in human lesions where there appears to be adsorption of plasma proteins and gradual deposition of collagen on the surface. Rarely, starch granules have been seen within the hyaline rings in human material and are present in pulse granulomas sometimes found in the lungs of infants and debilitated adults. The differences between the jaw, lung and experimental lesions may possibly be due to changes induced by long persistence of the foreign material in the tissues.

Excision is curative.

Sclerotic (dense) bone islands (idiopathic osteosclerosis)

Areas of sclerosis in the mandible are sometimes seen by chance in routine, particularly panoramic, radiographs or may be noticed for the first time after a surgical procedure. In the past, these have been interpreted as the result of low-grade infection and have sometimes been removed surgically. They are most frequent in the molar or premolar region and may be related to the apex of a tooth, but separated by the periodontal ligament, or more deeply in the jaw. Kawai *et al.* (1992) found them in 10% of 1203 Japanese outpatients: this is approximately twice the prevalence of these osteoscleroses in Westerners. These enostoses are normal variations in the bone pattern and microscopically appear, as their name implies, as islands of sclerotic but otherwise normal bone surrounded by normal trabeculae.

Fascial space infections (cervicofacial cellulitis)

Deep fascial space infections, of which the best known example is Ludwig's angina, are characterized by gross inflammatory exudate and oedema, together with fever and toxaemia which may be severe. Before the use of antibiotics the mortality was high and the disease is still life-threatening if treatment is delayed. The clinical variants and their current management have been reviewed by Chow (1992).

These infections have become rare in many parts of Britain, but appear to be considerably more common among Afro-Caribbeans. Such patients are fit, well-nourished young male adults with no apparent predisposing factors other than apical or periodontal abscesses. These patients do not have diagnosable immunological or haematological defects, though many have sickle cell trait. Their oral hygiene is possibly better than that of the general white population.

General clinical features
The characteristic features are diffuse, brawny swelling, pain, fever and malaise. The swelling is tense, tender, with a characteristic board-like firmness. The overlying skin is taut and shiny. Pain and oedema cause difficulty in opening the mouth and, often, difficulty in swallowing. Constitutional upset is severe with worsening fever, toxaemia and leucocytosis. The regional lymph nodes are swollen and tender.

Once oedema extends towards the glottis, as in Ludwig's angina particularly, or the tongue is forced upwards and backwards into the airway, there is increasing respiratory distress which, if not rapidly relieved, quickly results in asphyxia. Tracheostomy may then be necessary.

Aetiology and pathology

The organisms responsible are mainly odontogenic and include a variety of obligate anaerobes which Chow (1992) found to outnumber aerobes by a factor of 10 to 1 (Table 2.2).

Fasciae covering muscles and other structures are normally in close apposition. If these fascial planes are spread apart, a space is created. Such spaces contain little except loose connective tissue and are almost avascular. If virulent bacteria enter these fascial planes, inflammatory exudate is poured out from nearby vessels, but if it fails to localize the organisms it opens up the fascial space, carrying infection with it (Figure 2.7). Infection may thus spread through one or more fascial spaces until their natural boundaries are reached.

The main cause of cellulitis of the neck is infection arising from the region of the lower molars. Several fascial spaces are accessible from this area and the following factors contribute:

● the apices of the second and, more especially, the third molars are often close to the lingual surface of the mandible
● the mylohyoid attachment inclines downwards as it runs forward; the apices of the third molar are usually, and the second molar are often, below this line
● the posterior border of the mylohyoid is close to the sockets of the third molars; at this point the floor of the mouth consists only of mucous membrane covering part of the submandibular salivary gland.

When a virulent periapical infection of a lower third molar penetrates the lingual plate of the jaw, it is then at the entrance to several fascial spaces. Anteriorly there are the submandibular and sublingual spaces, while posteriorly are the parapharyngeal and pterygoid spaces. Infection in this area may rarely also spread from an acute pericoronitis, particularly when the deeper tissues are opened to infection by extraction of the tooth during the acute phase. Indresano *et al.* (1992) identified 21 patients, over a 6-year period, with deep space infections attributable to pericoronitis and reached the remarkable conclusion that, in the USA, as many as 15 000 serious or life-threatening infections a year might originate from third molar infections.

Cellulitis can be a complication of acute osteomyelitis of the jaws due to spread of an exceptionally virulent infection, but this is unlikely to be seen now.

In general, perioral cellulitis is only likely to develop when virulent and invasive organisms gain access to the fascial spaces. Since the predisposing causes do not often coincide, cellulitis is uncommon. Cellulitis in the region of the upper jaw is even more uncommon, but may develop in various sites as the result of infected local anaesthetic needles.

Table 2.2   Examples of bacteria isolated from perimandibular fascial space infections

ANAEROBIC BACTERIA

Porphyromonas gingivalis and Bacteroides species	*Escherichia coli* Klebsiella
	Pseudomonas aeruginosa
Fusobacteria including *Fusobacterium nucleatum*	*Staphylococcus epidermidis* and *S. aureus*
Peptostreptococci and peptococci	Proteus species
Eikenella corrodens	*Haemophilus influenzae* (children especially)

AEROBIC AND FACULTATIVE
BACTERIA

Beta-haemolytic
streptococci
Viridans streptococci
(*S. morbillorum,*
S. constellatus or
S. sanguis)

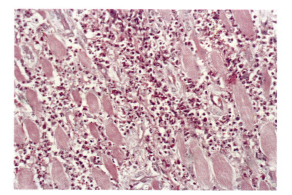

Figure 2.7   Acute cellulitis. The tissues are spread apart by the onward tracking of acute inflammatory cells and exudate

Sublingual cellulitis

The sublingual space lies between the mucous membrane of the floor of the mouth above, and the mylohyoid below and laterally. Medially, the space is bounded by the geniohyoid and genioglossus muscles, but in front of them the left and right sublingual spaces are continuous. A deep extension of the space lies between the genial muscles. Posteriorly, on either side, the sublingual space is open, communicating round the posterior border of the mylohyoid with the submandibular space below, and with the parapharyngeal space behind. The sublingual space contains the sublingual gland and related arteries and nerves.

Clinical features

The source of infection is usually a mandibular molar, but occasionally infection from a more anterior tooth may penetrate the lingual plate of bone. Sublingual cellulitis is characterized by gross swelling of the floor of the mouth. The mucosa is red or purplish and pushed upwards, level with the occlusal surfaces of the teeth, which indent it. Swallowing is difficult due to oedema of the muscles of the tongue, which becomes swollen and elevated, occasionally so severely as to threaten the airway.

Infection may remain localized in the sublingual space or may spread backwards towards the parapharyngeal, pterygoid or submandibular space.

Submandibular cellulitis

The submandibular space contains the submandibular salivary gland and is formed by the splitting of the deep cervical fascia above the hyoid bone. The submandibular space is bounded laterally and below by the superficial layer of the deep cervical fascia which extends from the hyoid bone to the mylohyoid and forms the superior and medial boundary of the space. The intercommunications of the three main fascial spaces in this area are shown by the deep process of the submandibular gland. This curves round the posterior border of the mylohyoid, juts into the entry to the parapharyngeal space and, by curving forward on to the superior surface of the mylohyoid muscle, extends into the sublingual space.

Clinical features

Submandibular cellulitis is typically caused by infection from the second or third molars. Painful brawny swelling is centred on the upper part of the neck, mainly along the lower border of the mandible. Infection may spread into the sublingual or parapharyngeal spaces as already indicated, to give rise to Ludwig's angina.

Ludwig's angina

Ludwig's angina is a severe form of cellulitis which usually arises from the lower second or third molars; it involves the sublingual and submandibular spaces bilaterally almost simultaneously and readily spreads into the parapharyngeal and pterygoid spaces.

The parapharyngeal space extends backwards from the lingual aspect of the third molar region, between the superior constrictor of the pharynx medially and the internal pterygoid laterally. Above the mylohyoid line the space is limited anteriorly by the pterygomandibular raphe. Below, the parapharyngeal space is bounded by the muscles arising from the styloid process. The carotid sheath lies within this space.

The pterygoid space lies lateral to the pharyngeal space. It is bordered laterally by the mandibular ramus and medially by the medial pterygoid muscle. Above, it communicates with the infratemporal fossa.

Clinical features

Ludwig's angina is characterized by rapid development of sublingual and submandibular cellulitis with painful brawny swelling of the upper part of the neck and the floor of the mouth on both sides. With involvement of the parapharyngeal space, the swelling tracks down the neck, and oedema can quickly spread into the loose connective tissue round the glottis.

Swallowing and opening the mouth become difficult, and the tongue may be pushed up against the soft palate. Oedema of the glottis causes increasing respiratory obstruction. The patient soon becomes seriously ill, with fever, respiratory distress, headache and malaise.

Respiratory obstruction is indicated by noisy breathing and restlessness, going on to violent efforts at respiration using the accessory muscles, and darkening cyanosis. A patient with cellulitis of the neck may die quickly from asphyxia, or later from the effects of spread of infection to the mediastinum via the carotid sheath.

Management

A patient with a brawny swelling of the mouth or neck, fever and malaise must be immediately admitted to hospital. The first essential is to secure the airway. If there is dyspnoea, an endotracheal tube should be inserted with the help of a fibreoptic bronchoscope. A specimen for culture should be obtained by fine-needle aspiration to avoid contamination by oral bacteria. The mainstay of treatment of cellulitis is vigorous use of antibiotics. Provided that the patient is not allergic, intravenous penicillin (not less than 600 mg given every 6 h) is the traditional treatment, but resistant bacteria are increasingly frequently encountered. To counter anaerobes, metronidazole (800 mg 8-hourly by i.v. infusion) can be given with penicillin or alone if the patient is allergic to the latter. A case has been made by Finer and Goustas (1992) for the use of ceftazidime, an injectable third-generation cephalosporin as initial treatment for severe infections. It has a wide spectrum of activity particularly against Gram-negative bacteria and is not nephrotoxic or ototoxic. However, metronidazole may also be needed.

The swelling should be incised early to relieve the pressure of exudate, particularly when the swelling is so large as to force the tongue into the airway. Little fluid is produced at first, but continues to dribble away. The neck should be laid open widely, all tissue spaces opened with sinus forceps and multiple corrugated drains inserted. Often through-and-through drainage is required with bilateral drains through the neck into the oral cavity.

General anaesthesia is particularly hazardous in the later stages of Ludwig's angina if the patient has not been intubated. If the patient is dependent on conscious effort to breathe, the airway is lost immediately a muscle relaxant is given and emergency tracheostomy becomes necessary. This may itself open up further tissue planes to infection. For this reason, surgical drainage should be undertaken early, before respiratory obstruction develops. Should anaesthesia be necessary at this stage, the patient can be given a gaseous induction without muscle relaxants and an attempt made at intubation, preferably using a fibreoptic bronchoscope. The surgeon must stand by ready to perform an emergency tracheostomy.

The tooth from which the infection started should be extracted as soon as the patient's condition allows.

Cavernous sinus thrombosis

Cavernous sinus thrombosis is a life-threatening complication that can rarely arise from an infected upper anterior tooth. Other sources include infected spots or boils on the upper lip or in the anterior nares. Infected thrombi in the anterior facial vein or, less frequently, in the pterygoid plexus of veins communicate with the cavernous sinus via either the ophthalmic veins or via the foramen ovale, respectively.

Clinical features

Gross oedema of the eyelid is associated with pulsatile exophthalmos due to venous obstruction. Venous stasis leads to cyanosis, and the superior orbital fissure syndrome (proptosis, fixed dilated pupil and limited eye movement) rapidly develops. The facial vein is dilated and the conjunctiva is oedematous. There is papilloedema with multiple retinal haemorrhages. The patient is seriously ill with rigors and a high swinging pyrexia. Initially one side is affected, but both sides become quickly affected if treatment is delayed. Blindness complicating cavernous sinus thrombosis secondary to dental infection has been reported by Ogundiya *et al.* (1989), who also reviewed earlier cases.

Management

Administration of antibiotics and drainage of pus are essential. Extraction of the causative tooth may spread the infection and should be delayed until the disease is controlled. Corticosteroids are recommended to prevent circulatory collapse secondary to pituitary dysfunction, but the use of anticoagulants is controversial as they may promote spread of the infection. There is a 50% mortality and of those who survive half may lose the sight of one or both eyes. Unusually early treatment of a patient reported by Ogundiya *et al.* (1989) allowed restoration of sight.

Necrotizing fasciitis

Necrotizing fasciitis is a rare but potentially lethal infection of subcutaneous tissues and deep fascia, associated with necrosis of the overlying skin due to thrombosis of nutrient vessels. It can arise from a dental infection and affect the face or neck where it can threaten the airway. Severe systemic toxicity is typically associated, but many patients are initially apyrexial. Most patients are young adults but in some, immunosuppression, diabetes mellitus or other deficiency states may be contributory. The infection was originally attributed to β-haemolytic streptococci. More recently other bacteria, including anaerobes such as Bacteroides species, have been isolated. In about 25% of cases the infection is odontogenic and Rubin and Cozzi (1987) reported fatal necrotizing mediastinitis complicating a dental infection.

Clinically, the rapid spread of tissue destruction is emphasized by Muto *et al.* (1992). Within 24–48 hours the area becomes red, oedematous and painful but soon becomes anaesthetic. The site, which may be well- or ill-demarcated, becomes dusky, purplish or black and by the fourth or fifth day necrosis of the skin appears. This necrotic tissue starts to separate within 8–10 days. Cases in Britain have recently been reported by Kaddour and Smelt (1992) and Gaukroger (1992), who have also reviewed earlier reports; all their patients were elderly women.

Management
Diagnosis depends on recognition of both fasciitis and cutaneous necrosis. However, surgical intervention and antimicrobial treatment should start before necrosis develops. A major danger is that in the early stages the infection can be mistaken for cellulitis and reliance placed solely on antibiotics.

Release of offensive brownish exudate with gas bubbles is indicative of tissue necrosis.

The airway should be protected by intubation and adequate hydration maintained. The area should be opened up and the extent of undermining of the skin determined by finger exploration. Drains should be inserted and parenteral antibiotics given as soon as material has been obtained for culture. Initial antimicrobial treatment should start with penicillin or a cephalosporin plus metronidazole, but changed if bacteriological findings dictate. Necrotic muscle and any other tissue should be excised and debridement maintained until the area is clean. If the problem is recognized and treated sufficiently early, little skin may need to be removed, but in many cases grafting is required after subsidence of the infection.

Cancrum oris (noma)

Cancrum oris is a gangrenous infection spreading outwards from the mouth to cause extensive facial destruction and, often, a fatal outcome.

The disease has virtually disappeared from the developed countries, but is still seen in countries, particularly parts of Africa, where malnutrition, poor oral hygiene and debilitating diseases are contributory. Two cases were reported by Griffin *et al.* (1983) in children who had been brought from Micronesia.

The disease predominantly affects children under the age of 10 years, and only those with impaired defences due to protein calorie malnutrition, anaemia or infections such as measles are susceptible.

The microbial cause appears to be the Gram-negative anaerobic fuso-spirochaetal complex of Vincent's infection (traditionally termed *Borrelia (Treponema) vincentii* and a fusiform bacillus which may be *Fusobacterium nucleatum*), probably in combination with other anaerobes such as Bacteroides species.

Cancrum oris starts within the oral cavity as an acute ulcerative gingivitis associated with extensive oedema but extends outwards, rapidly destroying soft tissues and bone (Figure 2.8). The gangrenous process starts as a painful, small, reddish-purple spot or indurated papule which ulcerates. The ulcer spreads to involve the labiogingival fold, adjacent

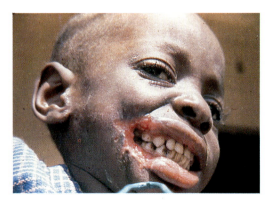

Figure 2.8   Cancrum oris. The soft tissue destruction is spreading towards the cheek from the angle of the mouth (By courtesy of Professor R.D. Emslie)

mucosa and underlying bone (Figure 2.9). Diffuse oedema of the face, fetor and profuse salivation are associated. As the overlying tissues become ischaemic, the skin turns blue-black. The gangrenous area becomes increasingly sharply demarcated and ultimately sloughs away. The slough is cone shaped, with its apex superficial so that the underlying destruction of hard and soft tissues is more extensive than external appearances suggest. As the slough separates, the bone becomes necrotic: sequestration and exfoliation of teeth follow.

Management
Underlying disease such as malnutrition, malaria, typhoid, tuberculosis and measles must be treated.

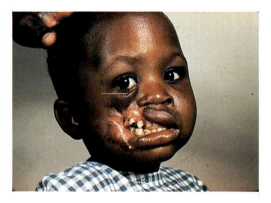

Figure 2.9   Cancrum oris. The acute infection has been controlled and there is healing at the margins of the extensive facial defect (By courtesy of Professor R.D. Emslie)

Parenteral rehydration, together with nasogastric tube feeding, may be needed. Blood transfusions and iron supplements are required when the haemoglobin is below 10 g/l. Without early treatment, the mortality is high.

A combination of penicillin and metronidazole will usually control the local infection. It gradually resolves in survivors, but is severely mutilating.

Soft tissue abscesses

An abscess may form as a result of direct spread from a periapical infection or be the result of localization of a fascial space infection. The cheek and palate are typical sites. The microbial causes are varied and ill-defined.

Buccal abscesses

An abscess affecting the cheek may be either medial or lateral to the buccinator. Infection from the apex of a molar tooth, after breaking through the buccal plate of either jaw, most commonly points on the buccal gingiva but occasionally spreads deep to the buccal sulcus. An abscess may thus form in the vestibule, medial to the buccinator muscle. If the apices of teeth are deep to the level of the attachment of the buccinator, infection can track across, reaching the lateral surface of the muscle (the buccinator space).

Clinically, there is pain, swelling, redness and tenderness of the cheek. There may be a history of acute toothache. The swelling, though not easily defined because of the thickness of the cheek, is more localized than that of cellulitis; systemic effects are slight. In the case of a vestibular abscess the intraoral swelling is prominent, obliterating the buccal sulcus; the cheek is oedematous and swollen. In the case of a buccinator space infection, the whole cheek is much thickened, red and hot externally. The angle of the mouth is pulled outwards. Later the swelling becomes fluctuant as pus localizes.

Recurrent buccal space abscesses have been described as a rare complication of Crohn's disease by Malins *et al.* (1991).

Palatal abscess

Infection may spread from a lateral incisor because of its backward-sloping root, or from the palatal root of a molar.

Clinically, the swelling is rounded, discrete and tender. It is usually close to the offending tooth, but occasionally infection may spread to the posterior border of the hard palate from a lateral incisor.

Submasseteric abscess

Sometimes infection around a lower third molar tracks backwards lateral to the mandibular ramus and pus localizes deep to the masseter attachment. Such an abscess deep to the thick masseter produces little visible swelling but is accompanied by profound muscle spasm and limitation of opening.

Management of a soft tissue abscess
Antibiotic therapy may be unnecessary if the abscess is small and well localized, as in the case of many vestibular or palatal abscesses. Otherwise 600 mg of penicillin should be given to hasten localization.

The infected tooth should be extracted or the root canal opened using general anaesthesia or regional analgesia well away from the site of infection, and pus must be drained by incision.

Actinomycosis

Actinomycosis is an uncommon, chronic, suppurative infection caused by a filamentous bacterium. It causes multiple abscesses and sinuses, followed by widespread fibrosis. The soft tissue in the region of the angle of the jaw is the most common site.

The causative organism is typically *Actinomyces israelii*, but other bacteria may occasionally be responsible. In culture, pathogenic actinomyces grow slowly on enriched media under anaerobic conditions to form a mass of branching filaments.

Though the infection is caused by organisms present in the normal mouth, it is not clear how it becomes established. Injuries, especially dental extractions or fractures of the jaw, can provide a pathway into the tissues and sometimes precede infection. Nevertheless the organisms are common in the mouth, but actinomycosis rarely follows extractions: most patients were previously healthy and it is uncommon even in patients with AIDS. The pathogenesis of actinomycosis is therefore unclear.

Clinical features
Men are predominantly affected, typically adults between the ages of 30 and 60 years. The complaint is usually of a chronic soft tissue swelling near the angle of the jaw in the upper neck. There may be a history of dental extractions, especially of lower molars, several weeks previously. The swelling is dusky red or purplish in colour, firm and slightly tender. The skin becomes fixed to the underlying tissues and eventually breaks down as the characteristic sinuses and discharge form. There is often difficulty in opening the mouth, but pain is minimal.

The lymph nodes are not affected, but may occasionally become involved by local spread of the actinomyces or by secondary infection.

Healing leads to scarring and puckering of the skin and, in the absence of treatment, a large fibrotic mass can form, covered by scarred and pigmented skin on which several sinuses open. However, such a picture is largely of historical interest. Currently the more usual clinical features are a persistent subcutaneous collection of pus or a sinus, unresponsive to conventional short courses of antibiotics.

Microscopy
Actinomyces israelii spreads by direct extension through the tissues and provokes chronic inflammation with suppuration. In the tissues, colonies of actinomyces form rounded masses of filaments, at the periphery of which radially-arranged club-shaped thickenings develop. Neutrophils mass round the colonies; pus forms centrally, chronic inflammatory cells surround the focus and an abscess wall of connective tissue is formed.

The abscess eventually points on the skin, discharging pus in which sulphur granules (colonies of actinomyces) may occasionally be visible (Figure 2.10). The abscess continues to discharge and the surrounding tissues become fibrotic. Nevertheless, the infection spreads to cause further abscesses. In the absence of effective treatment, the area may eventually become honeycombed with many abscesses and sinuses and widespread fibrosis, but this is unlikely to be seen now. The infection exceptionally rarely develops within the bone of the jaw.

Diagnosis

For bacteriological confirmation of the diagnosis a fresh specimen of pus is needed for culture. Sulphur granules are rarely obvious but may be seen when the pus is rinsed with sterile saline. A positive diagnosis can rarely be made in the absence of sulphur granules (Figure 2.11). It is also important to tell the laboratory that actinomycosis is suspected to enable the appropriate media to be used and the culture maintained long enough for the organisms to grow.

Frequently small amounts of penicillin have been given earlier. These are insufficient to control the infection but make bacteriological diagnosis difficult.

Management

The mainstay of treatment is penicillin, erythromycin or tetracycline: 2 g of oral penicillin a day should be given, and continued from 4 to 6 weeks

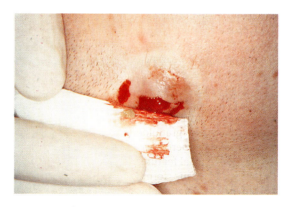

Figure 2.11   Actinomycosis. Incision of a persistent, solitary, dusky red nodule has released a large sulphur granule

or occasionally longer; pockets of surviving organisms may persist in the depths of the lesion to cause relapse after a short course of treatment. Abscesses should be drained surgically as they form. For patients allergic to penicillin, erythromycin is an effective alternative.

Complications

The most dangerous complication is spread of the infection to the lungs or elsewhere, but is rare. Actinomycosis sometimes primarily affects the lungs or ileocaecal region of the gut and in these situations may be fatal.

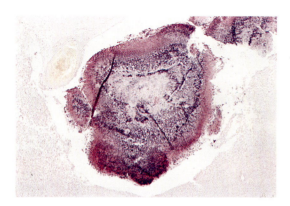

Figure 2.10   Actinomycosis. Gram staining of a sulphur granule shows the typical radial arrangement of the filaments at the periphery

The deep mycoses

The deep mycoses are rare in Britain, but are most likely to be seen in immunocompromised patients or in those who have come from endemic areas such as South America. Among immunodeficient patients, the chief underlying causes are diseases such as lymphoreticular diseases, diabetes mellitus or immunosuppressive treatment. AIDS patients are subject to a great variety of fungal infections (see Table 14.5) which may form the presenting symptom. Nevertheless, there are surprisingly few reports of oral lesions due to the deep mycoses among HIV-positive patients, though superficial candidosis is common.

Clinically, several of the deep mycoses can cause oral lesions at some stage, and often then give rise to a nodular and ulcerated mass, which can be tumour-like in appearance. The orofacial manifestations of the deep mycoses and their treatment have been reviewed by Scully and de Almeida (1992).

As to microscopic diagnosis, the deep mycoses frequently cause granulomatous reactions which may simulate tuberculosis to a greater or lesser degree. The crucial feature, if it can be found, is the characteristic tissue form of the fungus. Culture should be confirmatory, but since a deep mycosis is unlikely to be suspected clinically, fresh material is rarely available. The serology is sometimes informative, but it may be difficult to establish the diagnosis with certainty.

For life-threatening mycoses, intravenous amphotericin, 0.5–1 mg/kg/day is usually the first choice despite its toxicity, but where nephrotoxicity is too great a threat, amphotericin encapsulated in liposomes (1 mg/day increasing to 3 mg/day), fluconazole or itraconazole 200–400 mg/day are frequently effective and less toxic alternatives. Itraconazole is less well absorbed but highly tissue-bound. It has a broader spectrum of activity than fluconazole. Oral flucytosine is well absorbed, is synergistic with amphotericin, but resistance readily develops. However, there have been too few clinical trials to establish definitively the relative efficacy of the different antifungal drugs in specific deep mycoses. Intravenous amphotericin remains the mainstay for life-threatening infections, while fluconazole or itraconazole are mainly used for maintenance therapy.

Even when diagnosis cannot be confirmed by culture or serology, if the patient has been at risk of exposure as a result of residence in an endemic area, and the clinical and microscopic features are consistent with those of a mycosis, antifungal chemotherapy with a drug such as fluconazole may be justified. Response to such treatment will in turn help to confirm the diagnosis, and is likely to save the patient from further spread of the infection.

Histoplasmosis

Histoplasma capsulatum can cause localized or generalized disease, but is subclinical in perhaps 95% of cases.

Histoplasmosis is seen in the endemic areas of the Americas, Africa, South East Asia and Australia and can be secondary to immunodeficiency states, but is not naturally present in Britain. The main clinical types of infection are pulmonary, which may heal without symptoms, or disseminated and fatal. Oral lesions may develop in 30–50% of cases of disseminated disease. Virtually any part of the mouth can then be affected, but the lesions are not distinctive. Nodular, granulomatous, proliferative and ulcerative oral lesions of histoplasmosis are readily mistaken clinically for neoplasms. Extensive and painful tissue destruction can develop and palatal perforation is well recognized.

Microscopy

The lesions simulate tuberculosis to a variable degree, with granuloma formation and focal collections of epithelioid cells, together with Langhans-type giant cells, and there may be caseous necrosis. Alternatively, there may be diffuse sheets of inflammatory cells. The yeast forms, 2–4 μm in diameter, can sometimes be demonstrated, particularly in PAS or silver-stained sections, in epithelioid or giant cells, but are more likely to be numerous, in the absence of granuloma formation (Figures 2.12–2.14).

Antifungal treatment with intravenous amphotericin is essential to control pulmonary infection and prevent dissemination but itraconazole may also be effective.

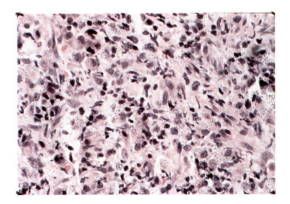

Figure 2.12 Histoplasmosis. Haematoxylin and eosin staining has failed to demonstrate the fungus and is uninformative

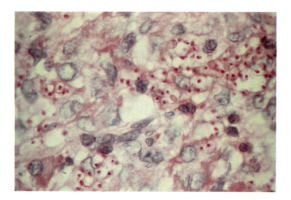

Figure 2.13   Histoplasmosis. PAS staining shows the yeast forms with their characteristic halos

Mucormycosis (phycomycosis, zygomycosis)

Mucormycosis is an invasive infection caused by any of the Phycomycetales, particularly Absidia, Mucor and Rhizopus. These common saprophytic moulds, which grow on decaying organic material, had long been thought to be entirely harmless. Mucor species have rarely been reported among the normal human flora.

Aetiology and pathology

The spores are probably inhaled, but infection mainly affects those with underlying disease, particularly poorly controlled diabetes mellitus or acute leukaemia, or those having immunosuppressive treatment.

The main forms of mucormycosis are pulmonary and rhinocerebral. Rhinocerebral mucormycosis typically starts in the maxillary antrum, particularly in young adult, poorly controlled diabetics. Invasion of surrounding tissues can cause necrotizing ulceration of the palate with a blackish slough and exposure of bone. Local pain and tenderness over the sinus and low fever are associated with nodular thickening of the antral lining and sometimes radiographic evidence of patchy destruction of the walls of several paranasal sinuses. There may also be nasal congestion or bloody discharge.

More important is spread to the orbit causing blurred vision, proptosis and limitation of movement of the eye. Spread to the brain is indicated by clouding of consciousness, cranial nerve palsies, loss of vision, coma and death, often within 2 weeks of the clinical signs.

Microscopy

Once infection has become established, the hyphae can be recognized in the tissues by their characteristically irregular width (3–20 μm) and by a crushed ribbon appearance (Figure 2.15). The hyphae are typically non-septate and show right-angled branching. They may be seen in haematoxylin and eosin stained sections, but more clearly when PAS or silver stains are used. The infection characteristically involves blood vessels with

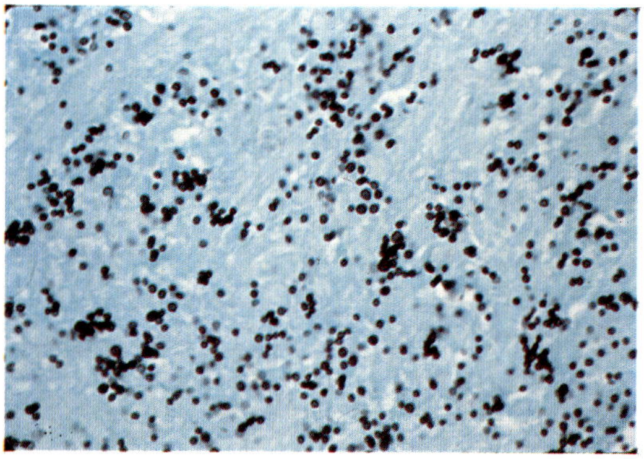

Figure 2.14   Histoplasmosis. Silver (Grocott) staining of the same specimen as in Figure 2.13 shows the fungus clearly

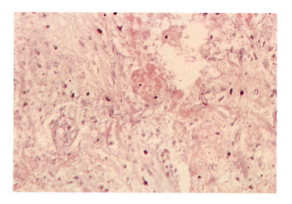

Figure 2.15   Mucormycosis. Haematoxylin and eosin staining of a solid mass of fungal hyphae shows the typical crushed ribbon appearance

thromboses and haemorrhages, an inflammatory response and tissue necrosis.

Diagnosis

When oral lesions are the first complaint, biopsy should enable the fungus and its characteristic pathological effects to be recognized, and allow relatively early diagnosis. If the only feature is sinusitis, biopsy is also important, but rapid diagnosis may be possible by examination of a wet smear of crushed fresh tissue stained with methylene blue. Such investigation is particularly important in a diabetic who appears to be developing ketotic coma unresponsive to insulin and other appropriate measures. Early loss of vision may help to differentiate rhinocerebral phycomycosis from pyogenic cavernous sinus thrombosis. No reliable method of immunological diagnosis is available.

Surgical debridement and antifungal treatment, usually with amphotericin, together with control of any diabetes are essential. Despite such treatment the mortality is high, especially in patients with leukaemia.

Aspergillosis

Aspergillus species (particularly *A. fumigatus*) are now a cause of opportunistic infections, rivalling candidosis in frequency as a complication of long-term antimicrobial or immunosuppressive treatment. Aspergillosis only rarely affects otherwise healthy patients.

Aspergillosis can have widely different manifestations. They include systemic aspergillosis and either pulmonary or disseminated infection in the immunosuppressed, allergic pneumonitis (an asthma-like disease) or rhinocerebral aspergillosis, or harmless aspergillomas (fungus balls) in the maxillary antrum. Zinreich *et al.* (1988) report the value of MRI to detect calcium and other metallic deposits characteristic of aspergillus infections of the sinuses.

Oronasal (rhinocerebral) aspergillosis

Rhinocerebral aspergillosis is a rare variant. It is usually caused by *A. flavus*, and particularly affects poorly controlled diabetics, though Martinez *et al.*

(1992) have described invasive maxillary aspergillosis after a dental extraction in a previously healthy patient. Pain, swelling of the face and nasal discharge may be early signs. Like rhinocerebral mucormycosis, aspergillosis tends to spread through the orbit to the brain, but spread is via tissue spaces rather than blood vessels, and is slower than in mucormycosis. Occasionally, infection extends through the palate to produce a necrotic brown or blackish ulcer. Painful, bleeding oral lesions have also been reported as a rare feature of disseminated aspergillosis.

Diagnosis is by recognition of the dichotomous hyphae in the tissues by microscopy, but the characteristic mop-like spore-bearing structures are rarely seen (Figures 2.16 and 2.17). Culture is therefore also essential and serology may be informative. Treatment is by surgical excision of infected tissue and intravenous amphotericin. Itraconazole is a possible alternative.

An aspergillomatous fungus ball is a rare cause of opacity of the antrum in a healthy person. The mass appears brown and dry and the hyphae are recognizable only by microscopy, though culture is confirmatory if fresh material is available. Following removal of the fungal mass, no treatment is necessary, provided that the patient remains healthy.

Cryptococcosis

The spores of *Cryptococcosis neoformans* are frequently spread by bird droppings, but infection is

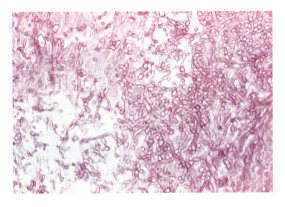

Figure 2.16 Aspergillosis. The hyphae show the typical septation and branching of aspergillus species (Haematoxylin and eosin)

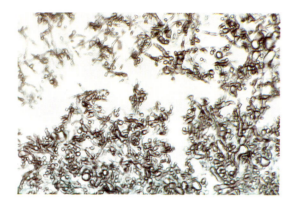

Figure 2.17 Aspergillosis. Grocott staining of the same specimen as in Figure 2.16 shows more clearly the even diameter of the hyphae and, in some cases, clubbing of their ends

often subclinical. Cryptococcosis can develop in normal persons but is usually secondary to immunosuppressive treatment, lymphomas or diabetes mellitus. In the USA, Diamond (1991) reported a prevalence of cryptococcosis in 5–15% of AIDS patients and it is the most frequent initial opportunistic infection.

Clinical features

The main forms of cryptococcosis are chronic meningitis, or pulmonary or disseminated infection. Oral lesions of cryptococcosis are reported to be uncommon and mainly a complication of widespread disease. In AIDS there may be fungaemia but an indefinite febrile illness.

An oral lesion has no distinctive clinical features, but appears as a granular swelling, a large necrotic ulcer or sometimes smaller ulcers.

Microscopy

Cryptococcosis causes granuloma formation with histiocytes, giant cells and lymphocytes, which may surround areas of necrosis. The organism is a spherical or ovoid spore surrounded by a characteristic halo formed by the large gelatinous capsule. It may be seen within giant cells or histiocytes or free in the tissues. It is helped by its unique ability among fungi to form melanin; Masson Fontana staining shows darkly staining budding yeasts.

Diagnosis can be confirmed by culture and positive latex agglutination or ELISA tests for capsular antigen.

Treatment with intravenous amphotericin together with flucytosine or fluconazole is successful in most cases, with a 90% survival rate. In AIDS patients, relapse is so common that continuous suppressive treatment with fluconazole or itraconazole must be given.

Blastomycosis (North American blastomycosis)

Males aged between 40 and 60 years are mainly affected with pulmonary or cutaneous disease. Lesions of the oral or nasal mucosa may be present in 25% of patients. Occasionally, oral lesions may be the first sign leading to the diagnosis, but are non-specific in character. They may be ulcerated or resemble actinomycosis; the regional lymph nodes are usually enlarged.

Microscopy

Blastomyces dermatiditis causes a chronic granulomatous reaction, usually with numerous macrophages and giant cells, but a tendency to suppuration. Within these lesions, the tissue phase of the organism may sometimes be seen as a large thick-walled yeast with single buds attached by a broad base.

Blastomycosis usually responds rapidly and completely to intravenous amphotericin and drainage of any abscesses, but fluconazole or itraconazole may be effective for less virulent infections.

Paracoccidioidomycosis (South American blastomycosis)

Infection by *Paracoccidioides brasiliensis* is endemic in and virtually confined to South America. Infection can be mucocutaneous, pulmonary or disseminated. Adult males are mainly affected, and frequently have oral lesions which, though often secondary to pulmonary or disseminated disease, are a common early sign. The fungus probably enters through gross or microscopic wounds, which may include periodontal tissues and extraction wounds. The lesions are frequently nodular and ulcerative, can affect any part of the mouth and sometimes extend on to adjacent skin. The ulcers may have a mulberry-like appearance with pin-point haemorrhages (de Almeida *et al.*, 1991) and the regional lymph nodes may be involved. Proliferative or papillomatous lesions resembling those on the skin (Figure 2.18) can also develop in the mouth but have rarely been reported.

Microscopy

Mucosal lesions are usually granulomatous, but with an acute inflammatory infiltrate and abscess formation. The tissue phase of the organism is a spherical yeast cell considerably larger than that of *Blastomyces dermatiditis*; multiple budding produces appearances described as Mickey Mouse or pilot wheel cells. These may lie free in the inflammatory infiltrate or within giant cells, but may not be readily found.

Paracoccidioidomycosis responds to amphotericin but itraconazole may also be effective.

Systemic infections by oral bacteria

The mouth is inhabited by a great variety of microbes, but has high levels of local immunity. As a result, bony wounds caused by multiple extractions or oral surgery usually heal without

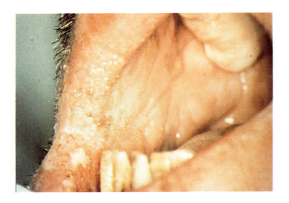

Figure 2.18 Paracoccidioidomycosis (South American blastomycosis). This papilliferous lesion is one of the possible clinical appearances

incident despite the innumerable pathogens present in periodontal pockets. The virulence of these bacteria is shown by the fact that human bites cause considerably more severe infections than animal bites. Moreover, oral bacteria escaping into the bloodstream of immunocompromised patients can cause severe metastatic infections or septicaemias, which can be fatal. Even *Leptotrichia buccalis*, long thought to be a harmless component of dental plaque, can cause septicaemia in immunodepressed patients.

A special example of a systemic infection of dental origin is infective endocarditis, which can follow dental operations, particularly extractions, and cause irreparable damage to heart valves or other organs.

Oral sources of bacteraemias

It is difficult to appreciate the sheer numbers of bacteria inhabiting the gingival margins when oral hygiene is poor, or the even vaster numbers present in periodontal pockets. By contrast, few bacteria inhabit the oral mucosa, and most are being constantly washed away by the saliva.

Sections of human teeth *in situ* show bacterial plaque in two dimensions, but *in vivo* plaque in a typical periodontal pocket consists of a solid mass of bacteria which usually forms a collar round the whole circumference of every tooth. As a result of the inflammation induced by these bacteria, they are in close contact with dilated, thin-walled blood vessels. Movement of the teeth during chewing, or more violently during extractions, repeatedly compresses and stretches or ruptures these vessels, so that bacteria can in effect be pumped into the bloodstream. Extractions appear, therefore, to be the precipitating factor in over 95% of cases of dentally related cases of infective endocarditis.

Chronic periapical lesions, by contrast, contain few bacteria, and it is difficult to obtain bacteria from them. Bacteria escaping from a necrotic pulp are immediately mopped up by inflammatory cells. Such few bacteria as are present are also well-isolated by the thick wall of granulation tissue that forms the bulk of the lesion. However, some physicians still regard periapical radiolucencies as 'dental abscesses' and a threat to patients' health. The 1920s idea of so-called focal sepsis has been difficult to eradicate from medical mythology.

Acute apical abscesses may contain many bacteria, but the numbers are still small in comparison with those filling periodontal pockets and unlike the latter usually only affect a single tooth and are unlikely to be an important source of systemic infection.

The chief effects of bacteraemias of dental origin in susceptible patients are:

- infective endocarditis
- lung and brain abscesses
- metastatic infections or septicaemias in immunodeficient patients.

Infective endocarditis

Little needs to be said here, other than that patients with congenital or acquired heart lesions are particularly at risk, and that the highest incidence of and mortality from this disease is in the elderly.

Only dental operations traumatizing the gingival tissues (extractions, scaling and mucogingival surgery) carry a significant risk of inducing infective endocarditis, because of the large numbers of bacteria that can be forced into the bloodstream from this region. Nevertheless, only 10–15% of cases of endocarditis follow dental operations. Many other dental procedures (even tooth-brushing) can cause bacteraemias, as can other medical procedures, such as endoscopy or intubation, but bacteraemia is *not* synonymous with infective endocarditis, and such minor bacterial showers do not justify antibiotic prophylaxis (Figures 2.19 and 2.20).

Root canal treatment hardly ever leads to endocarditis in clinical practice and antibiotic prophylaxis is not recommended for it.

Lung and brain abscesses

Some of these abscesses are due to oral anaerobic bacteria which are probably aspirated during sleep to cause a lung abscess and a secondary brain abscess. Isolated brain abscesses caused by oral bacteria are recognized but difficult to explain.

Immunodeficiency states

In severe immunodeficiency states, such as in organ transplant patients or those with lymphoreticular diseases, bacteraemias of oral origin can sometimes cause metastatic infections or septicaemias. Many of these are spontaneous and probably induced by

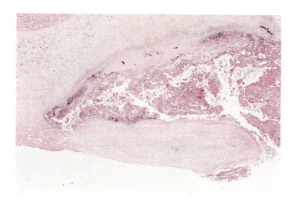

Figure 2.19   Infective endocarditis. Fibrinous vegetations have formed on the margins of the damaged valve

chewing; there is little evidence of dental operations precipitating bacteraemias in these patients, including those with AIDS.

However, if antibiotic cover for dental operations is felt to be desirable, , there neither is nor can be a definitive prophylactic regimen, as the causes are varied and unpredictable. A combination of amoxycillin 3 g plus metronidazole 400 mg by mouth, 1 hour before operations, may possibly offer some protection and can be repeated 6 hours later, if thought desirable.

Prosthetic joint replacements

These are susceptible to experimental blood-borne infections, but only when inocula are so heavy as to

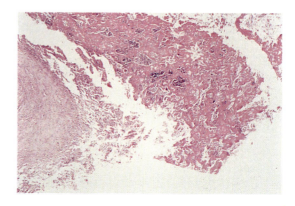

Figure 2.20   Infective endocarditis. A higher power view shows bacterial colonization of the fibrinous vegetations on the damaged valve

kill 50% of the animals. It is misleading to compare these experimental infections with the human situation. Despite the tens of thousands of such operations that have been carried out over the past 30 or more years in many countries, there have been virtually no authenticated cases where late prosthetic infection has been convincingly linked to dental treatment. The risks from antibiotic prophylaxis for dental procedures outweighs the benefits. Nevertheless, if an orthopaedic surgeon is adamant about the need for cover (as for infective endocarditis), it may be prudent to agree for the peace of mind of all concerned.

References

Chow, A.W. (1992) Life-threatening infections of the head and neck. *Clinical Infectious Diseases*, **14**, 991–1004

de Almeida, O.P., Jorge, J., Scully, C. *et al.* (1991) Oral manifestations of paracoccidioidomycosis (South American blastomycosis). *Oral Surgery, Oral Medicine and Oral Pathology*, **72**, 430–435

Diamond, R.D. (1991) The growing problem of mycoses in patients infected with the human immunodeficiency virus. *Review of Infectious Diseases*, **13**, 480–486

Finer, N. and Goustas, P. (1992) Ceftazidime versus aminoglycoside and (ureido)penicillin combination in the empirical treatment of serious infection. *Journal of the Royal Society of Medicine*, **85**, 530–533

Foster, J.H. (1992) Hyperbaric oxygen therapy: contraindications and complications. *Journal of Oral and Maxillofacial Surgery*, **50**, 1081–1086

Gaukroger, M.C. (1992) Cervicofacial necrotising fasciitis. *British Journal of Oral and Maxillofacial Surgery*, **30**, 111–114

Griffin, J.M., Bach, D.E., Nespeca, J.A. *et al.* (1983) Noma. Report of two cases. *Oral Surgery, Oral Medicine and Oral Pathology*, **56**, 605–607

Indresano, A.T., Haug, R.H. and Hoffman, M.J. (1992) The third molar as a cause of deep space infections. *Journal of Oral and Maxillofacial Surgery*, **50**, 33–35

Jansma, J., Vissink, A., Spijkervet, F.K.L. *et al.* (1992) Protocol for the prevention and treatment of oral sequelae resulting from head and neck radiation therapy. *Cancer*, **70**, 2171–2180

Kaddour, H.S. and Smelt, G.J.C. (1992) Necrotizing fasciitis of the neck. *Journal of Larygology and Otology*, **106**, 1008–1010

Kawai, T., Hirakuma, H., Murakami, S. *et al.* (1992) Radiographic investigation of idiopathic osteosclerosis of the jaws in Japanese dental outpatients. *Oral Surgery, Oral Medicine and Oral Pathology*, **74**, 237–242

Koorbusch, G.F., Fotos, P. and Goll, K.T. (1992) Retrospective assessment of osteomyelitis. Etiology, demographics, risk factors and management in 35 cases. *Oral Surgery, Oral Medicine and Oral Pathology*, **74**, 149–154

Malins, T.J., Wilson, A. and Ward-Booth, R.P. (1991) Recurrent buccal space abscesses. A complication of Crohn's disease. *Oral Surgery, Oral Medicine and Oral Pathology*, **72**, 19–21

Martinez, D., Burgueno, M., Forteza, G. *et al.* (1992) Invasive maxillary aspergillosis after dental extraction. *Oral Surgery, Oral Medicine and Oral Pathology*, **74**, 466–468

Marx, R.E. (1983) A new concept in the treatment of osteoradionecrosis. *Journal of Oral and Maxillofacial Surgery*, **41**, 351–357

Muto, T., Sato, K. and Kanazawa, M. (1992) Necrotizing fasciitis of the neck and chest. Report of a case. *International Journal of Oral and Maxillofacial Surgery*, **21**, 236–238

Ogundiya, D.A., Keith, D.A. and Mirowski, J. (1989) Cavernous sinus thrombosis and blindness as a complication of an odontogenic infection: report of a case and review of literature. *Journal of Oral and Maxillofacial Surgery*, **47**, 1317–1321

Ord, R.A. and El-Attar, A. (1987) Osteomyelitis of the mandible in children – clinical presentations and review of management. *British Journal of Oral and Maxillofacial Surgery*, **25**, 204–217

Robinson, P.G., Cooper, H. and Hatt, J. (1992) Healing after dental extractions in men with HIV infection. *Oral Surgery, Oral Medicine and Oral Pathology*, **74**, 426–430

Schneider, L.C. and Mesa, M.L. (1990) Differences between florid osseous dysplasia and chronic diffuse sclerosing osteomyelitis. *Oral Surgery, Oral Medicine and Oral Pathology*, **70**, 308–312

Rubin, G.M. and Cozzi, M.M. (1987) Fatal necrotizing mediastinitis as a complication of an odontogenic infection. *Journal of Oral and Maxillofacial Surgery*, **45**, 529–533

Scully, C. and de Almeida, O. (1992) Orofacial manifestations of the systemic mycoses. *Journal of Oral Pathology and Medicine*, **21**, 289–294

Shafer, W.G., Hine, M.K., Levy, B.M. *et al.* (1983) *A Textbook of Oral Pathology*, 4th edn, W.B. Saunders, Philadelphia

Van Merkesteyn, J.P.R., Bakker, D.J., van der Waal, I. *et al.* (1984) Hyperbaric oxygen treatment of chronic osteomyelitis of the jaws. *International Journal of Oral Surgery*, **13**, 386–395

Watson, W.L. and Scarborough, J.E. (1938) Osteoradionecrosis in intraoral cancer. *American Journal of Roentgenology*, **40**, 524–529

Zinreich, S.J., Kennedy, D.W., Malat, J. *et al.* (1988) Fungal sinusitis: diagnosis with CT and MR imaging. *Radiology*, **169**, 439–444

3

Cysts and cyst-like lesions of the jaws

Most jaw cysts fulfil the criteria of being pathological, fluid-filled cavities lined by epithelium. Only a few (simple and aneurysmal bone cysts) lack an epithelial lining or fluid contents, but occasionally a keratocyst has semi-solid contents of keratin. Cysts are the most common cause of chronic swellings of the jaws but few pose significant diagnostic or management problems to the competent surgeon.

The great majority of jaw cysts are odontogenic and usually radicular (periodontal) and can be recognized by the history and clinical and radiographic features. It is only rarely that the microscopic findings fail to confirm this assessment. However, it must always be borne in mind, as shown in Chapter 4, that ameloblastoma is the great deceiver. Important features of the main types of jaw cysts are summarized in Table 3.1 and the main points affecting the differential diagnosis of cysts from other cyst-like radiolucencies are summarized in Table 3.2.

Cysts of the jaws originate in several ways, as discussed in the text. However, inflammatory (periodontal) cysts, which are by far the most common, will be discussed first.

Relative frequency of different types of cyst
Several large series of cysts have been published and there is a moderate degree of agreement as follows:

Radicular	65–70%
Dentigerous	15–18%
Keratocysts	3–10%
Nasopalatine	2–5%

Keratocysts show the widest variation because of differences in diagnostic criteria in earlier series.

Mechanisms of cyst formation
The main factors responsible for cyst development include (in varying degree):

● proliferation of the epithelial lining and connective tissue capsule
● accumulation of fluid within the cyst
● resorption of the surrounding bone and incomplete compensatory repair.

Epithelial proliferation Young cysts in particular often show active proliferation with a thick irregular epithelium. In the case of radicular cysts, infection from the pulp chamber is the source of irritation. Oehlers (1970) confirmed that the majority of radicular cysts, regardless of size, regress without surgical treatment once infection has been eliminated from the root canal or the tooth extracted. However, a few large cysts (residual cysts) persist after extraction of the causative tooth. Though they may ultimately regress, in terms of practical politics it is quicker to remove them surgically.

As discussed later, persistent epithelial proliferation appears to be the major factor in the growth of keratocysts.

Hydrostatic effects of cyst fluids Radicular and many other types of cyst tend to grow expansively in a balloon-like manner. The hydrostatic pressure within cysts appears to be about 70 mm of water and is therefore higher than the capillary blood pressure.

Table 3.1 Major characteristics of jaw cysts

Cyst type	Site/relationship to teeth	M/F ratio	Age range	Radiographic features
Radicular periodontal	At apex of non-vital tooth	3:2	20–50	Unilocular
Residual	Causative tooth extracted	Equal	50+	Unilocular
Paradental	Related to inflamed third molar follicle	4:1	20–29	Unilocular, over roots of third molar
Dentigerous	Upper 3s. Lower 8s	2:1	10–40	Unilocular. Contains crown of tooth
Keratocyst (parakeratinized)	Frequently molar region. Impacted tooth in 50%±	2:1	40± (mean)	Multilocular
Keratocyst (othokeratinized)	Frequently molar region	3:2	34± (mean)	Usually unilocular. 'Dentigerous' in 40%±
Nasopalatine	Midline. Anterior maxilla	Almost equal	40± (mean)	Unilocular. Sometimes heart-shaped
Nasolabial	Soft tissues, deep to alae nasi	1:4	30–50 (peak)	Unilocular depression of bone of labial surface of maxilla
Median mandibular	Midline between roots of vital incisors	?	?	Unilocular. Teeth vital
Calcifying odontogenic cyst	Majority in incisor-canine region	Equal	1–30 (peak)	Usually unilocular, sometimes flecked with calcifications. Associated odontoma in 25%

Note: So-called globulomaxillary cyst is excluded for lack of evidence that it is an entity.

Earlier views were that cyst fluid contained mainly low molecular weight proteins and that the cyst wall, by acting as a semi-permeable membrane, maintained osmotic tension high enough to cause cyst expansion. More recent experiments have shown that cyst fluid is largely inflammatory exudate containing high concentrations of proteins, some (such as immunoglobulins) of high molecular weight together with cholesterol, breakdown products of erythrocytes, inflammatory cells, exfoliated epithelial cells, and fibrin. These findings are consistent with the usual presence of inflammation in cyst walls, as a consequence of which, capillaries in the cyst wall are more permeable and exude fluid into the cavity. The net effect is that hydrostatic pressure causes expansion of the cyst cavity.

Bone resorbing factors In vitro, cyst tissue in culture can be induced to release bone resorbing factors. These are predominantly prostaglandins E2 and E3. Various cysts and tumours possibly differ in the quantities of prostaglandins produced, but it is uncertain to what extent this affects the mode of growth of cysts. Collagenase may be found in the walls of keratocysts, but its contribution to cyst growth is also unclear.

Most cysts of the jaw show a similar pattern of slow expansive growth. They differ mainly in their relationship to a tooth; this and the radiographic features are usually an adequate guide as to their nature. Even when it is impossible to decide the precise nature of a cyst, this rarely affects treatment. However, it is essential to distinguish odontogenic keratocysts and cystic ameloblastomas from other cysts. These occasionally have identical radiological appearances and diagnosis ultimately depends on microscopy.

Table 3.2 Differential diagnosis of radiolucent cyst-like lesions of jaws

1.	Cysts	Odontogenic
		Non-odontogenic
2.	Tumours	Odontogenic
		Non-odontogenic (including metastases)
3.	Tumour-like lesions	Giant cell granuloma
4.	Hyperparathyroidism	Osteitis fibrosa cystica
5.	Cherubism	
6.	Stafne bone cavity	(Accessory salivary tissue)
7.	Solitary bone cyst	
8.	Aneurysmal bone cyst	
9.	Anatomical structures	(Antrum, nasal airways, incisive fossa)

Apical periodontal (radicular) cysts

Clinical features

The term *radicular cyst* is used here because of possible confusion between the different types of periodontal cysts. They are the most common cause of chronic major jaw swellings and the most common type of cyst of the jaws. They are rarely seen before the age of 10 years and are most frequent between the ages of 20 and 60 years. They are more common in men than women, roughly in the proportion of 3 to 2. More than three times as many cysts form in the maxilla as the mandible.

The vast majority of radicular cysts, like other cysts of the jaws, cause slowly progressive painless swellings. There are no symptoms until the cyst becomes large enough to be noticeable. If infected, the cyst becomes painful and may swell more rapidly partly due to peripheral inflammatory oedema.

The swelling is rounded and at first hard. Later, thinning of the bone may give rise to eggshell crackling on palpation. Finally, part of the wall can be resorbed entirely away leaving a soft, fluctuant, bluish swelling beneath the mucous membrane.

The dead tooth from which the cyst has originated is (by definition) present and its relationship to the cyst is usually obvious in radiographs.

Residual cysts

These were periapical cysts which have persisted after extraction of the causative tooth. Cysts of the jaws in older persons are usually residual cysts which are one of the most common causes of swelling of the edentulous jaw. They can cause trouble by interfering with the fit of dentures.

Residual cysts may slowly regress spontaneously if left untreated, and there is progressive thinning or even disappearance of their lining.

Lateral radicular cysts

Lateral radicular cysts are rare. They form at the side of the tooth as a result of the opening of a lateral branch of the root canal. Also rarely, the tooth is vital and the cyst appears to have resulted from inflammation in an adjacent gingival pocket; it then may be regarded as a type of paradental cyst.

Radiography

A radicular cyst appears as a rounded, clearly radiolucent area with a sharply defined outline intimately related to the apex of a tooth. There is sometimes a condensed peripheral radiopaque rim, but only if growth has been very slow and this is usually only seen in older patients.

The dead tooth from which a radicular cyst has arisen can be seen and may show an obvious carious cavity or discoloration due to pulpal devitalization. Adjacent teeth usually remain vital but may become displaced a little or, occasionally, slightly mobile. Very large cysts in the maxilla may extend in any available direction, become irregular in shape and readily transgress the midline.

Infection of a cyst causes the outline to become hazy as a result of increased vascularity and resorption of the surrounding bone.

Microscopy

All stages can be seen from a periapical granuloma containing a few strands of proliferating epithelium to an enlarging cyst with a hyperplastic epithelial lining and dense inflammatory infiltrate (Figure 3.1).

The epithelial lining The lining, derived from the epithelial rests of Malassez, is stratified squamous epithelium of variable thickness and is sometimes incomplete. Early, active proliferation of the lining epithelium is associated with inflammation and the epithelium may then be thick, irregular and hyperplastic or form rings and arcades to acquire a net-like appearance (Figures 3.2a,b). As cysts mature, the epithelial lining becomes thinner and flatter and inflammatory cells become progressively fewer.

Though the epithelium is stratified squamous in type, it is somewhat poorly formed and lacks a defined basal cell layer (Figures 3.3). Rarely, as a result of metaplastic change, the epithelium may keratinize or become respiratory in type with mucous and ciliated columnar cells, even in the mandible. Hyaline bodies may also be seen (Figures 3.4a,b).

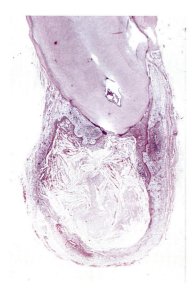

Figure 3.1 Periodontal (radicular) cyst. This early cyst with an intact epithelial lining is still attached to the extracted tooth from which it originated. Radiographically this appeared to be an apical granuloma

The cyst wall The capsule consists of collagenous fibrous connective tissue. During active growth the capsule is vascular and shows a moderately heavy inflammatory infiltrate adjacent to and infiltrating the proliferating epithelium.

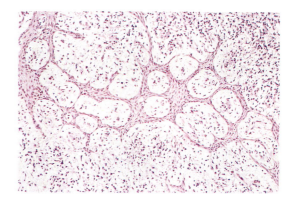

Figure 3.2(b) Radicular cyst. This reticular configuration of the proliferating epithelium can mimic the appearance of a plexiform ameloblastoma

Plasma cells are often prominent or predominant and indicate defensive antibody production against microbial products leaking from the tooth.

Round the capsule there is osteoclastic activity and resorption of the bone of the cyst wall. Beyond the zone of resorption there is usually active bone replacement. The net consequence is that the cyst expands but retains a bony shell, even after it has extended beyond the normal contours of the jaw. Nevertheless, resorption outpaces apposition to cause the bony wall to become progressively thinner, until it forms a mere eggshell, then ultimately disappears altogether. The cyst then starts to distend the soft tissues. Long-standing

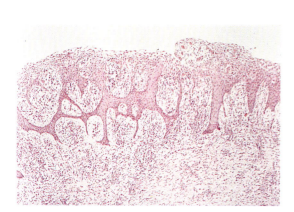

Figure 3.2(a) Radicular cyst. A typical appearance: arcades of proliferating epithelium are surrounded by inflammatory cells and small blood vessels extend close up under the surface

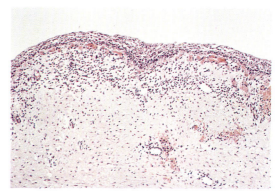

Figure 3.3 Mature radicular cyst. The thin lining lacks a basal cell layer and the inflammatory infiltrate is minimal

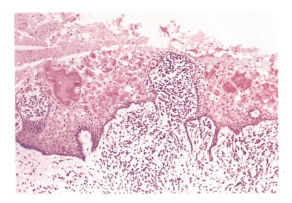

Figure 3.4(a)   Radicular cyst. Hyaline bodies have formed unusually large masses in this cyst lining

cysts are often characterized by a thin-flattened epithelial lining, a thick fibrous wall and minimal inflammatory infiltrate.

Clefts   Within the cyst capsule or contents there are often needle-shaped spaces or clefts left by cholesterol dissolved out during specimen preparation. Small clefts are enclosed within attenuated foreign body giant cells and associated with extravasated red cells and blood pigment. Clefts form in the cyst wall but may extend into the cyst cavity.

Cyst fluid   The fluid is usually watery and opalescent or sometimes thicker, more viscid and yellowish. Cholesterol crystals may give it a

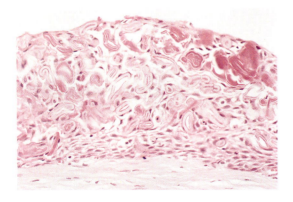

Figure 3.4(b)   Radicular cyst. At higher power, hyaline bodies are seen as refractile structures of varied form in the epithelial cyst lining

shimmering appearance and their characteristic notched rhomboidal shape may be seen under the microscope in a smear of the fluid. In sections, the protein content of the fluid is usually seen as amorphous eosinophilic material, often containing broken-down leucocytes, foam cells distended with fat globules and clefts.

Differential diagnosis

The different radiolucent lesions which must be considered in the differential diagnosis of cysts have been summarized in Table 3.2. The main practical consideration is to differentiate radicular and dentigerous cysts from unilocular keratocysts or ameloblastomas, as discussed later.

Resorption of the apices of adjacent teeth is suggestive of a neoplasm rather than a cyst but is not diagnostic. Rarely, a metastatic deposit may produce a sharply defined area of radiolucency, though usually the outline is ill-defined and irregular. Tumours also tend to be painful and to grow more rapidly than cysts. Nevertheless, it may be difficult or impossible to distinguish them from an infected cyst in radiographs, until at operation the solid nature of a tumour becomes obvious and microscopy confirms the diagnosis.

Aspiration   The cystic nature of a radiolucent area can be confirmed by aspirating its contents by a needle inserted through the wall, under aseptic conditions. However, this fluid will not distinguish one cyst from another, nor a cystic neoplasm from a true cyst. The presence of cholesterol crystals is of little diagnostic value. Rarely, a keratocyst may be filled with a semi-solid mass of squames and no aspirate is obtainable through a thin needle.

Treatment

Many different techniques have been advocated for the management of jaw cysts. Despite differences in detail they all depend on two basic principles – enucleation and wound closure, or marsupialization (decompression) with possible variations, namely:

● Enucleation with wound closure:
  (a) primary closure with or without bone grafting
  (b) secondary closure following initial marsupialization.

● Marsupialization (decompression):
  (a) incomplete removal of the lining and mar-
      supialization into the mouth or antrum
  (b) complete removal of lining and marsupial-
      ization into the mouth or antrum.

Despite these various options, only enucleation
and primary closure, without bone grafting, is
commonly carried out. Marsupialization into the
antrum may be used for large maxillary cysts with
incomplete bony walls separating them from the
antrum.

Enucleation and primary closure

This, the usual mode of treatment, is completely
satisfactory in the vast majority of cases.

Only the affected (dead) tooth may need to be
extracted or it may be root-filled and conserved.
Access is made by raising a mucoperiosteal flap
over the cyst and opening a window of adequate
size in the overlying bone. The cyst wall is then
carefully separated from the bone and the entire
structure removed intact. The cyst lining should
be sent complete in fixative, for histological
examination.

The edges of the cavity are smoothed off and free
bleeding stopped with swabs. The cavity is irrigated
to check for cyst remnants. Dusting it with
antibiotic powder to prevent infection of the clot
is probably unnecessary. The mucoperiosteal flap is
replaced and sutured in position to achieve a
watertight closure. The sutures should be left in
place for at least 10 days.

*Advantages and disadvantages of enucleation of
cysts* The cavity usually heals without complication and little after-care is necessary, and the
complete lining is available for examination to
confirm the diagnosis and to exclude a neoplasm.

Possible or theoretical disadvantages of enucleation include the following, but all are rare in
competent hands:

● The clot filling the cavity may become infected.
● Incomplete removal of the lining may lead to
  recurrence.
● Serious haemorrhage, either primary or secondary, may follow.
● Apices of vital teeth or other structures may be
  damaged. When teeth project into a cyst cavity,
  covered only by the cyst lining, removal of the

latter can damage the blood supply to, and kill,
the teeth. Similarly, the inferior dental nerve and
vessels may be directly associated with the cyst
lining.
● The antrum may be opened if enucleation of a
  large cyst of the maxilla is attempted.
● With exceptionally large cysts, removal of
  sufficient bone may excessively weaken the jaw
  and lead to fracture. Under these circumstances
  the cyst can be decompressed by temporary
  marsupialization. When enough new bone has
  formed, the cyst can then be enucleated.

Generally speaking, enucleation is completely
satisfactory and in competent hands can be applied
even to very large cysts. There are few contraindications and they are rarely absolute.

Marsupialization

The cyst's extent must be estimated as accurately as
possible using appropriately angled radiographs.
With these as a guide, the cyst is opened by
reflecting a mucoperiosteal flap, and a window
made as large as the local anatomy allows but not
such as to risk a fracture. The exposed cyst lining is
excised, the cavity washed out and the lining
sutured to the mucous membrane at the margins
of the orifice. The object is to produce a self-
cleansing cavity which becomes, in effect, an
invagination of the oral cavity. The cavity is
packed with ribbon gauze soaked in acriflavine
emulsion, BIPP or Whitehead's varnish, or a
temporary plug of gutta percha can be made. The
sutures and pack are removed after a week and a
permanent plug or extension to a denture is made
for the same purpose. Once the cavity has filled up
from the base and sides sufficiently to become self-
cleansing, the plug can be removed. The cavity
usually becomes closed by regrowth of the surrounding tissue and restoration of the normal
contour of the bone. The operation has disadvantages, as follows:

● the orifice may close, allowing the cyst to re-
  form
● the epithelial lining of the cyst may be friable or
  incomplete and cannot be sutured to the
  margins of the opening
● cleansing of the cavity depends on the patient,
  who has to be provided with a syringe to wash
  out the cavity after meals

- several visits are necessary to assess repair of the cavity and to decide when the plug can be removed
- the complete lining is not available for histological examination
- bony infilling may fail, particularly in the maxilla, and a permanent stagnating cavity is then left.

Paradental cysts

The paradental cyst is an uncommon inflammatory odontogenic cyst, first described by Craig (1976). It forms in relation to a partially erupted third molar tooth and is typically associated with pericoronitis. The cyst probably originates from the reduced enamel epithelium after unilateral expansion of the follicle as a result of inflammatory destruction of the adjacent alveolar bone. The cyst is attached to the amelocemental junction, usually on its buccal aspect, and rarely exceeds 2 cm in diameter. The microscopic features are not distinguishable from those of a radicular cyst but the tooth is vital. Most regard this cyst as an entity, but others term a variety of cysts developing beside a tooth, paradental.

Dentigerous (follicular) cysts

A dentigerous cyst surrounds the crown of an unerupted tooth and may displace it for a considerable distance. Dentigerous cysts are less common than radicular cysts, which preponderate in the ratio of at least 4 to 1. The lower third molars and upper canines are most often affected, but any permanent tooth can be involved.

Pathogenesis
Dentigerous cysts arise as a result of cystic change in the remains of the enamel organ after enamel formation is complete. Occasionally, the division between the remnants of the internal enamel epithelium and the external enamel epithelium forming the main cyst lining can be seen microscopically at the attachment of the cyst to the neck of the tooth. Though such a cyst appears to form between the layers of the reduced enamel epithelium, the layer which remains attached to the surface of the enamel is usually of negligible thickness and the enamel is virtually in direct contact with the cyst contents. The cyst lining originates from the major part of the reduced enamel epithelium and progressive growth of the cyst leads to dilatation of the dental follicle.

Factors which initiate dentigerous cyst development are not known. Inflammation does not play a significant role, but there is a strong association between failure of eruption of teeth and formation of dentigerous cysts. It is not merely that a dentigerous cyst may prevent a tooth from erupting, but dentigerous cysts predominantly affect maxillary canines and mandibular third molars which are particularly prone to failure of eruption.

Clinical features
Dentigerous cysts are uncommon in the first decade of life and are most often found between the ages of 20 and 50 years. They are more than twice as common in males as females.

Like other cysts, if uncomplicated they cause no symptoms until the swelling becomes obtrusive. Alternatively, a dentigerous cyst may be detected by chance in radiographs or when the cause is sought for a missing tooth. Infection causes the usual symptoms of pain and increased swelling.

Radiography
The appearance is characteristic, namely, a well-defined cyst containing the crown of a displaced tooth. The cavity is rounded and unilocular, but occasionally, trabeculation or ridging of the bony wall appears as pseudoloculation. The slow, regular growth of these cysts usually results in a sclerotic bony outline and a well-defined cortex. The affected tooth is often displaced a considerable distance and a third molar, for example, may be pushed to the lower border of the mandible or more rarely into the neck of the condyle. Occasionally, the tooth within a dentigerous cyst is a supernumerary. A dentigerous cyst in the lower third molar region may become very large and extend into the coronoid process and condylar neck. Rarely, a keratocyst may envelop the crown of the tooth, as may an ameloblastoma, and either of these may produce a radiographic appearance

exactly simulating a dentigerous cyst. Microscopy of the cyst lining is therefore essential.

Microscopy

The lining of dentigerous cysts typically consists of flattened stratified squamous epithelium in which mucous (goblet) cells are often present. The epithelium may rarely undergo metaplasia and keratinize. The structure of the cyst wall is otherwise similar to that of radicular cysts, but inflammatory changes are typically absent.

Management

Once the diagnosis has been established, it may occasionally be preferable to marsupialize a dentigerous cyst to allow the tooth to erupt if the tooth is in a favourable position and space is available. Alternatively, the tooth can be transplanted to the alveolar ridge or extracted, as appropriate, and the cyst enucleated. Usually, enucleation with removal of the tooth and primary closure is carried out.

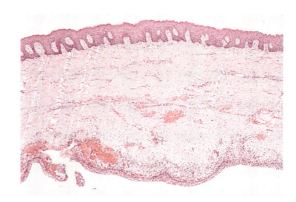

Figure 3.5 Eruption cyst. The thin epithelial lining, derived from the reduced enamel epithelium, is separated from the oral mucosa by connective tissue

Gingival cysts

Two types of gingival cyst are recognized, namely infantile (dental lamina cyst of the newborn) and adult types.

Eruption cysts

An eruption cyst occasionally forms in the gingiva overlying a tooth about to erupt. Eruption cysts are extraosseous but are probably superficial dentigerous cysts. They are uncommon and probably account for fewer than 1% of cysts.

Clinically, eruption cysts are seen in children and involve teeth having no predecessors namely, deciduous or permanent molars. The cyst appears as a soft, rounded, bluish swelling in the gingiva overlying the unerupted tooth.

Microscopically, an eruption cyst is lined by thin, poorly formed stratified squamous epithelium separated from the oral mucosa by connective tissue (Figure 3.5).

Management

The tissue overlying the crown of the tooth may be removed, but most eruption cysts probably burst spontaneously as the tooth erupts.

Dental lamina cyst of the newborn (Bohn's nodules)

Up to 80% of neonates have small nodules or cysts in the gingivae, which have arisen from epithelial rests of Serres, from the dental lamina. These may enlarge sufficiently to become clinically obvious as creamy coloured swellings, a few millimetres in diameter, but rupture spontaneously and heal in a matter of months. Similar lesions (Epstein's pearls) around the junction of the hard and soft palates arise from non-odontogenic epithelium but behave in a similar manner.

Microscopically, dental lamina cysts are lined by thin stratified squamous epithelium and contain layers of desquamated keratin (Figure 3.6).

Gingival cysts of adults

Gingival cysts are exceedingly rare but typically form in the free or attached gingiva, particularly

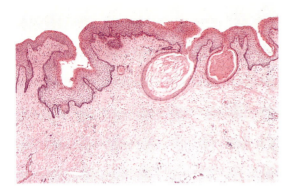

Figure 3.6 Gingival cysts in a child. Cystic change in several nodules (Bohn's nodules) of epithelium derived from the rests of Serres

after the age of 40 years. They are also thought to arise from the rests of Serres, but their late appearance is difficult to explain. Alternatively, they may result from traumatic implantation of superficial epithelium.

Clinically, gingival cysts appear to affect males and females equally. The cysts form dome-shaped swellings, usually less than 1 cm in diameter. They may sometimes erode the underlying bone and may then be difficult to differentiate from a lateral periodontal cyst.

Microscopically, gingival cysts are lined by very thin, flat, stratified squamous epithelium and may contain fluid or layers of keratin (Figure 3.7).

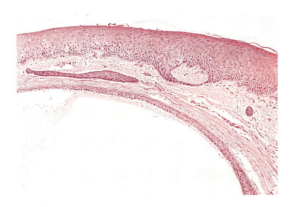

Figure 3.7 Gingival cyst of adulthood. The thin epithelial lining lies just deep to the gingival mucosa

Lateral periodontal cysts

These rare cysts are intraosseous and form in the bone beside a vital tooth. They are usually found in routine radiographs as they cause no symptoms unless they erode through the bone and extend into the gingiva. They differ from gingival cysts of adults in their situation and that they are twice as common in men as women.

The radiographic appearance is similar to that of other odontogenic cysts, apart from their position beside a tooth and near the crest of the alveolar ridge.

Microscopically, lateral periodontal cysts are lined by squamous or cuboidal epithelium, frequently only one or two cells thick, but sometimes with focal thickenings. Some of these cells may have clear cytoplasm and resemble those seen in the dental lamina.

Treatment
The cyst should be enucleated, but the related tooth can be retained if healthy.

Botryoid and sialo-odontogenic cysts

Botryoid odontogenic cyst

This rare entity, described by Weathers and Waldron (1973), is regarded as a multilocular variant of the lateral periodontal cyst. It typically affects the mandibular premolar to canine region in adults over the age of 50 years.

Microscopically, the loculae are separated by fine fibrous septa and lined by flattened non-keratinized epithelium which forms sporadic bud-like proliferations protruding into the cyst cavity. Interspersed among the epithelial cells are clear, glycogen-containing cells.

Sialo-odontogenic cyst

This may be a variant of the botryoid odontogenic cyst. However, sialo-odontogenic cysts have been reported over a wide age range. Of the 8 patients reported by Gardner *et al.* (1988), only three were over 50 and the youngest was 19 years.

Microscopy

Sialo-odontogenic cysts typically have:

1. An epithelial lining of variable thickness, but frequently much greater than that of a botryoid odontogenic cyst. It has a flat lower border with no inflammatory infiltrate.
2. An irregular or even papillary cystic surface to the epithelium, with a superficial layer of eosinophilic cuboidal cells and some ciliated cells (Figure 3.8).
3. Pools of mucicarmine-positive material and mucous cells in variable numbers within the epithelium.
4. Whorls or nodules of epithelial cells ('epithelial spheres') which may protrude into the cyst cavity as in a botryoid-odontogenic cyst (Figure 3.9).

Management

These cysts appear to be rather more aggressive than periodontal cysts. Two of them recurred among the 8 patients reported by Gardner *et al.* (1988), but one responded to a further enucleation, the other to curettage of the cavity. It seems important therefore to make sure that all traces of the epithelial lining are removed. Alternatively, the cyst can be resected, but it is uncertain whether such treatment is always necessary.

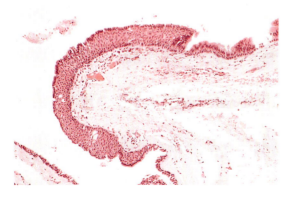

Figure 3.8 Sialo-odontogenic cyst. The lining is of greatly variable thickness and in its thickest part has a superficial layer of columnar cells

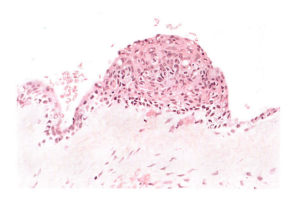

Figure 3.9 Sialo-odontogenic cyst. A plaque or 'epithelial sphere' of thickened epithelium is protruding into the cyst cavity

Odontogenic keratocysts

These cysts are uncommon, but are important because of their peculiarly infiltrative mode of growth and their strong tendency to recur after removal. Odontogenic keratocysts have been categorized as *orthokeratotic* and *parakeratotic* variants, as the latter, which form over 85% of keratocysts, have a considerably higher recurrence rate.

Despite the term *odontogenic keratocyst*, the majority of keratocysts, though they have a characteristic type of epithelial lining, fail to form significant amounts of keratin, while even radicular or dentigerous cysts can occasionally show metaplastic keratinization. However, the latter lack any significant tendency to recur after enucleation.

Keratocysts are thought to have arisen from parts of the dental lamina. Nevertheless, if this is so, it is difficult to reconcile the frequent appearance of keratocysts in middle age unless their growth is quite remarkably slow. The factors determining the development of these cysts are also unknown. In particular, keratocysts differ from other cysts in that proliferation of their lining rather than hydrostatic pressure is the main determinant of their growth. They also tend to extend by finger-like processes along the lines of least resistance, namely the cancellous spaces. Hence these cysts may be a considerable size before they expand the jaw and become clinically apparent. To accommodate this overgrowth, the cyst lining becomes much folded. Radioactive labelling suggests that, despite their slow growth, the lining may be proliferating more actively than cells of the oral mucosa. This epithelial proliferation is probably a factor determining the frequency with which keratocysts recur and the difficulties in eradicating them if allowed to extend into the soft tissue. As a consequence, the lesion has been likened to a 'benign cystic neoplasm'.

Clinical features

Keratocysts account for about 5% of jaw cysts. The parakeratotic variant is considerably more common in men than women. Most series record a peak incidence in the second and third decades, but other large series have shown peaks between the fifth and seventh decades. The variation in these reported findings may be partly accounted for by different diagnostic criteria and possibly also the findings may genuinely differ from one country to another.

They are often symptomless until the bone is expanded or they become infected. The main difference is that expansion of the jaw is much less than would be expected from the radiographic extent of the cyst. Hence there are often no clinical signs until the cyst is well advanced, and occasionally extensive cysts are found by chance on routine radiographs in asymptomatic patients.

The most common site, accounting for at least 80% of keratocysts, is the angle of the mandible, extending for variable distances into the ramus and forwards into the body. Extension of the cavity up the ramus, even into the neck of the condyle, is characteristic.

Keratocysts, once they have penetrated the cortex of the jaw, can continue to grow in the soft tissues and are then even more difficult to eradicate.

Radiography

Keratocysts appear as well-defined radiolucent areas. Parakeratotic cysts are typically multilocular or rounded with a scalloped margin. Orthokeratotic keratocysts are frequently unilocular. A multilocular keratocyst may be difficult to differentiate from an ameloblastoma radiographically, but the bony wall of a keratocyst is typically sclerotic and appears as a sharply demarcated cortex.

Rarely a keratocyst may envelop an unerupted tooth and simulate a dentigerous cyst. As they enlarge, keratocysts tend to displace the roots of adjacent teeth.

Microscopy

The cyst wall is thin and the lining has the following characteristic features:

1. The epithelium is of uniform thickness, typically about 7–10 cells thick without rete ridges.
2. The squamous epithelium has a clearly defined, palisaded layer of tall basal cells in the parakeratotic type, a prickle cell layer which forms the bulk of the epithelium, which is often much folded (Figure 3.10). In the orthokeratotic type the basal cell layer is cuboidal or flattened.
3. Keratin formation amounts to no more than a thin eosinophilic layer of parakeratin in the parakeratotic variant. In the orthokeratotic variant there is a well-defined granular cell layer and keratin formation may be so abundant as to fill the cyst cavity with semi-solid material (Figure 3.11).
4. Occasionally, daughter cysts or epithelial islands are present in the cyst wall, particularly when the patient has the jaw cysts, naevoid basal cell carcinoma (Gorlin–Goltz) syndrome (Figure 3.12).
5. The fibrous wall is thin and often loose or myxoid. Unlike other odontogenic cysts, the epithelial lining is weakly attached to and readily separates from the underlying connective tissue.

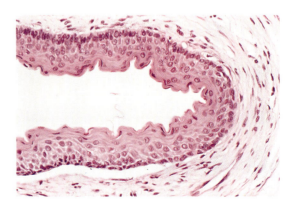

Figure 3.10 Odontogenic keratocyst – parakeratotic type. The well-formed epithelial lining is of uniform thickness. Other typical features are the palisading of the basal cell layer, the mere suggestion of parakeratosis and the finely corrugated surface

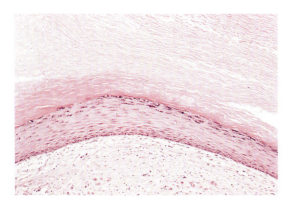

Figure 3.11 Odontogenic keratocyst – orthokeratinized type. Layers of keratin fill the cyst cavity. The granular cell layer is conspicuous but the basal cell layer is ill-defined

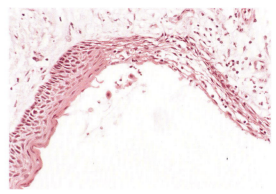

Figure 3.13 Odontogenic keratocyst. The typical parakeratotic lining is present on the left but on the right has lost its highly organized appearance, due to minor inflammation, and resembles that of a radicular cyst

6. Inflammatory cells are typically absent or scanty. If significant inflammation is superimposed, the characteristic appearances of the epithelium are lost, so that the lining resembles that of a radicular cyst (Figure 3.13). Confirmation then depends on finding uninflamed areas of typical epithelium.

The chief clinical and radiographic features of these two types of cysts are summarized in Table 3.3, but in essence the main differences are in the microscopic appearances and in the fact that the parakeratotic variant appears to have the strongest tendency to recur.

Recurrence

The overriding clinical problem with keratocysts is their strong tendency to recur after treatment, and recurrence rates of up to 60% have been reported. In a survey of 24 orthokeratotic cysts, Wright (1981) found only a single recurrence and that the parakeratotic variant was more likely to recur. His conclusions were abundantly confirmed by Crowley *et al.* (1992) who, in a survey of 449 keratocysts, found a recurrence rate of at least 46% in 387 parakeratinized cysts and only a single recurrence

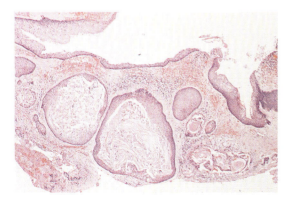

Figure 3.12 Odontogenic keratocyst. Unusually many daughter cysts are present in the wall and may be the source of recurrences. This appearance is more typical of the Gorlin–Goltz syndrome

Table 3.3 Important features of keratocysts

	Parakeratotic	*Orthokeratotic*
Relative frequency (approximately)	88%	12%
Sex:		
male = 61.5% overall	62%	57%
female = 38.5%	38%	43%
Age at presentation	34 yrs	40 yrs
Association with impacted tooth	48%	76%
Midline location	6%	16%
Pain	15%	9%
Radiographic appearance	Usually multilocular	Frequently monolocular
Recurrence	43%	4%

among 55 orthokeratinized cysts. Crowley *et al.* (1992) found that 2.2% of these cysts had linings partly ortho- and partly parakeratinized and that these had a similar recurrence rate to the entirely parakeratinized cysts.

The reasons for the high recurrence rate of parakeratinized cysts are not clear, but factors which may contribute include the following:

● keratocyst linings are thin and fragile and, particularly when the cysts are large, are very difficult to enucleate intact
● extension of the cyst into cancellous bone increases the difficulty of removing the lining
● keratocysts may have, in their periphery, satellite daughter cysts which may be left behind after enucleation of the main cyst
● evidence that the epithelial lining, particularly of parakeratinized cysts, is more vigorously proliferative than that of other cyst linings suggests that if a few epithelial cells remain they can readily form another cyst after enucleation of the main lesion
● if, as seems likely, keratocysts develop from remnants of dental lamina, then other remnants of dental lamina might contribute to the formation of a second lesion which appears to be recurrence.

The fact that recurrences have occasionally appeared several decades after the original operation suggests that new lesions of this sort can develop. However, the fact that cysts with mixed type linings have a recurrence rate consistent with the parakeratinized component suggests that the latter's proliferative capacity is a major determinant of recurrence.

The time of recurrence is very variable. It is typically within the first 5 years, but may, as already mentioned, be after many years. The parakeratinized variant is more likely to recur, but it seems probable, also, that the more conservative the enucleation the greater the likelihood of recurrence.

Rigorous treatment and, whenever possible, removal intact of every trace of the lining are likely to reduce the risk of recurrence, but there is not absolute certainty of a complete cure and rarely recurrence of keratocysts has been reported in bone grafts after excision. Clearly, it is important to warn patients of the possible need for further operations and they should be followed up with regular radiological examinations at intervals for an indefinite period.

Treatment

It is desirable to confirm the diagnosis of keratocysts before operation, to dispel any doubts as to whether the lesion is an ameloblastoma. The quickest and most reliable method is by biopsy. However, once the cavity has been opened, careful inspection is usually adequate to settle the diagnosis in most cases.

Once the diagnosis has been confirmed, treatment should be by complete enucleation. This is usually difficult as the lining is friable (particularly if inflamed), but treatment should be thorough, even aggressive, to try to ensure that every fragment of cyst lining has been removed. Because of these difficulties, recommendations have ranged from simple enucleation with prolonged follow-up, to jaw resection and reconstruction, but several studies have found that the recurrence rate of keratocysts is not significantly affected by the mode of treatment. The present consensus, based on several recent series, is that the cyst should be opened widely, the lining carefully enucleated and then the bony margins cut back by at least 5 mm all round with an acrylic burr. Though it appears that the orthokeratotic variant is less likely to recur, there is probably no justification for less thorough treatment than for the parakeratotic type. Prolonged radiographic follow-up is essential and recurrences are treated in a similar manner as they develop. This is the policy advocated by the present authors.

Syndrome of multiple jaw cysts, skeletal anomalies and multiple basal cell carcinomas

This syndrome, often called the Gorlin–Goltz syndrome, is inherited as an autosomal dominant trait and has the following main features:

1. Multiple keratocysts of the jaws in approximately 85% of patients.
2. Multiple, early onset basal cell carcinomas of the skin in over 50% of patients (Figure 3.14).
3. Skeletal anomalies (usually of a minor nature) such as bifid ribs and abnormalities of the vertebrae.
4. Characteristic facies with frontal and temporoparietal bossing and a broad nasal root in about 70% of patients.

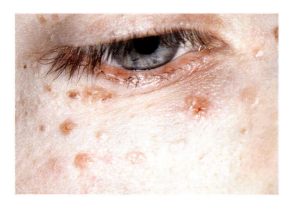

Figure 3.14 Gorlin–Goltz syndrome. Multiple basal cell carcinomas (basal cell naevi) surround the eye

5. Intracranial anomalies frequently include a characteristic lamellar calcification of the falx cerebri, an abnormally shaped sella turcica and occasionally intracranial tumours.

Many other findings have been reported and the effects on the patient depend on the syndrome's predominant manifestation. Thus in some cases there are innumerable basal cell carcinomas which can be disfiguring or troublesome in other ways. Though termed 'naevoid', these tumours differ from typical basal cell carcinomas only in their early onset and have been reported even in a child of 2.

Other patients have a great many jaw cysts necessitating repeated operations.

Microscopy
The cysts, in the great majority of patients, are of the parakeratotic type but more frequently have daughter cysts or islands of epithelium in the walls (Woolgar *et al.*, 1987). Like keratocysts in normal persons, they are more common in the body or ramus of the mandible.

Management
Patients should be warned of the possible need for repeated operations to remove jaw cysts and of other features of the syndrome. Referral to a dermatologist or other specialists may also be necessary.

The cysts must be managed like other keratocysts and enucleated intact if possible. If large, pre-liminary marsupialization to allow shrinkage of the cyst, before enucleation, has been recommended. If neglected, these cysts can give rise to any of the complications of other jaw cysts.

Primordial cysts

Odontogenic keratocysts were originally termed 'primordial cysts', but the term has been revived to describe what appears to be a different entity. However, not all pathologists recognize the latter and regard the terms primordial and keratocysts as synonymous.

The existence of these rare cysts, as mentioned earlier, is somewhat controversial. They have been categorized as a form of follicular cyst and are believed to result from cystic degeneration of the stellate reticulum before the start of enamel formation. A tooth (usually a lower third molar) is therefore missing.

Clinically, primordial cysts are usually found early in life, often during a routine radiographic examination, when they are seen as a sharply defined unilocular area of radiolucency close under the crest of the alveolar ridge. Growth of these cysts is slow and produces little expansion of the bone.

Microscopically, these cysts are lined by stratified squamous epithelium which may or may not keratinize, and there are cords or strands of odontogenic epithelium in the cyst wall. However, primordial cysts may be indistinguishable from the keratocysts described above – hence the doubt about their being a distinct entity.

Treatment of primordial cysts should be the same as for keratocysts, namely, thorough enucleation and curettage of the bony wall.

Calcifying odontogenic cyst

The calcifying odontogenic cyst frequently has a propensity for continued growth and forms a solid tumour in about 14% of cases.

Clinically, almost any age can be affected, but the peak incidence is between the ages of 10 and 19 years. There is no sex predilection and the maxilla or mandible are equally frequently affected (Buchner, 1991). The lesion most often forms anterior to the first molar, particularly in the incisor/canine region. Though typically intraosseous, approximately 20% of cases form in the gingival mucosa and may merely indent the underlying bone. On radiographs, the appearance is usually that of a cyst, but it may be multilocular or flecks of calcification may be seen. Erosion of the roots of adjacent teeth is an occasional feature.

Microscopy

The lining consists of squamous epithelium with cuboidal or ameloblast-like basal cells which may be palisaded (Figure 3.15). This epithelium is sometimes many cells thick and can contain areas resembling stellate reticulum. The most striking feature, however, is abnormal keratinization, producing areas of swollen, eosinophilic cells whose cytoplasm and nuclei become progressively paler (ghost cells) and eventually disappear to leave hyaline masses. The extent of this change may be such as to fill the cyst cavity. The ghost cells typically calcify in patchy fashion and in areas where this keratin-like material comes into contact with the connective tissue capsule, it excites a foreign body reaction.

Management

Though calcifying odontogenic cysts have a potential for continued growth, Buchner (1991) could find few reports of recurrence after enucleation.

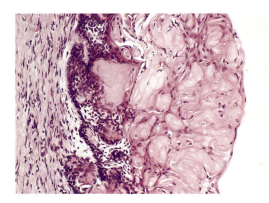

Figure 3.15 Calcifying odontogenic cyst showing a peripheral layer of ameloblast-like cells and, on the right, masses of pale-staining ghost cells towards the lumen

Enucleation should therefore be considered as the first choice, but follow-up should be maintained for a decade.

Nasopalatine, incisive canal and related cysts

These uncommon cysts form in the midline of the anterior part of the maxilla. The nasopalatine, median palatine, palatine papilla and median alveolar cysts are probably all variants of the same entity, but differ slightly in their relation to the postulated line of the nasopalatine canal.

Pathogenesis

Nasopalatine canal cysts arise from the epithelium of the nasopalatine ducts in the incisive canal. In cats, for example, there is an organ of smell communicating with the mouth through the palatine canal, and cats inhale through the mouth when identifying an odour. In man, only vestiges of a primitive organ of smell in the incisive canal can be found, in the form of incomplete epithelium-lined ducts, cords of epithelial cells or merely epithelial rests.

Clinical features

Nasopalatine cysts are slow-growing and resemble other jaw cysts clinically, apart from their site. Occasionally, they cause intermittent discharge with a salty taste. If neglected, they can grow large enough to produce a swelling in the midline of the anterior part of the palate or perforate the palate anteriorly and form a prolabial swelling. If very superficial, they give rise to the so-called palatine papilla cyst.

Radiography shows a well-defined rounded, ovoid or occasionally heart-shaped radiolucent area, and a well-defined, often sclerotic margin in the anterior part of the midline of the maxilla. These cysts are usually symmetrical but may be slightly larger to one side.

The anterior palatine fossa must be distinguished from a small nasopalatine cyst. The maximum size of a normal fossa is up to 6 or 7 mm.

Microscopy

The lining of nasopalatine cysts is variable in character, but is usually either stratified squamous epithelium or ciliated columnar (respiratory) epithelium or both together. A few scattered chronic inflammatory cells are often seen beneath the epithelium in some parts of the cyst wall, but are not a prominent feature. Mucous glands are often also present in the wall.

A characteristic feature is the frequent presence of neurovascular bundles in the wall. These are the long nasopalatine nerve and vessels which pass through the nasopalatine canal and are often removed with the cyst (Figure 3.16).

Treatment

Nasopalatine cysts should be enucleated and recurrence is then unlikely. With exceptionally large examples, enucleation brings with it the risk of perforation of the nasal floor or formation of a palatal fistula. The site of these cysts also makes possible damage to the nerve supply to, with resulting anaesthesia of, the anterior palate or devitalization of the anterior teeth. The upper aspect of these rare, large nasopalatine cysts (or other anterior maxillary cysts) can be exposed by a Le Fort I down-fracture osteotomy to gain access to the floor of the nose and this enables complete enucleation to be carried out.

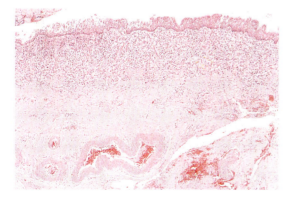

Figure 3.16 Nasopalatine canal cyst. The cyst lining (above) consists predominantly of respiratory epithelium, while below there are prominent vessels and nerves from the nasopalatine canal

Globulomaxillary cyst

This exceedingly rare lesion has been traditionally ascribed to proliferation of sequestered epithelium along the line of fusion of embryonic processes. It is now accepted that this view of embryological development is incorrect and there is no evidence that epithelium becomes buried in this fashion. Most so-called globulomaxillary cysts appear to be lateral periodontal cysts or keratocysts.

Nasolabial cyst

This exceedingly rare cyst is in the soft tissues outside the bone, deep to the nasolabial fold. The aetiology is unknown. The lining is pseudostratified columnar epithelium often with some stratified squamous epithelium. If allowed to grow sufficiently large, the cyst produces a swelling of the upper lip and distorts the nostril. Characteristically, the nasolabial fold is obliterated. Tangential radiographs often reveal a saucer-like concavity underlying the cyst (Figure 3.17).

Treatment of a nasolabial cyst is usually by simple excision, but occasionally may be complicated if the cyst has perforated the nasal mucosa and discharged into the nose.

Median mandibular cyst

This cyst was thought to be a fissural cyst which originated from entrapped epithelium during fusion of the halves of the mandible or a developmental cyst that resulted from inclusion of epithelium trapped in the central groove of the mandibular process in the 10–14 mm embryo. These concepts are untenable. The mandible forms as a single unit within the mandibular process, there is no fusion and it is not possible for epithelium to become entrapped. The median mandibular cyst may be a primordial cyst that develops from a supernumerary tooth bud or remnants of the dental lamina, but many are found to be other types of cyst on microscopy. The cyst forms in the symphyseal region and is asymptomatic unless infected. Typically, the adjacent teeth are vital.

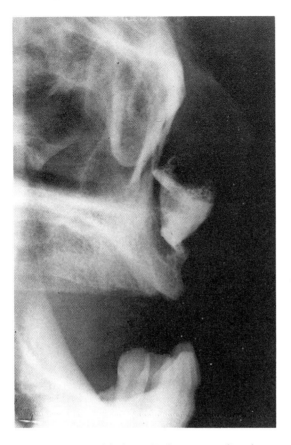

Figure 3.17 Nasolabial cyst. Radiopaque medium has been injected to show clearly the ovoid form and situation of this cyst

The treatment of choice for median mandibular cysts is enucleation, but care must be taken not to endanger the vitality of the related anterior teeth. If, therefore, the cyst is exceptionally large, marsupialization may be necessary.

Cyst-like lesions without epithelial lining

Simple (solitary: haemorrhagic) bone cyst

Simple bone cyst is a preferable term to *solitary* as they can be multiple. It is a bone cavity, but has no epithelial lining and often no fluid content.

The pathogenesis of solitary bone cysts is unknown. The idea that these cysts ('traumatic' or 'haemorrhagic' bone cysts) resulted from injury to, and haemorrhage within, the bone of the jaw, followed by a failure of organization of the clot and of bony repair, is untenable. There is no evidence that a blow, insufficient to cause a fracture, can cause extensive bleeding within the bone nor that anything other than normal repair would follow. Blood-filled bone cavities in the jaws are left by the enucleation of cysts, but solitary bone cysts do not arise as a complication. Further, a common form of treatment for solitary bone cysts is to open them and to allow bleeding into the cavity. Normal healing usually follows.

Clinical features
Simple bone cysts are mostly seen in teenagers, and are rare after the age of 25 years. They mainly form in the mandible, but are typically painless and frequently a chance radiographic finding, particularly when panoramic radiographs are taken. Significant expansion of the jaw is unusual. Females are affected more often than males in a ratio of about 3 to 2.

Radiography
These cavities form rounded, radiolucent areas which generally tend to be less sharply defined than odontogenic cysts, and have two distinctive features (Figure 3.18):

● the area of radiolucency is typically much larger than the size of any swelling suggests
● the cavity can arch up between the roots of the teeth and may, as a consequence, be first seen on a bite-wing radiograph.

They may also extend across the midline of the anterior mandible.

Microscopy
The cavity has a rough bony wall and such lining as there is may be thin connective tissue or only a few red cells, blood pigment or osteoclasts adhering to the surface of the bone.

There are often no cyst contents, but there may sometimes be a little fluid.

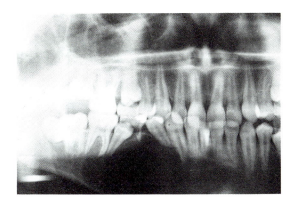

Figure 3.18 Simple ('traumatic') bone cyst. In this 13-year-old child the cyst has extended high into the alveolar ridge, as is particularly characteristic of these lesions. Its exceptionally large size illustrates how far these lesions can grow before expanding the jaw and becoming clinically apparent

Treatment

It may only be necessary to open the cavity to confirm the diagnosis. The characteristic lack of cyst fluid and the unlined bony wall are then usually enough to indicate the diagnosis, but it is preferable if possible to remove some of the connective tissue lining for confirmatory purposes. Opening of the cavity is followed by healing, probably as a result of bleeding, but natural regression is also a possibility. The fact that progressive solitary bone cysts are not seen in elderly patients also suggests that these lesions can resolve spontaneously. Spontaneous bone regeneration was seen by Saito *et al.* (1992) in two excised specimens.

Aneurysmal bone cyst

Aneurysmal bone cysts are traditionally included with other jaw cysts, but are cysts mainly in terms of their radiographic appearance. They rarely affect the jaws. Nothing is known of the aetiology and the most acceptable possibility is that the aneurysmal bone cyst is a vascular malformation, but they are secondary to other bone lesions in a significant minority of cases.

Clinical features

Most patients are between 10 and 20 years of age and there is a slight female preponderance. The mandible is usually affected.

The main manifestation is usually a painless swelling and a radiolucent area, which may be balloon-like or occasionally show a suggestion of trabeculation or loculation. It may expand rapidly.

Microscopy

The aneurysmal bone cyst consists of a highly cellular mass of blood-filled spaces which has been likened to a blood-filled sponge (Figure 3.19). Despite this appearance, the blood-filled spaces lack an endothelial lining identifiable by immuno-cytochemistry or electron microscopy. Alles and Schulz (1986) therefore suggest that the appearance is due to extravasation of red cells from the septal capillaries which lack a basal membrane to their endothelium. However, the extreme cellularity, mitotic activity and frequent presence of giant cells may lead to confusion with a sarcoma (Figure 3.20). It is essential that this mistake should not be made and the patient subjected to unnecessarily radical and possibly hazardous treatment.

An ossifying fibroma or other bone tumour may be associated. In 123 aneurysmal bone cysts below the head and neck region, Martinez and Sissons (1988) found that 36 were part of some other bone

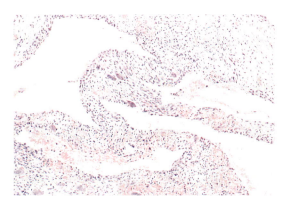

Figure 3.19 Aneurysmal bone cyst. The sponge-like mass consists of large blood-filled spaces, separated by cellular fibroblastic septa containing occasional multinucleated giant cells

lesion, particularly a giant cell tumour or chondro-blastoma.

Treatment of an aneurysmal bone cyst usually consists of thorough curettage, but excision may be preferable as the lesion occasionally recurs. The blood appears to be static, and in contrast to juvenile angiofibroma (Chapter 13), which can appear considerably less vascular microscopically, there is little risk of haemorrhage. Cryotherapy is an alternative approach, but experience of its value is limited.

Stafne's idiopathic bone cavity

Stafne's bone cavities are symptomless and only found by chance in radiographs. They may be mistaken for cysts in the mandible.

They are seen as clearly demarcated round or oval radiolucencies, nearly always below the inferior dental canal in the premolar, molar or angle regions of the mandible. These cavities are concave depressions in the lingual aspect of the mandible and contain accessory lobes of the submandibular salivary gland. Very occasionally, a similar lesion is seen above the inferior dental canal and these are found to contain accessory sublingual gland tissue. Even more rarely, similar enclaved islands of salivary tissue may be found in other parts of the mandible. Intraosseous salivary gland

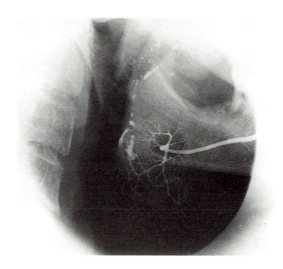

Figure 3.21 Stafne bone cavity. The round, well-defined radiolucent area near the angle of the mandible is typical and the sialogram shows the relationship to the submandibular gland

tumours which probably arise from this ectopic tissue are discussed in Chapter 12.

No treatment is necessary for Stafne's idiopathic bone cavities and their diagnosis may be confirmed by sialography (Figure 3.21).

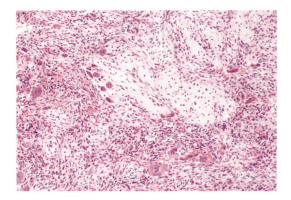

Figure 3.20 Aneurysmal bone cyst. The area on the left contains many giant cells and resembles a giant cell granuloma. On the right there is osseous metaplasia

Cystic neoplasms

Cysts frequently form within ameloblastomas but are usually microscopic. In a few cases such a cyst can expand rapidly (probably by hydrostatic pressure) and, as a result, envelop the tumour. In some cases the gross specimen therefore appears to be a cyst in which the tumour forms no more than mural thickenings. Once fluid has accumulated within such cysts, the epithelial lining becomes flattened and may be indistinguishable from that of a non-neoplastic cyst histologically. Radiographically too, an ameloblastoma may sometimes exactly simulate a dental or dentigerous cyst. It is not surprising, therefore, that the idea has spread that neoplasms can arise within cyst linings.

Though this is an uncommon cause of confusion, it emphasizes the importance of enucleating cysts completely. This makes the whole lining available for examination to exclude the presence of any neoplastic tissue.

Neoplastic change in cyst linings

Rarely, carcinomas can arise from the epithelial lining of cysts. Eversole *et al.* (1975) considered that 36 cases in the world literature were authentic. These are currently termed *primary intraosseous carcinoma ex odontogenic cyst* and are discussed in Chapter 4.

Benign mucosal cysts of the antrum

The benign mucosal cyst of the antrum is sometimes referred to as a mucocele or retention cyst. With the widespread use of panoramic radiography, it has become apparent that these cysts are common. Many authors have reported a 5% incidence in orthopantomograms surveyed at random. The peak incidence is in the third decade and 1.5 times more males than females are affected.

Symptoms are nearly always absent until the patient becomes aware of a sensation of fullness of the side of the face, numbness or nasal obstruction.

Radiography
Antral cysts are usually single and appear as smooth, spherical or dome-shaped opacities with either a narrow or a broad base. They vary in size from 10 mm to lesions filling most of the antral cavity. Characteristically, the thin cortical line of the antral floor remains intact and is not displaced.

Radiographic follow-up shows that many of these cysts persist for a long time without enlarging, while others resolve spontaneously.

Microscopically, antral mucous cysts may either be secretory (retention) cysts and lined by respiratory (Figure 3.22) or less well differentiated epithelium, or non-secretory and, like a mucous extravasation cyst of the oral mucosa, be lined by fibroblasts.

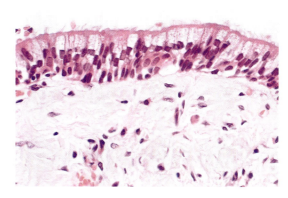

Figure 3.22 Mucosal cyst of the maxillary antrum. The cyst is lined by columnar ciliated epithelium resembling the antral lining from which it has arisen

Surgical intervention of antral mucosal cysts is only necessary if they cause symptoms. They may be removed via a Caldwell–Luc approach or endoscopically through the lateral wall of the nose.

Sublingual dermoids

Dermoid cysts lined by epidermis and skin appendages are found in the floor of the mouth lingual to the mandible, usually in the midline (Figure 3.23). They produce swellings of the floor of the mouth and neck. It has been postulated that they arise from epithelium trapped between the two embryonic lingual swellings which enlarge backwards from the mandibular arch to form the anterior two-thirds of the tongue.

Enucleation is curative and recurrence rare.

References

Alles, J.U. and Schulz, A. (1986) Immunocytochemical markers (endothelial and histiocytic) and ultrastructure of primary aneurysmal bone cysts. *Human Pathology*, **17**, 39–45

Buchner, A. (1991) The central (intraosseous) calcifying odontogenic cyst: an analysis of 215 cases. *Journal of Oral and Maxillofacial Surgery*, **49**, 330–339

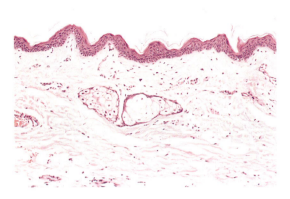

Figure 3.23   Dermoid cyst. The lining consists of epidermis and contains sebaceous tissue in the wall

Crowley, T.E., Kaugars, G.E. and Gunsolley, J.C. (1992) Odontogenic keratocysts: a clinical and histologic comparison of the parakeratin and orthokeratin variants. *Journal of Oral and Maxillofacial Surgery*, **50**, 22–26

Craig, G.T. (1976) The paradental cyst. A specific inflammatory odontogenic cyst. *British Dental Journal*, **141**, 9–14

Eversole, L.R., Sabes, W.R. and Rovin, S. (1975) Aggressive growth and neoplastic potential of odontogenic cysts. *Cancer*, **35**, 270–282

Gardner, D.G., Kessler, H.P., Morency, R. *et al.* (1988) The glandular odontogenic cyst: an apparent entity. *Journal of Oral Pathology*, **17**, 359–366

Martinez, V. and Sissons, H.A. (1988) Aneurysmal bone cyst. A review of 123 cases including primary lesions and those secondary to other bone pathology. *Cancer*, **61**, 2291–2304

Oehlers, F.A.C. (1970) Periapical lesions and residual dental cysts. *British Journal of Oral Surgery*, **8**, 103–113

Saito, Y., Hoshima, Y., Nagamine, T. *et al.* (1992) Simple bone cyst. A clinical and histopathologic study of fifteen cases. *Oral Surgery, Oral Medicine and Oral Pathology*, **74**, 487–491

Weathers, D.R. and Waldron, C.A. (1973) Unusual multi-locular cysts of the jaws (botryoid odontogenic cysts). *Oral Surgery, Oral Medicine and Oral Pathology*, **36**, 235–241

Woolgar, J.A., Rippin, J.W. and Browne, R.M. (1987) A comparative histological study of odontogenic keratocysts in basal cell naevus syndrome and control patients. *Journal of Oral Pathology*, **16**, 75–80

Wright, J.M. (1981) The odontogenic keratocyst: orthokeratinized variant. *Oral Surgery, Oral Medicine and Oral Pathology*, **51**, 609–618

4

Odontogenic tumours and tumour-like lesions

Odontogenic tissues, both ectodermal and mesenchymal, can give rise to true neoplasms, hamartomas (odontomas) and combinations of neoplasm and hamartomatous proliferation. Rather than trying to deal with these lesions in strict academic or histogenetic order, they are described in groups which have features in common.

Ameloblastoma

The ameloblastoma arises from odontogenic epithelium: it forms in the jaws or, exceedingly rarely, in the immediately adjacent soft tissues. It is the most common neoplasm of the jaws and its most striking histological feature is the ameloblast-like cells.

Clinical features

Most ameloblastomas are first recognized in patients aged between 30 and 60 years. They are rare in children. Eighty per cent form in the mandible; of these, 70% develop in the molar region, and often involve the ramus. They are symptomless until the swelling becomes noticeable. Small tumours may occasionally first be seen in routine radiographs. Even large tumours rarely cause paraesthesia or pain. If neglected, the tumour can perforate the bone and, ultimately, spread into the soft tissues making subsequent excision difficult.

Very rarely (fewer than 1% of cases), amelo-blastomas form superficially to the alveolar ridge and cause little or no bone erosion. Extraosseous ameloblastomas typically affect middle-aged patients and resemble fibrous nodules clinically: their prominence usually leads the patient to seek treatment before they grow beyond 2 cm in diameter (El-Mofty *et al.*, 1991).

Radiography

At least 85% of ameloblastomas form rounded, well-defined, multilocular, cyst-like radiolucent areas with well-defined margins. Variants are a honeycomb pattern of radiolucency, a soap-bubble appearance, a monolocular well-defined cavity (unicystic ameloblastoma) or rarely a few large radiolucent areas with small daughter cysts nearby. The bony margins are typically scalloped (Figures 4.1 and 4.2).

There is buccal and lingual expansion. The latter, seen on an occlusal radiograph, is not pathognomonic of ameloblastoma (Figure 4.3). The roots of adjacent teeth are frequently resorbed.

Differentiation of typical ameloblastomas from keratocysts, other tumours of the jaws or hyperparathyroidism by radiography alone is not possible, though the appearances are often highly suggestive.

About 13% of ameloblastomas are unicystic. They are more likely to be seen in persons under 20 years old, particularly involve the posterior part of the body of the mandible and may surround the crown of a displaced molar tooth. The radiolucent area is frequently well circumscribed, with the result that the tumour may not be distinguishable radiographically from a radicular, dentigerous or other non-neoplastic cyst.

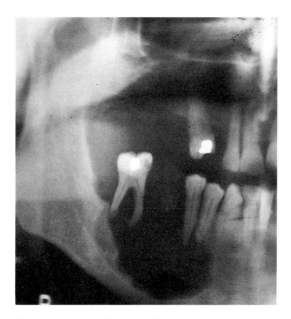

Figure 4.1   Ameloblastoma. This example shows one of many possible radiographic appearances, namely a well-defined, rounded area of radiolucency with scalloped margins but without obvious resorption of involved teeth

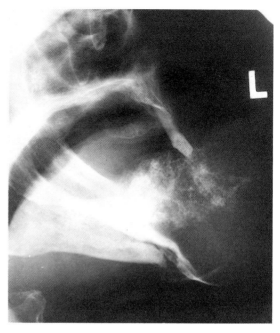

Figure 4.2   Ameloblastoma. This neglected tumour, in a 26-year-old vagrant, had destroyed a large part of the anterior mandible, invaded the soft tissues and projected forward as a gross swelling

Microscopy

Several subtypes have been described and some of these variations may be seen within limited areas of a single tumour. However, it has not been confirmed that these microscopic variations affect the behaviour.

Follicular ameloblastomas are the most readily recognizable pattern and consist of islands or trabeculae of epithelial cells in a connective tissue stroma (Figure 4.4). These epithelial processes consist of a core of loosely arranged polygonal or angular cells, resembling stellate reticulum, surrounded by a well-organized single layer of tall, columnar, ameloblast-like cells with nuclei at the opposite pole to the basement membrane (Figure 4.5). In other specimens, or other parts of the same tumour, the peripheral cells may be cut obliquely or be more cuboidal and resemble basal cells.

Cyst formation is common and varies from microcysts within a predominantly solid to a predominantly cystic tumour. Cysts may develop either within the epithelial islands (see Figure 4.6) or as a consequence of cystic degeneration of the connective tissue stroma.

In unicystic ameloblastomas, the cystic area expands to surround the remainder of the tumour. The latter has the structure of a typical ameloblastoma, but the lining of the cystic area becomes flattened and can closely resemble that of a non-neoplastic cyst. However, ameloblast-like columnar cells can sometimes be seen in the basal layer of the cyst lining or the latter may show budding or actual infiltration of the fibrous wall. Biopsy of the cyst wall alone may, nevertheless, lead to it being misdiagnosed as a simple cyst. This cystic overgrowth of amelobastomas, with obliteration of the normal microscopic features of the tumour in the flattened cyst wall, is the reason for earlier beliefs that ameloblastomas can originate in non-neoplastic cysts. Only rare examples of this phenomenon have been authenticated. As a consequence, all cystic lesions should be enucleated, and the entire cyst wall, particularly any mural thickenings, examined for tumour. However, Saku *et al.* (1991) report that cystic as well as solid

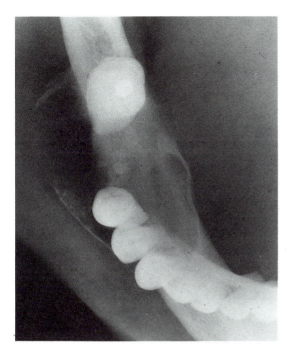

Figure 4.3 Ameloblastoma. The occlusal view shows buccal and lingual expansion and a faint suggestion of loculation

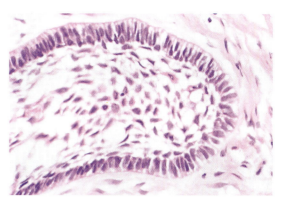

Figure 4.5 Ameloblastoma. High power showing palisaded basal layer and nuclei polarized away from the prominent basement membrane zone

ameloblastomas bind the lectins UEA-1 and BSA-1, enabling them to be differentiated from non-neoplastic odontogenic cysts which do not.

Plexiform ameloblastomas consist largely of thin trabeculae bordered by ameloblast-like or columnar cells, in a loose, vascular sparsely cellular con-

nective tissue stroma. Cyst formation is common and frequently due to stromal degeneration.

Acanthomatous ameloblastomas show squamous metaplasia of the central core of epithelium of tumours which otherwise resemble the more common follicular type (Figure 4.7). Keratin formation may be prominent and the tumour may be mistaken for a squamous cell carcinoma.

Granular cell ameloblastomas are rare. They usually resemble the more common follicular type, but the epithelium, particularly in the centres of the tumour islands, forms sheets of large eosinophilic granular cells resembling those of other granular cell tumours (Figure 4.8). This change may be so extensive that the peripheral columnar cells are replaced and the nature of the

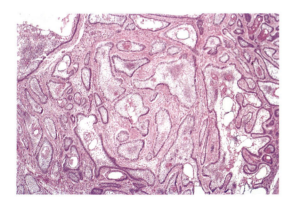

Figure 4.4 Ameloblastoma. Low power showing follicular ameloblastoma in a fibrous stroma

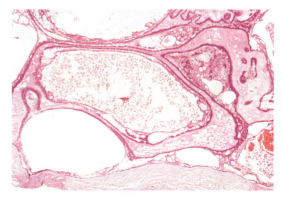

Figure 4.6 Ameloblastoma showing cystic degeneration of the central stellate reticulum-like area

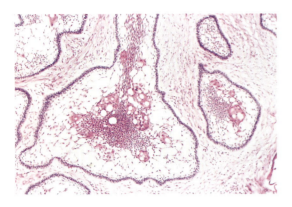

Figure 4.7   Ameloblastoma with squamous metaplasia in the stellate reticulum-like area and microcystic degeneration

tumour may be difficult to recognize from a small biopsy specimen. Granular cell formation was thought to be an ageing or degenerative change but can be seen in ameloblastomas in young persons.

Desmoplastic ameloblastomas consist of only small islands of neoplastic epithelium, with few ameloblast-like cells, in a dense collagenous stroma. There is little or no cyst formation and this variant may be difficult to recognize as an ameloblastoma. It is unusual in that it has a strong tendency to form in the anterior part of the jaw and particularly in the maxilla. Most specimens are detected before they exceed 2 cm in diameter.

Basal cell ameloblastomas are the most uncommon variant and consist of more darkly staining cells

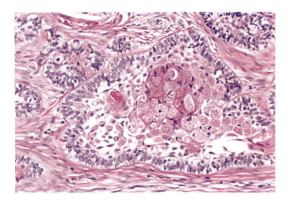

Figure 4.8   Ameloblastoma with granular cells in the centre of the follicle

predominantly in a trabecular pattern with little evidence of palisading at the periphery. Rare examples of extraosseous basal cell ameloblastomas have been mistaken for basal cell carcinomas.

These histological variations do not seem to affect the tumour's behaviour, except in so far as Hartman (1974), from a survey of 20 granular cell ameloblastomas, has suggested that they were more likely to recur than other types.

Management

The diagnosis should be confirmed by biopsy, but may only be made after operation in the case of cystic ameloblastomas, where tumour tissue may be found only in a limited area of mural thickening.

Treatment depends on the type and site of the tumour, but is usually by wide excision, preferably taking up to 1 cm of clinically normal bone around the margin. Curettage leads to recurrence, though this may not be evident for several years. Excision can be curative, but may involve resection of the jaw and bone grafting. However, ameloblastomas are slow growing, typically infiltrate cancellous bone and only later invade compact bone. It may therefore be possible to preserve the lower border of the mandible, if free of tumour, to continue the dissection subperiosteally, and avoid complete resection and bone grafting. Bony repair follows, and a good deal of the jaw re-forms. Any residual tumour may take many years to recur, and regular radiographic follow-up should be carried out. A further limited operation can then be carried out if necessary. This approach is generally less unpleasant for the patient, who must be warned of the necessity of regular follow-up and of the possibility of further surgery. However even with *en bloc* resections, recurrence rates of up to 25% have been reported in the past.

The chief risk with mandibular ameloblastomas is extension into the soft tissues, when it becomes difficult to define the tumour margins and vital structures may be approached.

Maxillary ameloblastomas can present considerable problems and, because of their proximity to the base of the skull and vital structures, are potentially lethal. Bredenkamp *et al.* (1989) reported 5 such cases of which only 2 were known to be alive and disease-free after periods of 14 months to 5 years. Four earlier cases were also reviewed: all had died or were presumed dead from their disease.

Maxillectomy should be regarded as the first requirement. Radical excision at the earliest possible stage is essential, as effective reoperation is unlikely to be possible and there is no satisfactory surgical protocol for the management of extensive tumours involving the base of the skull. Chemotherapy has not been shown to be of any value. Postoperative radiotherapy may slow the progress of recurrences, but is little more than palliative and has not been shown to be of any value as the primary treatment.

Unicystic ameloblastomas, by contrast, appear to have a considerably better prognosis. They are frequently enucleated as cysts before their neoplastic nature is appreciated, but even with this form of treatment, recurrence rates may be only 10–20%. The need for reoperation is determined by thorough examination of the specimen. Extension of the tumour through the fibrous cyst wall is an indication that recurrence is likely, but operation may be delayed until this appears. A local excision is frequently then adequate, but prolonged observation is essential.

Primary extraosseous ameloblastomas can be managed by local excision and though recurrence rates may be up to 25%, reoperation with wider local excision should be curative. By contrast, soft tissue extensions of intraosseous ameloblastomas require wide excision. However, the difficulties in defining their margins make them difficult to manage.

Odontoameloblastoma

This rare neoplasm is essentially an ameloblastoma combined with an odontoma.

Clinically, the chief differences from an ameloblastoma is that it affects children and that the calcified odontomatous tissues are clearly visible in radiographs. However, its behaviour is that of an ameloblastoma, namely progressive infiltration and local destruction of surrounding tissues. The treatment is also the same as for an ameloblastoma. Too few cases have been reported to be certain about

the ultimate prognosis, but rigorous long-term follow-up is clearly essential.

Malignant ameloblastoma and ameloblastic carcinoma

Both of these are exceptionally rare tumours and many pathologists may not see either in a lifetime's practice.

Malignant ameloblastoma is a histologically typical ameloblastoma which, nevertheless, has given rise to pulmonary metastases. These have retained the same microscopic appearances as the primary. Few of the reported cases have been adequately authenticated, and it has also been argued that even of the genuine cases some, at least, have resulted from aspiration implantation. If so, local excision of the secondary deposit should be curative.

Ameloblastic carcinoma refers to a tumour which initially has the microscopic features of an ameloblastoma, but which behaves in an aggressively malignant fashion, losing differentiation and metastasizing (Figure 4.9). In the later stages the microscopic appearances can resemble a squamous cell carcinoma. Exceptionally rarely, the progressive loss of differentiation can be seen in successive specimens from the same patient and, when this

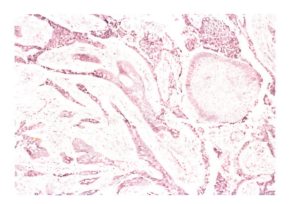

Figure 4.9 Ameloblastic carcinoma. There is a single typical island with palisaded basal cells surrounded by cords of infiltrating tumour. This arose from a typical follicular ameloblastoma which then became atypical histologically and showed widespread local and systemic dissemination

happens, provides convincing evidence of the tumour's histogenesis. Also rarely, hypercalcaemia can be associated.

The problems of management are, therefore, those of an intraosseous carcinoma and if it has already metastasized, the prognosis is correspondingly poor.

Primary intra-alveolar carcinoma

Primary intra-alveolar carcinoma is a rare tumour which can arise in an odontogenic cyst. Müller and Waldron (1991) considered that this accounted for the majority of cases and traced 81 reported examples. The peak incidence is in the sixth and seventh decades and males are affected twice as frequently as females. Most cases have originated in residual cysts in the posterior mandible, but some have originated in keratocysts. Accelerated growth and pain are typical features, but neither may be obtrusive in the early stages. Radiographically, neoplastic change may be suspected in a cyst with a ragged margin, but sometimes the diagnosis is not made until after enucleation. Microscopically, the tumour is typically a well-differentiated squamous cell carcinoma.

Primary intraosseous carcinomas with no evidence of origin in odontogenic cysts are even more rare. They may originate from odontogenic rests, but it may be difficult to exclude the possibility that a carcinoma has entirely overgrown a cyst lining. To *et al.* (1991) reported 3 cases but felt that several of 24 earlier cases were of dubious validity. They noted that, in 50% of them, diagnosis had been delayed by treatment of teeth thought to be causing the symptoms.

Clinically and radiographically, true primary intraosseous carcinomas cannot be reliably distinguished from infected cysts or other malignant tumours.

The diagnosis of primary intra-alveolar carcinoma can only be made by excluding (a) bone invasion by a mucosal carcinoma, (b) intraosseous salivary gland carcinoma (Chapter 12), (c) a metastasis, or (d) ameloblastic carcinoma.

From the viewpoint of management and prognosis, such distinctions are likely to be of considerably less significance than the extent of the tumour or the presence of metastases. However,

metastases are slow to develop and are typically in the regional lymph nodes.

Treatment is preferably by radical excision, but many cases have been enucleated initially as cysts. If then carcinomatous change is found, radical excision should be carried out. The prognosis then appears to be relatively good and the 5-year survival rate appears to be 30–40%. However, data is limited by the rarity of this disease and the brevity of follow-up in many cases.

Adenomatoid odontogenic tumour

This uncommon lesion, previously known as adenoameloblastoma, is completely benign, and probably a hamartoma. It has little in common with the ameloblastoma in behaviour, and also has no glandular component.

Clinical features
Adenomatoid odontogenic tumour affects young people, either in late adolescence or as young adults, and is rare in older persons. Females are more frequently affected, in the ratio of 2 to 1. The tumour is most frequently found in the anterior maxilla and forms a very slow-growing swelling if not noticed by chance on a radiograph. It frequently has the appearances of a dental or dentigerous cyst and its nature may be unsuspected until found to be solid at operation. In an analysis of 499 examples retrieved from the world literature, Philipsen *et al.* (1991) found that tumours containing a tooth (follicular variant) were three times as common as those that did not (extrafollicular variant), were recognized earlier at a mean age of 17 years and affected females twice as frequently as males. The extrafollicular variant was recognized at a mean age of 24 and over 50% of all types were diagnosed between the ages of 13 and 19 years. A rare extraosseous variant resembles a fibrous epulis clinically and accounted for less than 3% of cases.

Microscopy
There is a well-defined capsule and most specimens are only a few centimetres in diameter (Figure 4.10). The mass consists of whorls, strands

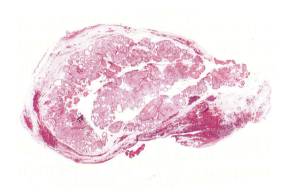

Figure 4.10   Adenomatoid odontogenic tumour. Low power view shows a discrete tumour mass with central cystic space and extensive calcification

Calcifying epithelial odontogenic tumour (CEOT)

This rare tumour, with bizarre cellular features, is often also referred to, for simplicity, as a Pindborg tumour after he first described it in 1955. Though exceedingly rare, this tumour is important, partly because of its unusual structure and because it has been mistaken, particularly in the past, for a poorly differentiated carcinoma.

Clinical features

Adults are mainly affected at an average age of about 40 years. The typical site is in the posterior body of the mandible which is twice as frequently involved as the maxilla.

Symptoms are usually lacking until a swelling becomes apparent. Radiographs show a translucent area with poorly defined margins and, usually, increasing calcification with areas of radiopacity within the tumour as it matures.

and sheets of epithelium, among which are micro-cysts, resembling ducts cut in cross-section and lined by columnar cells similar to ameloblasts (Figure 4.11). These microcysts may contain homo-geneous eosinophilic material. Fragments of amor-phous or crystalline calcification may be seen among the sheets of epithelial cells.

Microscopy

The tumour consists of sheets or strands of polygonal, slightly eosinophilic epithelial cells in a connective tissue stroma. The outlines of the epithelial cells are often distinct and intercellular bridges may be clearly seen. A striking feature is the gross variation in nuclear size including giant, frequently hyperchromatic nuclei and multi-nucleated cells (Figure 4.12). Though mitoses are

Management

These lesions shell out readily and enucleation should be curative. There appear to be no authenticated recurrences.

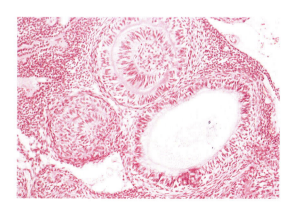

Figure 4.11   Adenomatoid odontogenic tumour. Low power view showing duct-like microcysts and cells forming spheroidal solid structures

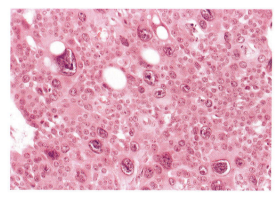

Figure 4.12   Calcifying epithelial odontogenic tumour showing a sheet of polyhedral cells and widespread pleomorphism

rare, there is an alarming resemblance to a poorly differentiated carcinoma. However, unlike most epidermoid carcinomas, inflammatory infiltration of the stroma is typically absent.

Within the tumour, there are typically homogeneous hyaline areas, with the staining characteristics of amyloid, which may calcify (Figure 4.13). These calcifications form concentric masses in and around the epithelial cells, particularly those which appear to be degenerating, and may form large masses. Rarely, dentine or tooth-like structures may form but ameloblast-like cells are not seen.

The presence of amyloid is regarded by some as a criterion of diagnosis of calcifying epithelial odontogenic tumours. However, amyloid can be present in other epithelial tumours such as basal cell carcinomas, and it seems no more reasonable to regard a tumour product such as this as an essential feature than to dismiss the diagnosis of melanoma because of the absence of melanin production.

Calcifying epithelial odontogenic tumours are not encapsulated, are locally invasive and their behaviour seems to be similar to that of ameloblastomas.

A clear cell variant of CEOT tumour has been described, but may be difficult to distinguish from the clear cell odontogenic tumour discussed below.

Management
Diagnosis depends on histological examination and to make sure that there is no confusion with a poorly differentiated carcinoma.

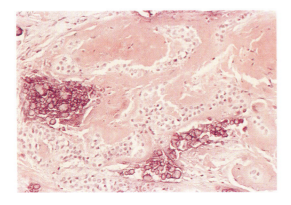

Figure 4.13 Calcifying epithelial odontogenic tumour with extensive amyloid-like deposits and areas of calcification. Congo red stain

Complete excision of the tumour with a border of normal bone appears to be curative. If excision is inadequate, recurrence follows.

Clear cell odontogenic carcinoma

This rare neoplasm was first described by Hansen *et al.* (1985). It is locally invasive and destructive; lymph node and pulmonary metastases have been reported by Bang *et al.* (1989).

Clinically, most cases have been in elderly patients (60–74 years) and have caused symptoms such as mild pain or tenderness, or loosening of teeth. The tumour causes expansion of the jaw and a ragged area of radiolucency. Two of the three first reported cases were in the maxilla.

Microscopy
The tumour is poorly circumscribed and consists of clear cells, uniform in size with a central nucleus and a well-defined cell membrane. They form large sheets, interrupted by relatively thin strands of dense fibrous tissue stroma, in which there is no inflammatory infiltrate. There may also be lesser, dense areas of small basaloid epithelial cells with scanty cytoplasm.

A variable number of the epithelial cells may have a finely fibrillar rather than completely clear cytoplasm and may contain diastase-labile, PAS-positive granules. There may be some nuclear pleomorphism but no more than occasional mitoses.

Differential diagnosis
Significant numbers of clear cells are rarely found in the CEOT, which also has a considerably more pleomorphic cellular picture than clear cell odontogenic carcinoma. The latter also lacks the calcifications and amyloid formation typical of CEOT.

Intraosseous salivary gland tumours are a well-recognized entity, though their rare clear cell variants (Chapter 12) do not appear to have been reported in the jaws and in any case salivary gland tumours affect the mandible. The most important tumour that needs to be distinguished from a clear cell odontogenic tumour is a metastasis of a renal cell carcinoma and, though these usually also involve the mandible, the differential diagnosis (Chapter 12) needs to be considered as it so seriously affects the prognosis.

Management

The behaviour of these tumours is potentially more aggressive than that of the CEOT. Wide excision may be effective in the short term, but recurrences or metastases or both have followed several years later.

Odontogenic ghost cell tumour (calcifying odontogenic cyst, Gorlin cyst)

The odontogenic ghost cell tumour is a rarity and though recognized in the jaws by Gorlin and colleagues only in 1964 (Gorlin *et al.*, 1964), its cutaneous counterpart (benign calcifying epithelioma of Malherbe) was described in 1880 and is currently termed a pilomatrixoma. Though most frequently cystic (Chapter 3), this lesion can rarely be solid and has a potential for continued growth. The term *odontogenic ghost cell tumour* is therefore preferable. Its clinical features are similar to those of the cystic variant.

Microscopy

The appearances have much in common with the cystic variant, but tend to resemble an ameloblastoma in that processes of ameloblastoma-like odontogenic epithelium infiltrate a connective tissue stroma and frequently surround stellate reticulum-like cells (see Figure 3.5). There are variable numbers of ghost cells and deposits of dentinoid. In approximately 10% of cases, odontomas or other odontogenic tumours are associated.

Management

The capability for continued growth leads to recurrence after incomplete removal. Excision is required and is effective.

Odontogenic ghost cell carcinoma

The malignant variant of the odontogenic ghost cell tumour is rare. An example which metastasized to lungs and other sites to cause the death of the patient was reported by Grodjesk *et al.* (1987) who reviewed previous reports of aggressive behaviour of these tumours.

Clinically this carcinoma grows more rapidly than the benign variant.

Microscopically, the cell types in the benign and malignant ghost cell tumours are similar, but in the latter, the epithelial cells are pleomorphic, and the nuclei are frequently hyperchromatic, show mitotic activity and are retained in some of the ghost cells.

Wide excision of odontogenic ghost cell carcinoma and careful follow-up is necessary, but there is as yet no definitive protocol for the treatment of these rare tumours.

Squamous odontogenic tumour

The squamous odontogenic tumour, first described by Pullon *et al.* (1975), is another rare entity.

Clinically, the squamous odontogenic tumour mainly affects young adults and involves the alveolar process of either the maxilla or mandible, close to the roots of erupted teeth which it may loosen. It can also expand the jaw. Radiographically also, squamous odontogenic tumour can mimic severe bone loss due to periodontal disease, or can produce a cyst-like area of radiolucency.

Microscopy

The characteristic features are circumscribed, rounded or more irregular islands of squamous epithelium in a fibrous stroma (Figures 4.14 and 4.15). Foci of keratin or parakeratin and calcifications or globular eosinophilic structures may form in the epithelial islands.

Management

This tumour appears generally to be benign, though invasion of adjacent structures by maxillary

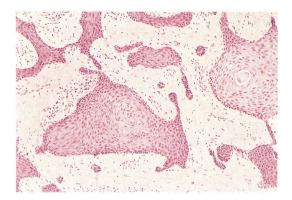

Figure 4.14 Squamous odontogenic tumour showing islands of squamous cells without peripheral palisading in a moderately cellular fibrous stroma

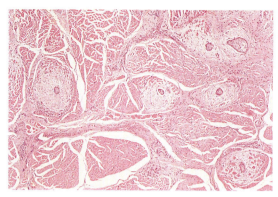

Figure 4.16 Squamous odontogenic tumour showing islands of tumour cells in the surrounding muscle

lesions (Figure 4.16) has been reported (Goldblatt *et al.*, 1982). Curettage or conservative resection and extraction of any teeth involved appears frequently to have been effective treatment, but some, particularly in the maxilla, may require wider resection.

Ameloblastic fibroma

This rare tumour is somewhat similar histologically to the ameloblastoma.

Clinically, ameloblastic fibroma, unlike most ameloblastomas, usually affects young adults or adolescents, but the radiographic appearances may be very similar, namely a multi- or unilocular cyst, most frequently in the posterior part of the body of the mandible. Otherwise, ameloblastic fibromas are slow-growing and usually asymptomatic, apart from eventual expansion of the jaw.

Microscopy

This neoplasm has both epithelial and connective tissue components. The epithelium consists of ameloblast-like or more cuboidal cells surrounding others resembling stellate reticulum or are sometimes more compactly arranged (Figures 4.17 and 4.18). The epithelium is sharply circumscribed by a

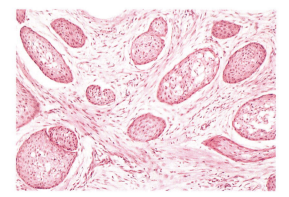

Figure 4.15 Squamous odontogenic tumour – higher power view

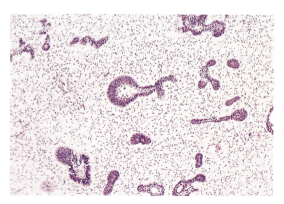

Figure 4.17 Ameloblastic fibroma showing proliferating cords of odontogenic epithelium in a richly cellular mesodermal stroma

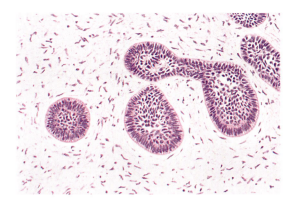

Figure 4.18 Ameloblastic fibroma. The epithelial elements resemble a well-structured ameloblastoma with peripheral palisaded nuclei and central stellate reticulum-like zone. The stroma is cellular mesoderm and resembles the developing dental papilla

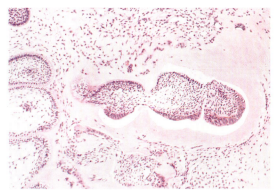

Figure 4.19 Ameloblastic fibroma with induction to form tooth-like material. Such tumours are termed ameloblastic fibro-odontomas

basal membrane and forms islands, strands or cauliflower-like proliferations in a loose but cellular, fibromyxoid connective tissue, which forms little collagen and resembles the immature dental papilla.

An exceedingly rare granular cell variant, in which large eosinophilic granular cells replace the fibromxyoid connective tissue component, has been described and termed *granular cell ameloblastic fibroma*.

Ameloblastic fibro-odontoma

This lesion consists of an ameloblastic fibroma together with mixed calcifying or calcified dental tissues (Figure 4.19). Clinically, it is essentially similar to an ameloblastic fibroma, but radiographs typically show the opaque odontomatous tissues in a circumscribed but otherwise radiolucent area.

Management
The ameloblastic fibroma and fibro-odontoma are benign, and though they may separate readily from their bony walls, Trodahl (1972) reported a recurrence rate of over 40% in the material submitted to the Armed Forces Institute of Pathology. Conservative resection with a margin of sound bone therefore appears to be the treatment of choice.

In the past there has been confusion between the ameloblastic fibro-odontoma and the odonto-ameloblastoma. The latter, as described earlier, is an aggressive tumour for which more radical surgery is essential.

Ameloblastic sarcoma (ameloblastic fibrosarcoma)

Ameloblastic sarcoma is an exceedingly rare malignant counterpart of ameloblastic fibroma – itself a rare tumour.

Clinical features
Wood *et al.* (1988) found reports of 43 cases. In these, the mandible was twice as frequently affected as the maxilla. Young adults of either sex were equally affected, though the reported age incidence ranges from 13 to 78 years.

Some cases appear to arise in ameloblastic fibromas. They initially have similar symptoms, but recur and become obviously aggressive. Others are obviously malignant from the start, grow rapidly and cause either pain or swelling or both.

Radiography
Typically an ill-defined area of radiolucency may be associated, in maxillary lesions, with extension into

the antrum to produce an opacity as well as destruction of the walls.

Microscopy

The essential features are islands of epithelium with the same features as those of the ameloblastic fibroma, but surrounded by highly cellular and pleomorphic fibrous tissue (Figure 4.20). Pleomorphism may be gross and mitoses frequent, but there can be all grades of transition from the benign variant, so that it may be difficult to be certain, histologically, whether or not the mesenchymal component is malignant. In some areas, the sarcomatous element can overwhelm the epithelial component, but in the absence of the latter, the diagnosis cannot be confirmed.

Management

The ameloblastic fibrosarcoma is aggressive, with invasion of adjacent soft and hard tissues, including the base of the skull. Wide radical excision seems to offer the most promising approach as, in many of the reported cases treated more conservatively, there have been multiple recurrences, and sometimes death from local spread of the tumour. However, it is not certain whether this tumour metastasizes. Successful treatment by chemotherapy has been claimed, but its value has not been widely confirmed.

Odontogenic myxoma

The myxoma is peculiar to the jaws. Myxoid tumours elsewhere in the skeleton are the result of myxomatous degeneration in fibrous tumours. Myxomas of the jaws, by contrast, show a close structural resemblance to dental mesenchyme, occasionally contain epithelial rests, affect the tooth-bearing areas of the jaws and a tooth is frequently absent. Growth of this tumour is often rapid at first.

Clinically, young people are predominantly affected, though the age incidence is wide. A fusiform swelling of the jaw and loosening of teeth are typical. Radiographically, there is a radiolucent area with scalloped margins or a soap-bubble appearance which may be similar to that of an ameloblastoma.

Microscopy

Myxomas consist of spindle-shaped or angular cells with long, fine, anastomosing processes (Figure 4.21). Moshiri *et al.* (1992) reported positive reactions to antibodies to vimentin and actin and negative reactions to S-100 protein: ultrastructural studies also suggested that myxoma cells were myofibroblasts. These cells are scantily distributed in loose mucoid intercellular material. Small amounts of collagen fibres may also be formed and there may be small, scattered epithelial rests (Figure 4.22). The tumour margins are ill-defined and peripheral bone is progressively resorbed.

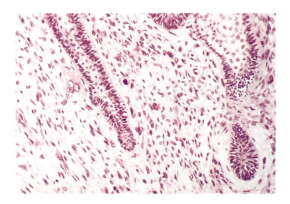

Figure 4.20   Ameloblastic fibrosarcoma. The epithelial component is benign but the mesenchymal tissue shows gross pleomorphism and mitoses

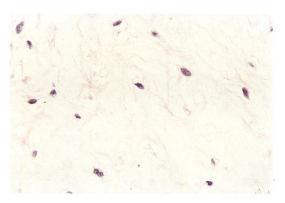

Figure 4.21   Odontogenic myxoma showing rounded and stellate cells in pale staining mucoid stroma

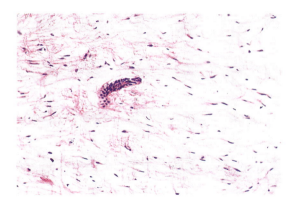

Figure 4.22 Odontogenic fibromyxoma with small island of odontogenic epithelium

Occasional variants on these appearances are mainly due to formation of greater amounts of collagen when the lesion may be termed a fibromyxoma.

Management

Myxomas are benign, but can infiltrate widely so that recurrence after excision is common. Wide excision is desirable in the hope of preventing recurrence, but is not always successful. Irradiation and other methods used to destroy residual tumour tissue have not proved to be of significant value. In spite of aggressive treatment, some tumours can persist for more than 30 years (Cawson, 1972) after the original operations. By this time the tumour may appear inactive and be symptomless.

Rare variants, with a more cellular and pleomorphic microscopic picture, can behave aggressively and may be categorized as myxosarcomas. However, though locally destructive, myxosarcomas appear to have little potential for metastasis.

Odontogenic fibroma

The odontogenic origin of this rare endosteal tumour is confirmed by the presence of epithelial rests, but they are not invariably found.

Clinically, odontogenic fibroma more frequently affects the mandible, but there seems to be no significant predilection for either sex or any age. It forms a slow-growing, asymptomatic mass and usually, therefore, remains unrecognized until it causes a swelling. Alternatively, it may be seen by chance in a radiograph as a sharply defined, rounded area of lucency in a tooth-bearing area.

Microscopy

The odontogenic fibroma consists of spindle-shaped fibroblasts with variable amounts of collagen fibres which may have a whorled arrangement. Strands of epithelium resembling the rests of Malassez may be present in very variable amounts (Figure 4.23).

Management

The odontogenic fibroma does not infiltrate or adhere to the surrounding bone which merely undergoes pressure resorption. It shells out from the bone so that conservative excision is curative.

Cemental tumours and dysplasias

Cementum, being a modified form of bone, is subject to changes comparable to the dysplasias of bone or to neoplastic change. Cemental tumours and dysplasias are a group of lesions in which there is continued proliferation of cementum, but they form a difficult group with characteristics that are

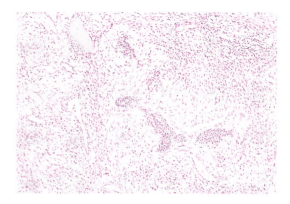

Figure 4.23 Odontogenic fibroma showing odontogenic rests in a cellular fibroblastic stroma

sometimes controversial. In making a diagnosis, account should be taken of the clinical and radiographic features, the microscopic features and the behaviour. These lesions are relatively uncommon, so that there is too little knowledge to reach any firm conclusions about all of them. Four main types are usually described, but some cases do not fit precisely into these categories. They are all rare except in Blacks.

Cementoblastoma

This is probably a benign neoplasm, which forms a mass of cementum-like tissue as an irregular or rounded mass attached to, and often resorbing, the root of a tooth.

Clinically, cementoblastomas are mainly seen in young adult males, typically below the age of 25 years. The tumour is usually slow growing and most frequently attached to a mandibular first molar root. The jaw is not usually expanded, but occasionally a cementoblastoma can produce gross bony swelling and pain.

Radiography

There is a radiopaque mass with a thin but well-defined radiolucent periphery, attached to the roots of a tooth. The mass is usually densely radiopaque, but may appear mottled. It is typically rounded, but may be more irregular. Resorption of the roots to which the mass is attached is common, but the tooth remains vital (Figure 4.24).

Microscopy

The mass consists of cementum which typically contains many reversal lines, and has a pagetoid appearance (Figure 4.25). Cells are enclosed within the hard tissue like osteocytes in bone, while in the larger irregular spaces in the calcified tissue are many osteoclast- and osteoblast-like cells (Figure 4.26). At the periphery and in areas of active growth, there is a broad zone of unmineralized tissue, and the mass has a fibrous capsule.

These appearances are similar to those of an osteoblastoma and they are only distinguishable by the cementoblastoma's relationship to teeth. However, if not recognized by its clinical and other features, the highly active cellular elements may be mistaken for an osteosarcoma.

Management

Cementoblastomas are benign and if the related tooth is extracted and the mass completely excised, there should be no recurrence. If incompletely removed, the mass will continue to grow. More aggressive variants, for which more radical treatment may be needed, have also been described (Figure 4.27).

Cemento-ossifying fibroma

No practical distinction can be made between so-called cementifying and ossifying fibromas.

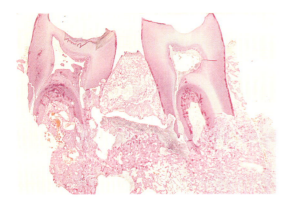

Figure 4.24 Cementoblastoma. Low power showing extensive destruction of the roots of associated molar teeth

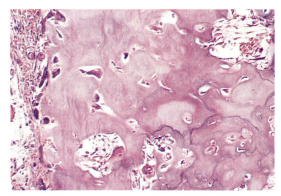

Figure 4.25 Cementoblastoma showing pagetoid basophilic reversal lines and hyperchromatic cells

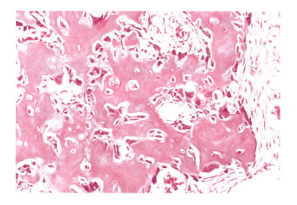

Figure 4.26 Cementoblastoma: cellular area with pleomorphic, hyperchromatic cells

Clinically, these uncommon tumours are well circumscribed and characterized by slow expansile growth, usually in the mandibular premolar or molar region. The most common complaint is a painless swelling, unless seen by chance in a routine radiographic examination. They can affect patients over a wide age range, but most commonly between 20 and 40 years, with a reported female predilection.

Radiography

These tumours usually have well-defined borders, and are radiolucent or with varying degrees of calcification (Figure 4.28). Calcifications tend to be concentrated at the centre of the lesion and some specimens appear largely radiopaque with a narrow radiolucent rim (Figures 4.29 and 4.30). Sometimes there is divergence or occasionally resorption of related roots. Large mandibular tumours are rare but can cause a characteristic downward bowing of the lower border of the jaw.

Microscopy

Cemento-ossifying fibromas consist of spindle-shaped fibroblasts, with a widely variable degree of cellularity (Figures 4.31 and 4.32). Some specimens show moderate amounts of collagen, while others may have less intercellular matrix and the cells may be in whorled or storiform patterns.

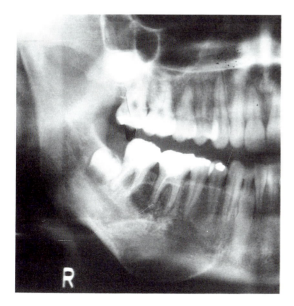

Figure 4.27 Cementoblastoma. This was an exceptionally large and aggressive example. The area of greater radiolucency between the roots of the second and third molars is due to penetration of the lingual cortex by the tumour

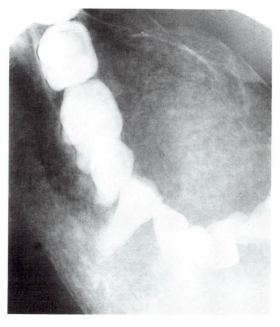

Figure 4.28 Cemento-ossifying fibroma. An unusually large example showing a speckled appearance due to multiple small calcifications

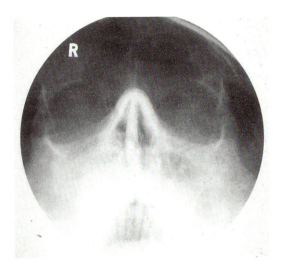

Figure 4.29   Cemento-ossifying fibroma. The conventional occipitomental radiograph shows a diffuse, ill-defined area of radiopacity

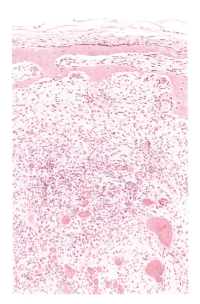

Figure 4.31   Cemento-ossifying fibroma. Only a few cementicle-like calcifications have formed in an early, predominantly fibrous tumour

The types of calcifications within the tumour also vary widely. Trabeculae of woven bone with osteoblastic rimming are often prominent and frequently form an interconnecting reticular pattern. Thicker trabeculae of lamellar bone as well as dystrophic calcifications may also be seen. Specimens which have a predominance of acellular ovoid or spherical calcifications resembling cementicles (Figure 4.33) are commonly termed cementifying fibromas. These nodules are minute at first, but gradually grow, fuse and ultimately form a dense mass. However, similar amorphous spherical calcifications can be found in fibro-osseous lesions of the skull or other bones far distant from any odontogenic tissue. In any case, most so-called cementifying fibromas show admixed spherical calcifications and bone trabeculae, so that the different patterns of calcification are clearly only minor variants of the same pathological process.

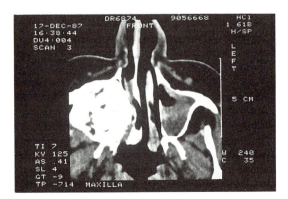

Figure 4.30   Cemento-ossifying fibroma. The CT scan of the same patient as in Figure 4.29 shows it to be well-defined and obliterating the maxillary antrum

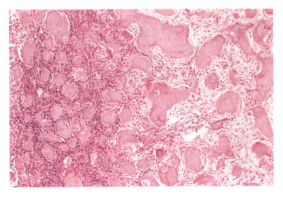

Figure 4.32   Cemento-ossifying fibroma. The variations in fibrous stroma and calcifications can be seen in immediately adjacent areas

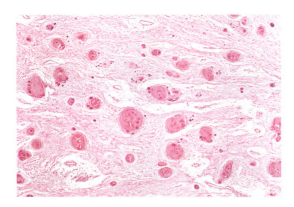

Figure 4.33 Cemento-ossifying fibroma. Concentrically laminated spheroidal cementicles lie in a sparsely cellular fibrous stroma

Histologically, cemento-ossifying fibroma may be indistinguishable from many cases of fibrous dysplasia except by the clinical and radiographic findings. Important differences are that ossifying fibroma more frequently affects the mandible, is well circumscribed and can have a fibrous capsule. Fibrous dysplasia, by contrast, merges with normal bone at its margins. It can also extend to the alveolar margin, but in so doing does not fuse with or otherwise distort the roots of teeth. Microscopically, the trabeculae in fibrous dysplasia, though variably shaped, tend to be slender and arcuate or branched with osteoblasts throughout their substance. This contrasts with the more conspicuous osteoblastic rimming typical of ossify-ing fibroma, where the bone is typically lamellar rather than woven.

A biopsy of an ossifying fibroma also may not be distinguishable microscopically from periapical cemental dysplasia or from other localized cemento-osseous lesions. The latter, which are often found in the mandible at the site of previous extractions, have little or no potential for continued growth and are probably reactive rather than neoplastic.

Though there may be conceptual arguments for distinguishing small ossifying fibromas from cemento-osseous dysplasias, it is not of practical surgical importance.

Management

Cemento-ossifying fibromas may have a definable capsule and can usually be enucleated. Occasionally, large tumours which have distorted the jaw require local resection and bone grafting. The prognosis is good and recurrence rare. However, if an associated tooth is extracted, a densely calcified cemento-ossifying fibroma can become a focus for chronic osteomyelitis. If this happens, complete excision becomes necessary.

Periapical cemental dysplasia

As its name implies, this lesion is probably dysplastic and seems to lack any potential for progressive growth.

Periapical cemental dysplasia affects women, particularly the middle-aged, 10–15 times more frequently than men: it is also more common in Blacks. It usually affects the mandibular incisor region, but can affect several sites or be generalized. It is asymptomatic, but can be seen in radiographs in its early stages as rounded radiolucent areas simulating periapical granulomas, but the related teeth are vital. Increasing radiopacity starts centrally until the masses become densely radiopaque, and all stages of development may be seen in multiple lesions.

Microscopy

The appearances resemble those of cemento-ossifying fibroma (see Figures 4.33 and 4.34). In the early stages, cellular fibrous tissue contains

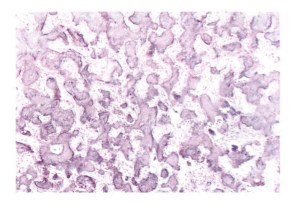

Figure 4.34 Periapical cemental dysplasia with multiple irregular trabulae of immature cementum in moderately cellular fibroblastic stroma

foci of cementum-like tissue which grows and fuses to form a solid, bone-like mass.

Management

The main consideration is to distinguish early lesions from periapical granulomas by routine dental investigation. Once this has been confirmed, further treatment is usually unnecessary.

Florid cemento-osseous dysplasia (gigantiform cementoma)

Women of middle age, particularly Blacks, are mostly affected. The calcifications are frequently symmetrical, may involve all four quadrants and are asymptomatic unless infected. There is a rare familial type.

Radiography

Gigantiform cementoma appears as radiopaque, irregular masses without radiolucent borders and in the past these have been interpreted as diffuse sclerosing osteomyelitis. However, any infection of these lesions is a secondary event.

Microscopy

The masses consist of densely calcified material resembling secondary cementum and containing few lacunae (Figure 4.35) and are sometimes fused to the roots of teeth.

Treatment is difficult in that complete removal of these lesions may require more extensive surgery than their nature justifies and observation by regular follow-up with radiographs at intervals is more appropriate. If infection supervenes, as a result of extraction of an associated tooth or from any other source, chronic osteomyelitis may develop in the dense calcified tissue. In such circumstances the mass may eventually sequestrate or the entire lesion may need to be excised to allow the infection to resolve.

Odontomas

Odontomas are hamartomas or malformations of dental tissues not neoplasms. Even when the morphology is grossly distorted, as in complex odontomas, the pulp, dentine, enamel and cementum form in correct anatomical relationship with one another. Like teeth, they do not develop further, once fully calcified. They also tend to erupt, but once exposed to the saliva can become carious and lead to abscess formation. Odontomas may also prevent normal teeth from erupting, or displace them. Cyst formation is another occasional complication.

Odontomas affect the maxilla slightly more frequently than the mandible and are frequently detected in early adolescence, in routine radiographs.

Compound odontomas

These consist of many separate, small denticles. The malformation may be produced by repeated divisions of a tooth germ or by overgrowth of, and multiple budding-off from, the dental lamina with the formation of many tooth germs (Figures 4.36 and 4.37).

The denticles are embedded in fibrous connective tissue, and have a fibrous capsule. Inflammatory or cystic changes may involve the mass.

Clinically, a compound odontoma most frequently forms in the anterior part of the jaws, where it usually gives rise to a painless swelling.

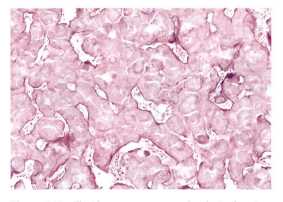

Figure 4.35 Florid cemento-osseous dysplasia showing a homogeneous mass of relatively acellular cementum and poorly cellular stroma

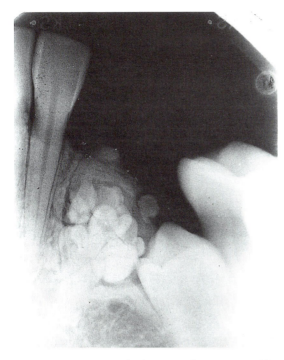

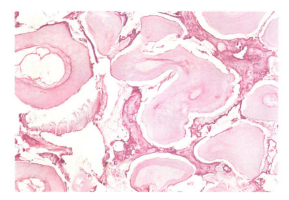

Figure 4.37 Compound odontoma. The poorly formed denticles cut at different angles appear to have little morphological resemblance to teeth, but are of the same structure

Figure 4.36 Compound odontoma. This type is readily recognizable by the multiplicity of densely radiopaque denticles

The denticles may be seen radiologically as separate calcified bodies.

The mass should be enucleated surgically as a potential source of obstruction to erupting teeth.

mistaken for a sequestrum or an area of sclerotic bone.

Histologically, the mass consists of enamel, dentine and cementum, together with pulp and periodontal ligament in varying amounts (Figure 4.38). The arrangement is disordered, but frequently has a radial pattern. The pulp is usually finely branched so that the mass is perforated by small vascular channels like a sponge. If seen before calcification starts, the mass may be mistaken for one of the several types of mixed odontogenic tumours.

The odontoma should be removed by as conservative surgery as possible.

Complex odontoma

This odontoma consists of an irregular mass of hard and soft dental tissues, having no morphological resemblance to a tooth and frequently forming a cauliflower-like mass of hard dental tissues.

Clinically, this malformation is usually seen in young persons, but may escape diagnosis until late in life. Typically, a hard painless swelling is present, but the mass may start to erupt and its many stagnation areas encourage infection.

Radiographically, when calcification is complete, an irregular radiopaque mass is seen with areas of dense radiopacity due to the enamel. Should the mass become infected, the calcified tissues may be

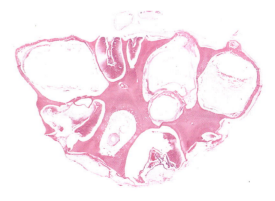

Figure 4.38 Complex odontoma showing a disorganized mass of dentine and cementum. The enamel has been dissolved out during decalcification but basophilic remnants of immature enamel matrix persist

Other types of odontomas

In the past, complex classifications have been devised to include such anomalies as dilated, gestant (invaginated) and geminated odontomas. Frequently, part of these malformations is obviously tooth-like. Dilated and gestant odontomas arise by invagination of cells of the enamel organ or of the epithelial sheath of Hertwig, which actively proliferate to expand the developing tooth, or extend through the opposite pole. Gestant odontomas range in severity from a cingulum pit in an otherwise normal upper lateral incisor to the so-called dens in dente.

These malformations require to be removed as potential obstructions to the eruption of other teeth, as a focus for infection or for cosmetic resions.

Enamel pearls are uncommon, minor abnormalities, which are formed on otherwise normal teeth by displaced ameloblasts or by proliferation of these cells beyond the normal limit of the amelocemental junction.

The pearl may consist only of a nodule of enamel attached to the dentine, or may have a core of dentine which sometimes contains a horn of pulp. Enamel pearls are usually rounded, a few millimetres in diameter, and often form near the bifurcation of first molar roots. An enamel pearl can cause a stagnation area at the gingival margin, but its removal may expose the pulp and necessitate extraction.

References

Bang, G., Koppang, H.S., Hansen, L.S. *et al.* (1989) Clear cell odontogenic carcinoma: report of three cases with pulmonary and lymph node metastases. *Journal of Oral and Pathological Medicine,* **18,** 113–118

Bredenkamp, J.K., Zimmerman, M.C. and Mickel, R.A. (1989) Maxillary ameloblastoma. A potentially lethal neoplasm. *Archives of Otolaryngology and Head and Neck Surgery,* **115,** 99–104

Cawson, R.A. (1972) Myxoma of the mandible with a 35 year follow-up. *British Journal of Oral Surgery,* **10,** 59–63

El-Mofty, S.K., Gerard, N.O., Farish, S.E. *et al.* (1991) Peripheral ameloblastoma: clinical and histologic study of 11 cases. *Journal of Oral and Maxillofacial Surgery,* **49,** 970–974

Goldblatt, L.I., Brannon, R.B. and Ellis, G.L. (1982) Squamous odontogenic tumor. Report of five cases and review of the literature. *Oral Surgery, Oral Medicine and Oral Pathology,* **54,** 187–196

Gorlin, R.J., Pindborg, J.J., Redman, R.S. *et al.* (1964) The calcifying odontogenic cyst: a new entity and possible analogue of the cutaneous epithelioma of Malherbe. *Cancer,* **17,** 723–729

Grodjesk, J.E., Dolinsky, H.B., Schneider, L.C. *et al.* (1987) Odontogenic ghost cell carcinoma. *Oral Surgery, Oral Medicine and Oral Pathology,* **63,** 576–581

Hansen, L.S., Eversole, L.R., Green, T.L. *et al.* (1985) Clear cell odontogenic tumor – a new histologic variant with aggressive potential. *Head and Neck Surgery,* **8,** 115–123

Hartman, K.S. (1974) Granular-cell ameloblastoma. A survey of twenty cases from the Armed Forces Institute of Pathology. *Oral Surgery, Oral Medicine and Oral Pathology,* **38,** 241–253

Moshiri, S., Oda, D., Worthington, P. *et al.* (1992) Odontogenic myxoma: histochemical and ultrastructural study. *Journal of Oral Pathology and Medicine,* **21,** 401–403

Müller, S. and Waldron, C.A. (1991) Primary intraosseous squamous carcinoma. Report of two cases. *International Journal of Oral and Maxillofacial Surgery,* **20,** 362–365

Philipsen, H.P., Reichert, P.A., Zhang, K.J. *et al.* (1991) Adenomatoid odontogenic tumor: biologic profile based on 499 cases. *Journal of Oral Pathology and Medicine,* **20,** 149–158

Pullon, P.A., Shafer, W.G., Elzay, R.P. *et al.* (1975) Squamous odontogenic tumor. Report of six cases of a previously undescribed lesion. *Oral Surgery, Oral Medicine and Oral Pathology,* **40,** 616–630

Saku, T., Shibata, Y., Koyama, Z. *et al.* (1991) Lectin histochemistry of cystic jaw lesions: an aid for differential diagnosis between cystic ameloblastoma and odontogenic cysts. *Journal of Oral Pathology and Medicine,* **20,** 108–113

To, E.H.W., Brown, J.S., Avery, B.S. *et al.* (1991) Primary intraosseous carcinoma of the jaws. Three new cases and a review of the literature. *British Journal of Oral and Maxillofacial Surgery,* **29,** 19–25

Trodahl, J.N. (1972) Ameloblastic fibroma. A survey of cases from the Armed Forces Institute of Pathology. *Oral Surgery, Oral Medicine and Oral Pathology,* **33,** 547–558

Wood, R.M., Markle, T.L., Barker, B.F. and Hiatt, W.R. (1988) Ameloblastic fibrosarcoma. *Oral Surgery, Oral Medicine and Oral Pathology,* **66,** 74–77

5

Non-odontogenic tumours of the jaws

It is not always possible to be certain whether some tumours of the jaws have arisen from osseous or dental connective tissues, but such a distinction is usually of little surgical significance. Many of these tumours are particularly rare in the jaws and considerably more common in other parts of the skeleton.

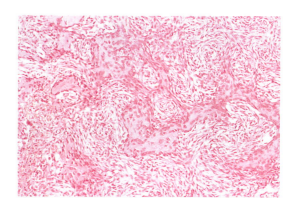

Figure 5.1 Juvenile (aggressive) ossifying fibroma showing highly cellular matrix and woven bone

Ossifying (cemento-ossifying) fibroma

No distinction is drawn between ossifying and cementifying fibroma, as discussed in the previous chapter.

'Juvenile active (aggressive)' ossifying fibroma

This designation has been given to some rarely reported ossifying fibromas, mainly found in the maxilla of younger patients. They have been locally aggressive and showed a tendency to recur. A more cellular ('active') variant of ossifying fibroma may be difficult to distinguish from an osteoblastoma and should probably be categorized as such.

However, there are no reliable criteria for distinguishing these lesions from more typical cemento-ossifying fibromas (Figure 5.1).

Osteoma and other bony overgrowths

Neoplasms of either compact or cancellous bone are less common than localized overgrowths (exostoses). Exostoses consist of lamellae of compact bone, but exceptionally large specimens may have a core of cancellous bone. Small exostoses may form irregularly on the surface of the alveolar processes and specific variants develop on the palate (torus palatinus) or mandible (torus mandibularis). They differ from other exostoses only in their characteristic sites of development and symmetricallity.

Torus palatinus may start to develop in early adult life, but is not usually noticed until middle age.

The common site is towards the posterior of the midline of the hard palate and the swelling is rounded and symmetrical, sometimes with a midline groove. If the swelling is large enough to interfere with the fitting of a denture or is otherwise obtrusive, it should be removed.

Tori mandibularis form on the lingual aspect of the mandible opposite the mental foramen. They are typically bilateral, forming hard, rounded swellings. Their behaviour and management is the same as that of torus palatinus.

Compact and cancellous osteoma

The compact osteoma consists of lamellae of bone sometimes arranged like the layers of an onion but not in Haversian systems (osteones). This neoplasm therefore consists of dense bone containing occasional vascular spaces (Figure 5.2), and is very slow growing.

The cancellous osteoma consists of trabeculae of bone, between which are marrow spaces, surrounded by a lamellated cortex (Figure 5.3).

Osteomas should be excised only if they become large enough to cause symptoms or make the fitting of a denture difficult.

Gardner's syndrome

Gardner's syndrome comprises multiple osteomas of the jaws, polyposis coli with a high malignant potential, and often other abnormalities such as

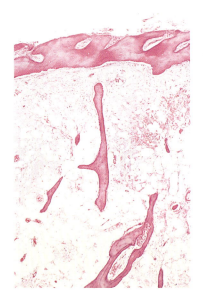

Figure 5.3   Cancellous osteoma with thin bony trabeculae in sparsely cellular fatty stroma

dental defects and epidermal cysts. It is inherited as an autosomal dominant trait.

The osteomas of the jaws are typically multiple and may be ranged along the alveolar ridge, along the borders of the mandible or form endosteal radiopacities. However, the importance of this syndrome is that most of those affected die of bowel cancer by the age of 50. Though some members of the family do not have polyposis coli, the finding of multiple osteomas of the jaws should prompt examination for bowel disease.

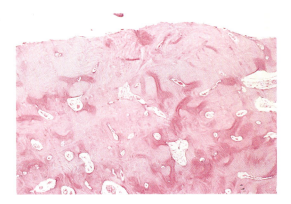

Figure 5.2   Compact osteoma consisting of dense, vital bone with few osteones

Osteochondroma (cartilage-capped osteoma)

This bony overgrowth grows by ossification beneath a cartilaginous cap. Osteochondromas are rare in the maxillofacial skeleton, but in this area the condyle and coronoid process are most frequently affected. There, it can interfere with joint function and limit opening of the mouth. The bony overgrowth will be evident in radiographs, but the cartilaginous cap may not be obvious. Almost any age can be affected, but the mean age of patients is in the fifth decade.

Microscopy

The appearance is not unlike that of an epiphysis with a cap of hyaline cartilage overlying slowly proliferating bone (Figure 5.4). The cartilage cells are sometimes regularly aligned but the cartilage is sometimes more irregular and may contain minute foci of ossification. As age advances the cartilaginous cap becomes progressively thinner and the mass consists increasingly of bone which is usually mostly cancellous and contains fatty or haemopoietic marrow. The cortex and medulla of the mass are continuous with those of the underlying bone.

Management

There is doubt as to whether osteochondromas are true neoplasms or developmental anomalies. Those that arise from the condyle cannot readily be distinguished from condylar hyperplasia. Typically, but not invariably, growth of the tumour ceases with skeletal maturation. Complete excision, together with the overlying periosteum, is curative but in the axial skeleton approximately 3% have undergone sarcomatous change (Henry *et al.*, 1992).

Multiple osteochondromatosis

This rare genetic anomaly is an autosomal dominant trait, but males are somewhat more frequently affected.

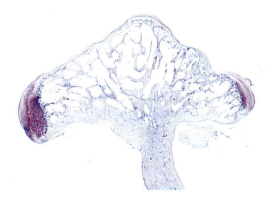

Figure 5.4 Osteochondroma. A pedunculated tumour stained with Masson's trichrome to demonstrate the partial cartilaginous cap

Osteochondromas usually appear in early infancy, particularly on the limbs, and may eventually be numbered in hundreds, but the face and jaws are usually spared. Growth of the lesions stops at the end of puberty but chondrosarcomatous change, later in life, may take place in 10–25% of cases.

Soft tissue osteochondromas

The tongue is the most frequently affected site for these rare tumours where they form firm painless swellings. They respond to excision.

Osteoid osteoma and osteoblastoma

These tumours or tumour-like lesions are not histologically distinguishable, but differ clinically and radiographically. They may not therefore be separate entities but variants of the same disorder. They are both rare in the jaws and more common in other bones. Most patients are below the age of 30 years and males are affected twice as often as females.

Osteoid osteoma

The mandible is affected approximately twice as frequently as the maxilla: the typical complaint is of pain which is characteristically worse at night but variable in nature and severity; it is usually troublesome rather than disabling. The pain is characteristically relieved by aspirin, and can occasionally precede radiologically detectable changes. Osteoid osteomas which are less than 2 cm in diameter appear to have limited growth potential.

Radiographically, osteoid osteoma is considerably more frequently cortical than medullary in site and typically shows a nidus of radiolucency surrounded by densely sclerotic bone. In a minority the nidus becomes calcified.

Microscopically, diagnosis depends on finding the nidus, though it may be no more than 1 or 2 mm in diameter. If the whole specimen is available, the nidus may be identifiable grossly as a greyish or reddish core which may be soft or granular. The nidus consists of osteoid and woven bone which is in trabeculae of irregular length and width, and rimmed by osteoblasts (Figure 5.5). The trabeculae may also show a pagetoid (jigsaw puzzle, 'mosaic') pattern of reversal lines. The connective tissue matrix is highly vascular with many small thin-walled vessels, fibroblasts and multinucleated giant cells.

Management

Excision of the complete nidus, though usually minute, is necessary; otherwise recurrence is likely. The problem of finding the nidus is made easier by smallness of the whole mass, which can be removed entirely. The condition is benign and surgical excision is curative.

Osteoblastoma

Osteoblastomas are even more rare than osteoid osteomas, particularly in the head and neck region, but in this area the mandible is also the most frequent site. As with osteoid osteoma, those aged under 30 years are affected, and males predominate in the ratio of 2 to 1. The chief complaint of dull aching pain is not usually nocturnal, and is said frequently not to respond to aspirin. More important is that osteoblastomas have a potential for progressive growth, can produce swelling of the jaw and may loosen adjacent teeth.

Radiographically, an osteoblastoma appears as a rounded area of radiolucency, usually in the medulla and containing variable amounts of mineralization. Unlike osteoid osteoma, there is no nidus, perilesional sclerosis is usually slight and the mass is larger (2–10 cm diameter). However, the radiographic features are variable and can mimic osteosarcoma or other malignant tumours in up to 25% of cases and show a sun-ray appearance or Codman's triangles.

Microscopically, the appearances of osteoblastoma are the same as those of, and cannot reliably be distinguished from, the nidus of osteoid osteoma.

Management

The osteoblastoma is benign and responds to conservative excision, but recurrence is likely if this is inadequate. There have been isolated reports of malignant change in osteoblastoma, but such lesions may have been low-grade osteosarcomas from the start. However, even 'malignant osteoblastomas' appear only to be locally aggressive and, unlike osteosarcoma, appear to have little or no potential for metastasis.

As mentioned earlier, cementoblastoma is also histologically similar to, and can be regarded as a counterpart of, osteoblastoma. If it is related to the root of a tooth and the microscopic findings are appropriate, it seems reasonable to regard it as a cementoblastoma. In addition, a cementoblastoma may be distinguishable microscopically by peripheral radiating columns of cementum surrounded by large cementoblasts. However, the surgeon may justifiably regard such distinctions as of little practical significance.

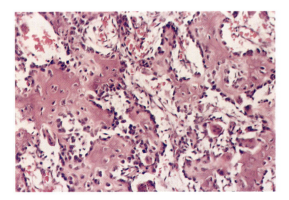

Figure 5.5 Osteoblastoma showing osteoid trabeculae with many osteoblasts within them, and scattered osteoclastic giant cells in a vascular stroma

Giant cell granuloma of the jaw

Most central giant cell lesions of the jaws are hyperplastic and can clearly be distinguished from neoplasms by their behaviour. The name is misleading as there is no granuloma formation in the histological sense; a more appropriate term is *central giant cell lesion of the jaws*. The earlier name 'giant cell reparative granuloma' also derives from an unproven hypothesis (also applied to solitary bone cysts) that it was a reaction to trauma followed by intramedullary haemorrhage. No evidence supports this idea and giant cell hyperplasia does not follow bleeding into bone after a fracture or enucleation of a cyst. Moreover, these lesions often grow rapidly, and far from being 'reparative' are locally destructive.

Though the giant cell granuloma is the main type of giant cell lesion affecting the jaw, it is uncommon. Its important and distinctive feature is that although it may grow rapidly and simulate a neoplasm clinically, wide excision is unnecessary and regression usually follows mere curettage.

It is probable that this lesion is a developmental disorder and similar collections of giant cells can be seen in fibrous dysplasia and related conditions such as cherubism.

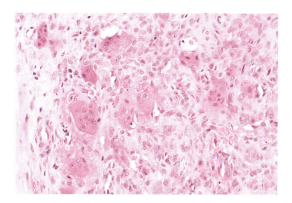

Figure 5.6 Giant cell granuloma showing many multinucleated giant cells in a stroma of plump, spindle-shaped cells

Clinical features

Central giant cell granuloma is usually seen in young people under 20 years old and in females twice as frequently as males. The usual site is the mandible, anterior to the first molars, where the teeth have had deciduous predecessors. There is frequently only a painless swelling, but growth is sometimes rapid, and there may occasionally be pain or paraesthesia of the lower lip. Radiographs show a rounded cyst-like area of radiolucency often with a suggestion of loculation or a soap-bubble appearance. The roots of related teeth can be displaced or, less frequently, resorbed. Occasionally the mass can break through the bone, particularly of the alveolar ridge, to produce a soft tissue swelling. Diagnosis depends on biopsy, but needs to be supplemented by blood chemistry to exclude hyperparathyroidism, as discussed later.

Microscopy

Giant cell granuloma forms a lobulated mass of proliferating connective tissue containing many giant cells (Figure 5.6). It is frequently highly vascular, so that signs of bleeding and deposits of haemosiderin are often seen. In some cases there is considerable fibroblastic proliferation and in others there is prominent osteoid and bone formation, particularly near the periphery.

There are no changes in blood chemistry, but the histological features are indistinguishable from hyperparathyroidism. These giant cells have been shown by Flanagan *et al.* (1988) by their response to calcitonin, their activity in tissue culture and by osteoclast-specific monoclonal antibodies to be indistinguishable from osteoclasts. Whitaker and Waldron (1993) have described in detail more aggressive variants which recurred after initial curettage. These patients ranged in age from 30 months to 67 years. In 6 of these cases the microscopy was that of a typical giant cell tumour of bone which generally showed larger, more evenly distributed giant cells with absence of osteoid centrally or peripherally. Nevertheless, of the 4 cases where the outcome after a year or more was known, 2 responded to a second curettage.

Differential diagnosis of central giant cell lesions

- Hyperparathyroidism. The histological appearances are identical. Blood chemistry should be carried out and a raised serum calcium and alkaline phosphatase indicate hyperparathyroidism (Chapter 6).
- Fibrous dysplasia. A limited biopsy may show foci of giant cells, but the radiographic and histological features, and behaviour, are distinctive (Chapter 6).
- Cherubism. The microscopic features may be indistinguishable from giant cell granuloma, but the lesions are symmetrical and young children are affected (Chapter 6).

- Giant cell tumour (osteoclastoma) is an aggressive neoplasm which affects long bones, but may not be distinguishable with certainty by microscopy alone, from a giant cell granuloma. Osteoclastomas occasionally form in such bones as the temporal or sphenoid, but it is questionable how many of the few reported cases of these neoplasms in the jaws can be authenticated, and in their report of a primary malignant giant cell tumour of the jaw, Mintz *et al.* (1981) claimed it to be the first documented case. This tumour metastasized to the lungs and a lymph node.
- Aneurysmal bone cysts may contain many giant cells, but their other histological features (Chapter 3) and, in particular, the multiple blood-filled spaces, should enable the distinction to be readily made.

Management
Curettage of giant cell granulomas is adequate and wide excision is usually unnecessary; small fragments that may be left behind rarely require further treatment and appear to resolve spontaneously. A minority of these tumours are more aggressive, recurrence follows incomplete removal and further surgery becomes necessary. Frequently, further curettage appears to be adequate and wider excision is rarely required.

Osteosarcoma

This highly malignant tumour is the most common primary neoplasm of bone, but is overall rare. Approximately 7% of osteosarcomas may be found in the jaws and according to Garrington *et al.* (1967) their annual incidence in the USA is 1 per 1.5 million persons.

Most cases of osteosarcoma have no identifiable cause apart from the few which have followed irradiation. Osteosarcoma is also a recognized complication of Paget's disease of bone but hardly ever in the jaws.

Clinically, osteosarcoma of the jaws characteristically affects patients considerably later than in the long bones, namely at a mean age of 30–39 years and occasionally in elderly persons.

Rarely, it may develop much later as a result of irradiation many years previously. Males are slightly more frequently affected than females. The mandible, and in particular the body, is more frequently affected than the maxilla.

A typical picture is that of a firm swelling which grows in a few months and becomes painful. The teeth may be loosened and there may be paraesthesia or anaesthesia in the mental nerve area. Metastases to the lungs may develop early. However, the fact that some patients have symptoms for many months before diagnosis suggests that some of these tumours may be slow growing.

Radiography
The appearances are varied. In the early stages there may be only subtle changes with only slight variation in the trabecular pattern, but an early feature (Garrington *et al.*, 1967) may be symmetrical widening of the periodontal ligament space around one or several teeth as a result of tumour infiltration. This finding is not specific, but in association with pain, swelling or other radiographic changes is highly suggestive of osteosarcoma.

Later, irregular bone destruction usually predominates over bone formation. Bone formation in a soft tissue mass is highly characteristic of osteosarcoma. A sun-ray appearance at the surface or Codman's triangles at the margins due to elevation of the periosteum and new bone formation may be seen on appropriate radiographs, but are uncommon and not specific to osteosarcoma. The extent of the tumour can be shown by CT scanning.

Microscopy
Osteosarcomas originate from bone cells which have the potentiality to produce a highly pleomorphic picture in which bone formation does not necessarily predominate. The tumour cells are variable in size and shape, many are large and hyperchromatic, and mitotic figures may be prominent, particularly in the more highly cellular areas of the tumour. Cells resembling osteoblasts, fibroblasts and cartilage cells can be recognized; giant cells may be conspicuous, but many cells are of indeterminate appearance.

Formation of osteoid is the main criterion of diagnosis of osteosarcoma, but it may be small in amount and difficult to distinguish from collagen (Figure 5.7). Inability to detect osteoid appears to be a factor limiting the evaluation of aspiration cytology. Cartilage and fibrous tissue are usually also present. Predominantly fibroblastic variants appear to have a somewhat better prognosis than the more common osteoblastic type.

The amount of these tissues may vary widely in different parts of the tumour, but in jaw osteosarcomas there is frequently extensive cartilage formation and limited areas of osteoid formation. A small biopsy may, therefore, show malignant cartilage, and can lead to a mistaken diagnosis of chondrosarcoma. Overall, the general picture is one of uncontrolled and irregular cell activity.

A rare variant known as small cell osteosarcoma has a close resemblance to Ewing's sarcoma but for the fact that it forms osteoid. Another uncommon variant appears histologically to be a low-grade tumour and consists largely of spindle-shaped cells and limited osteoid formation. These low-grade intramedullary osteosarcomas are difficult to differentiate histologically from benign lesions such as fibrous dysplasia, desmoplastic fibroma or ossifying fibroma. However, they are infiltrative and pursue a relentless course.

Management
Diagnosis depends on biopsy which may need to be repeated if there is any doubt. Chest radiographs should also be taken, as secondary deposits may be present when the patient is first seen. Fine needle aspiration has been reported by White *et al.* (1988) to give an 80.4% accuracy in the diagnosis of osteosarcoma. Serum alkaline phosphatase levels are raised in about 50% of cases and particularly with those tumours where new bone formation predominates.

Osteosarcomas of the jaws are rapidly invasive, but tend to metastasize to the lungs less frequently or later than those of the long bones. Metastasis to regional nodes may be seen in fewer than 10% of cases. Nevertheless, approximately 50% of osteosarcomas of the jaw recur locally within a year of initial treatment. Only 4 out of 66 patients reported by Clark *et al.* (1983) developed metastases, but most died from uncontrollable local disease. With aggressive surgery, supplemented as necessary by radiotherapy and sometimes chemotherapy, Tran *et al.* (1992) claimed a 49% 10-year survival rate for 15 osteosarcomas mainly of the maxilla or mandible, but deaths continued even after the decade.

Early radical excision of osteosarcoma of the jaws is essential. This involves mandibulectomy or maxillectomy, together with wide excision of any soft tissue extensions of the tumour. However, osteosarcomas often extend within the medulla for some distance beyond the radiographic margins, so that recurrence of the tumour in the excision margins is a major problem. Excision may be combined with pre- or postoperative radiotherapy by such means as high-dose interstitial needling, and adjuvant chemotherapy is increasingly widely used. Immunotherapy has proved to be disappointing.

The prognosis depends mainly on the extent of the tumour at operation and deteriorates with spread to the soft tissues, to the base of the skull, or with recurrence after excision which may happen in over 50% of cases.

Juxtacortical osteosarcoma

Juxtacortical osteosarcoma is a rare variant which, like endosteal osteosarcoma, mainly affects the limbs but can occasionally involve the jaws. Its chief importance is its better prognosis, as reviewed by Millar *et al.* (1990), who reported 4 cases but were able to find only 8 previous reports.

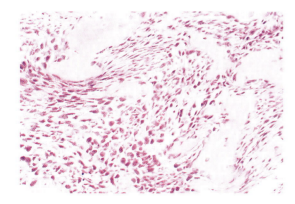

Figure 5.7 Osteosarcoma showing tumour bone in a cellular stroma of pleomorphic, malignant osteoblasts

Clinically, juxtacortical osteosarcoma typically affects the mandible, and the average age of patients is about 35 years. It may cause dull aching pain and forms a slow-growing mass on the surface of the jaw or in the adjacent parosteal tissue. The mass is typically rounded with a broad base.

Radiographically, juxtacortical osteosarcoma characteristically has an opaque base and is more lucent superficially. The pattern of and amount of opacity and radiolucency varies widely.

Microscopy

Juxtacortical osteosarcoma characteristically shows a deep zone of benign-looking, parallel trabeculae of bone separated by fibrous tissue: mitotic activity and cellular abnormalities are frequently difficult to find (Figure 5.8). The more superficial and, particularly, the radiolucent zones are likely to show more obvious neoplastic activity and cellular pleomorphism consistent with osteosarcoma. A minority of specimens show obviously sarcomatous features throughout.

The terms *periosteal* and *parosteal osteosarcoma* result from an attempt to subdivide the variants of this tumour, when affecting the long bones, on the basis of differing radiographic and microscopic features. It is suggested that the periosteal type is a separate entity and tends to be a high-grade tumour with more obviously malignant features. Even so, its prognosis is appreciably better than for endosteal osteosarcoma. However, this subclassification does not appear as yet to be justifiable for jaw tumours.

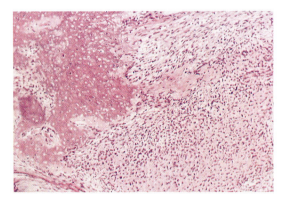

Figure 5.8   Parosteal osteosarcoma showing a subperiosteal mass of bony trabeculae merging with cellular tumour stroma

Management

It is obviously essential to establish the diagnosis firmly as early as possible by adequate biopsy of the superficial radiolucent areas.

Wide excision, including underlying bone, is desirable, though recurrence has even followed hemimandibulectomy. Of the 4 cases reported by Millar *et al.* (1990), all were disease free 1–16 years later and of the 8 earlier cases, 5 were recurrence free for periods of 6–11 years.

Chondroma

The chondroma is a particularly rare tumour of the jaws. Many pathologists, including the present authors, believe that the majority of so-called chondromas of the jaws ultimately prove to be malignant. In any case, chondrosarcomas in the maxillofacial region are considerably more frequent than chondromas. However, chondromas are described here in deference to those who hold other views.

Chondromas are far more frequently found (though still rare) in the nose or nasal sinuses and hence can occasionally be found in the maxilla rather than the mandible. Clinically, true chondromas are small and likely to be no more than chance findings.

Microscopically, chondromas consist of hyaline cartilage, but the cells are irregular in size and distribution (Figure 5.9). Calcification or ossification may develop within the cartilage.

Treatment is by wide excision, including an adequate margin of normal tissue all round, because of the difficulty in distinguishing benign from malignant tumours and the probability that a chondroid tumour is malignant.

Chondrosarcoma

Chondrosarcomas of the jaws affect adults at an average age of about 45 years. The maxilla is the site in 60% of cases, most frequently in the anterior alveolar region, but there is no special site of predilection for mandibular tumours.

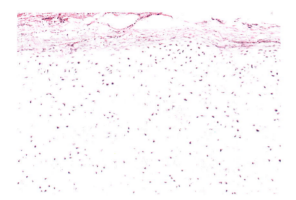

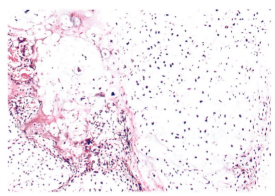

Figure 5.9 Chondroma. A circumscribed encapsulated mass of hyaline cartilage contains predominantly mononuclear chondrocytes

Figure 5.10 Chondrosarcoma showing cellular cartilage with pleomorphic chondrocytes, many of which have multiple nuclei

There is wide variation in the reported relative frequency of chondrosarcomas and osteosarcomas of the jaws. These differences probably result from varying histological criteria for distinguishing chondrosarcomas from chondrogenic osteosarcomas. From a practical viewpoint this distinction may be important, as chondrosarcomas of the jaws appear to have a worse prognosis than osteosarcomas (Garrington and Collett, 1988a,b).

Pain, swelling or loosening of teeth associated with an area of greater or lesser radiolucency are typical features. Radiographically, chondrosarcoma of the jaws can be well or poorly circumscribed, or may appear multilocular. Though radiolucency is typical, calcifications are frequently present and may be widespread and dense. Symmetrical widening of the periodontal ligament space around affected teeth may be seen (Hackney *et al.*, 1991).

The radiographic margins are an unreliable guide to the extent of the tumour which can infiltrate between the bone trabeculae without causing their resorption.

Microscopy

The product of the neoplastic chondrocytes ranges from comparatively well-formed cartilage (grade I tumours), which are the most frequent grade in the jaws, to myxoid tissue (grade III). The chondrocytes show the pleomorphism characteristic of these sarcomas (Figure 5.10); they may be binucleate but show no mitotic activity in grade I tumours. Grade II tumours form myxoid tissue as well as

cartilage and there are occasional mitoses among the chondrocytes. The amount of calcification in the neoplastic cartilage corresponds with the radiographic appearances and can be punctate or loose and fluffy in appearance.

Behaviour and management

Chondrosarcomas of the maxillofacial region are aggressive; local recurrence or persistent tumour is the main cause of death. Fewer than 10% of these tumours (usually grade III tumours) metastasize; the lungs or other bones are then the usual sites of distant spread. Metastasis to lymph nodes is very rare.

Chondrosarcomas must be widely excised as early as possible. The first operation is critical, as inadequate excision is likely to lead to recurrences beyond the original area of operation with inevitable problems of management. A major difficulty as mentioned earlier is the ability of the tumour to extend in the cancellous spaces a considerable distance beyond the radiographic margins. Another is the ability of chondroid tumours to seed and grow in the soft tissues of the operation site. Chondrosarcomas only occasionally respond to radiotherapy, and chemotherapy appears to be of little value.

The prognosis of chondrosarcomas of the maxillofacial region is generally worse than for other sites because of the difficulties of adequate excision in this area. The 5-year survival rate is from 40% to 60% and depends on the tumour stage and grade, and on the extent of the original excision. Maxillary tumours have an even worse prognosis than mandibular, but in the 37 cases reported by Garrington and Collett (1988) there were no survivors from chondrosarcoma of either jaw after 15 years.

Mesenchymal chondrosarcoma

Mesenchymal chondrosarcoma is considerably more uncommon than chondrosarcoma but a relatively high proportion of them (15–35%) are in the craniofacial region. A minority form in the soft tissues.

Clinically, mesenchymal chondrosarcoma has a wide age distribution. It presents no specific signs or symptoms but rapidly developing pain and swelling, sometimes with loosening of teeth, are typical.

Radiographically, there is an area of radiolucency, usually speckled with calcifications. There is only partial circumscription and no peripheral sclerosis.

Microscopy

The overall appearance is that of a highly cellular tumour in which only small foci of tissue are recognizable as poorly formed cartilage; however there are striking variants.

Typically, the bulk of the tumour consists of sheets of irregularly ovoid or sometimes spindle-shaped, darkly staining cells with little cytoplasm, with occasional or numerous mitoses. Scattered about are generally small, poorly circumscribed foci of cartilage in which there may be calcification. These foci may be scanty or occasionally form the bulk of the tumour and some areas of the tumour may be highly vascular.

One variant (haemangiopericytoma-like mesenchymal chondrosarcoma) consists of sheets of small mesenchymal cells surrounding cleft-like vascular spaces (Figure 5.11). Cartilage can sometimes be very scanty in such tumours. In another variant, the vascular component forms sinusoids within the tumour.

Management

Mesenchymal chondrosarcoma is highly malignant and the frequency of metastases is high. Spread,

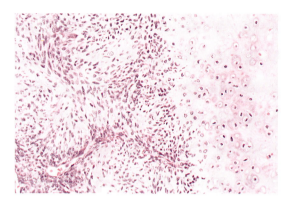

Figure 5.11   Mesenchymal chondrosarcoma showing cellular, haemangiopericytoma-like area on the left and an island of well-differentiated cartilage on the right

usually to the lungs but sometimes to lymph nodes, frequently follows local recurrences.

Early radical surgery followed by combined chemotherapy is therefore required. However, its value is as yet uncertain and either local recurrences or metastases can appear 10 or more years after treatment. There are no reliable microscopic guides to prognosis.

Chondromyxoid fibroma (fibromyxoid chondroma)

This rare tumour occasionally forms in the mandible. Lustman *et al.* (1986) found 10 earlier reports and added three more. Twelve of these were in the mandible and Damm *et al.* (1985) reported another example in the maxilla. Though so few cases have been seen in the jaws, the importance of this tumour is that it is benign but can be mistaken microscopically for a chondrosarcoma.

Clinically, most patients are below the age of 30 and symptoms are frequently slight or absent. However, chondromyxoid fibroma can sometimes simulate a malignant tumour and can cause pain, swelling of the jaw or loosening of teeth.

Radiographically, this tumour is likely to appear as radiolucent areas with irregular but, typically, sclerotic margins and trabeculation or an appearance suggesting loculation. Opacities are rarely seen in the tumour area.

Microscopy

The typical features are lobules of myxoid tissue with more cellular and compact peripheries, and surrounded by fine but highly vascular fibrous tissue septa. In excision specimens the surrounding bone may be seen to be sclerotic.

The cells of the myxoid areas are variable in shape, but many are angular or stellate with long slender processes, or may be within lacunae. The more closely packed peripheral cells tend to be more rounded and may have an epithelioid appearance. Cartilage can occasionally form up to 75% of the tumour but may be present only in minute amounts, and calcifications are seen in a minority of cases. Cyst formation and areas of haemorrhage may be seen (Figure 5.12).

Findings which may add to the impression of malignancy are cells with large hyperchromatic nuclei and osteoclast-like giant cells. Features helping to distinguish this tumour from a chondrosarcoma are an earlier age of onset, its sclerotic margins and frequent lack of calcifications or calcifications of a different type from those seen in chondrosarcomas.

Management

Chondromyxoid fibroma can recur if excision is inadequate. Like other chondroid tumours it can grow in the soft tissue as a result of seeding of tumour cells at operation. However, it is doubtful whether sarcomatous change has been authenticated. The tumour should be excised with as wide as possible a margin of normal tissue.

Chondroblastoma

Chondroblastoma is a benign tumour but involves the maxillofacial region even more rarely than chondromyxoid fibroma. Out of 495 cases reviewed by Kurt *et al.* (1989), only 7 were in the mandible but 23 were in the temporal bone.

Clinically, the median age of presentation of these tumours in the head and neck region is approximately 40 and males have been affected twice as frequently as females. Characteristic radiographic appearances in the long bones are a rounded area of radiolucency with a thin sclerotic border which may sometimes show a scalloped pattern and varying amounts of calcification. These appearances may be less well defined in the jaws.

Microscopy

The chondroblastoma is highly cellular. Rounded cells, with well-defined outlines, eosinophilic or amphophilic cytoplasm and an epithelioid appearance are the main component. Multinucleate giant cells are common and range from those with only two or three nuclei, to large osteoclast-like cells (Figures 5.13 and 5.14). They are usually associated with areas of haemorrhage or necrosis and secondary aneurysmal bone cyst formation has been seen in up to 25% of cases. The frequency of giant cells in these tumours is indicated by its earlier names of 'calcifying giant cell tumour' or 'epiphyseal chondromatous giant cell tumour'.

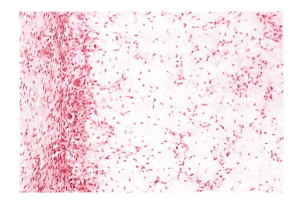

Figure 5.12 Chondromyxoid fibroma showing a lobule of spindle-shaped or stellate cells in a myxochondroid matrix with small multinucleated cells

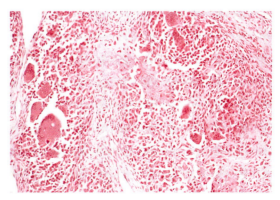

Figure 5.13 Chondroblastoma showing polyhedral chondroblasts together with multinucleated giant cells in a cellular, chondroid matrix

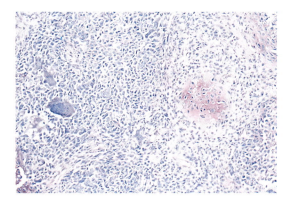

Figure 5.14   Chondroblastoma stained to show chondroid areas more clearly (Taylor's blue)

Chondroid areas can be sharply defined or merge imperceptibly into the epithelioid areas. A net-like pattern of calcification extending between the cells or punctate calcifications are characteristic. Calcification in the cartilaginous areas may be seen, but ossification is rare and myxoid areas are absent.

Management

As indicated earlier, information about chondroblastomas of the jaws is scanty. Curettage, followed if necessary by bone grafting, has frequently been successful, but up to 30% of cases may recur. If aneurysmal bone cyst is associated, curettage alone is inadequate and its combination with cryosurgery is probably more effective. There is in either case a good response to radiotherapy for otherwise uncontrollable or surgically inaccessible lesions.

Ewing's sarcoma

Ewing's sarcoma comprises 10–15% of all primary sarcomas of bone, but fewer than 3% are in the jaws. It predominantly affects the legs or pelvis, but of those that affect the head and neck region the mandible is affected twice as frequently as the maxilla.

The histogenesis of Ewing's sarcoma has long been controversial, but immunocytochemistry has shown that the cells stain for neural markers such as neuron-specific enolase. Moreover, the tumour cells may form rosette-like patterns as seen in neuroblastoma and retinoblastoma. Though Ewing's sarcoma cells may stain for vimentin and have been thought to be pluripotential, it is generally accepted that this tumour is of neuro-ectodermal origin and shares cytogenetic abnormalities with primitive neuroectodermal tumour (Dehner, 1993).

Clinically, the majority of patients are white males, usually aged from 5 to 20 years, and rarely over 30 years.

Typical symptoms are bone swelling and often pain, progressing over a period of months. Teeth may become loosened and the overlying mucosa ulcerated. Fever, leucocytosis, raised ESR and anaemia indicate a poor prognosis.

Radiographically, Ewing's sarcoma appears as an irregular osteolytic lesion with or without cortical expansion. The onion-skin appearance due to the periosteal reaction, sometimes seen in long bones, is rare in the jaws. The clinical and radiographic findings in 105 reported cases have been reviewed by Wood *et al*. (1990).

Microscopically, Ewing's sarcoma cells resemble but are about twice the size of mature lymphocytes, having a darkly staining nucleus, surrounded by a rim of cytoplasm, which is typically vacuolated. The tumour cells are in diffuse sheets or in loose lobules, separated by septa. Grouping of tumour cells round blood vessels, and areas of haemorrhage and necrosis, may be seen (Figures 5.15 and 5.16).

Important diagnostic features are the presence of intracellular glycogen in approximately 75% of cases (Figure 5.17), but absence of reticulin from the stroma.

Ewing's sarcoma may be difficult to differentiate from metastatic neuroblastoma or malignant lymphoma unless intracellular glycogen is present. Alcohol fixation is useful for increasing the reliability of staining for glycogen. Small cell osteosarcoma may also appear similar but for small foci of osteoid.

Management

The most common sites for metastases are the lungs and other bones. Since Ewing's sarcoma is so rare as a primary tumour in the jaws, the possibility that such a tumour is a metastasis from another bone may need to be investigated by a skeletal

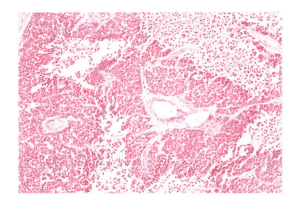

Figure 5.15 Ewing's sarcoma. Sheets of small round cells surround blood vessels and there is extensive necrosis

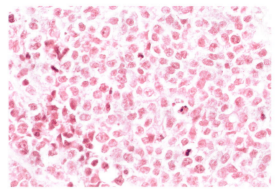

Figure 5.16 Ewing's sarcoma. A high mitotic rate is seen at higher power

survey. Lymph nodes are involved in 10–20% of cases.

Currently, the initial treatment of choice is probably as wide excision as possible, together with megavoltage irradiation and multi-agent chemotherapy. This combination treatment appears to have improved the 5-year survival rate from about 10% to 60% or more. However, there is a significant increase in second (particularly lymphoreticular) tumours as a consequence of the chemotherapy and there is insufficient information as to the effectiveness of multimodal treatment of Ewing's sarcoma of the jaws.

Extraskeletal osteosarcoma, chondrosarcoma and Ewing's sarcoma

These sarcomas can rarely also develop in the soft tissues where they must be distinguished from a variety of pseudosarcomatous lesions or other sarcomas (Chapter 13).

Desmoplastic fibroma

Desmoplastic fibroma of the jaws is a fibromatosis, a term which describes tumour-like fibrous proliferations which infiltrate the surrounding

tissues like a fibrosarcoma, but never metastasize (Chapter 13).

Clinically, the majority (75%) of patients are below the age of 30 and 50% are between the ages of 10 and 20 years. The mandible, usually at the junction between the ramus and body, is the most common site in the head and neck region. Of 49 previously reported lesions affecting the jaws reviewed by Hashimoto *et al.* (1991), only 6 were in the maxilla.

The main manifestation is a gradually enlarging swelling but occasionally there is aching pain. Radiographically, desmoplastic fibroma gives rise to a well-circumscribed area of lucency which has a honeycomb or trabeculated appearance, and usually has a partial or complete sclerotic rim.

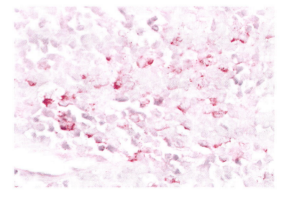

Figure 5.17 Ewing's sarcoma. PAS staining shows the intracellular glycogen typical of this tumour

Roots of related teeth may be resorbed and, rarely, the margins suggest infiltration of the surrounding bone.

Microscopy

The mass consists of fibroblasts and collagen fibres forming broad bundles. These fibrous bundles interlace to some degree, but do not form the streaming or herring-bone appearances seen in fibrosarcomas. The nuclei of the fibroblasts show no atypia, but may be more plump and vesiculated than normal and contain 2 or 3 minute nucleoli. Mitotic activity is virtually absent. The margins are less well circumscribed than suggested by the radiographic appearances and merge with the surrounding bone.

Management

Desmoplastic fibroma is progressive but, as mentioned earlier, does not metastasize. Because of its infiltrative character, curettage or local excision is followed by recurrence in up to 30% of cases. Excision with an adequate margin of normal bone is therefore required and wider excision still is necessary for lesions which have extended into the soft tissues. However, mutilating surgery is not justified as any recurrences are purely local and can be controlled when they appear. Malignant change has been reported after radiotherapy which is therefore contraindicated.

Fibrosarcoma of bone

Fibrosarcomas of bone account for less than 5% of primary malignant bone tumours. The most common sites are the metaphyseal region of the medulla of a bone of the leg. In approximately 20% of cases, fibrosarcoma is secondary to some other bone lesion such as Paget's disease or a giant cell tumour, or a complication of previous radiotherapy of a soft tissue lesion.

Approximately 15% of fibrosarcomas of bone are in the head and neck region, with a predilection for the skull or jaws. The mandible, particularly the body, is affected more frequently than the maxilla in the ratio of 3–4 to 1. Males are slightly more frequently affected than females; most patients are between 30 and 40 years of age, but there is a wide age distribution.

Clinically, fibrosarcoma of the jaws causes pain, swelling and loosening of teeth. Radiographically it causes an ill-defined lucent area with no distinctive features or, rarely, a relatively well-circumscribed area of radiolucency.

Microscopically, fibrosarcoma of bone appears similar to its soft tissue counterpart (Chapter 13) with long interlacing fascicles of spindle-shaped fibroblasts and some collagen formation. The chief difficulty in differential diagnosis is with desmoblastic fibroma described earlier.

Management

The treatment is radical surgical excision, possibly supplemented by radiotherapy. The tumour may metastasize to the lungs or other bones, but though data on fibrosarcomas of the jaws is limited, they are thought to have a better prognosis than osteo- or chondrosarcomas. About 30% of fibrosarcomas arise from the periosteum and appear to have a better prognosis than intramedullary fibrosarcomas. Five-year survival rates for fibrosarcomas of the bones of the head and neck range from 27% to 40%. The prognosis is affected by the extent of the tumour at operation and the degree of dedifferentiation. Fibrosarcomas of bone secondary to other diseases generally also have a worse prognosis.

Malignant fibrous histiocytoma

Fibrous histiocytomas range, in behaviour, from benign to malignant and, in many parts of the body, lesions earlier reported as fibrosarcomas or other sarcomas have been found on reassessment to be malignant fibrous histiocytomas. These tumours are predominantly soft tissue tumours (Chapter 13) but a minority are intraosseous. Block *et al.* (1986) were able to find reports of 16 cases affecting the maxilla and added another.

Clinically, malignant fibrous histiocytomas of the jaws do not show any distinctive features to distinguish them from other sarcomas. Pain, swelling and loosening of teeth are typical effects.

The microscopic features are described in Chapter 13.

Management

Fibrous histiocytomas, even if histologically benign, should be widely excised. One patient reported by Besly *et al.* (1993) required exenteration of the orbit. The possibility of lymph node involvement should also be considered and neck dissection carried out if necessary. The prognosis appears to be remarkably poor, and (apart from 1 patient lost to follow-up) of the 16 patients reviewed by Block *et al.* (1986), the longest known period of disease-free survival was only 27 months and 8 quickly died from their tumours or had metastases. Adjuvant radiotherapy or chemotherapy or both have frequently been given but their value is uncertain. Factors which may affect the prognosis are discussed in Chapter 13.

Haemangioma of bone

Solitary haemangiomas form less than 1% of tumours of bone, but a high proportion are in the head and neck region. Of these, about 30% are in the jaws, the mandible being involved twice as often as the maxilla. Women are twice as frequently affected as men, but the tumour can be seen at virtually any age.

Clinically, a haemangioma of the jaw gives rise to progressive painless swelling. When the overlying bone becomes sufficiently thinned, the swelling may become pulsatile, teeth may be loosened and there may be profuse bleeding, particularly from the gingival margins involved by the tumour. Some behave aggressively with rapid erosion of surrounding bone.

Radiographically, a haemangioma appears as a generally rounded or pseudoloculated area of radiolucency with ill-defined margins and often a soap-bubble appearance (Figure 5.18).

Microscopy

Haemangiomas of bone are essentially similar to their soft tissue counterparts (Chapter 13). They are usually cavernous (Figure 5.19) and rarely capillary or mixed, but arteriovenous tumours are most likely to bleed severely.

Figure 5.18   Subtraction angiogram of an extensive haemangioma of the mandible

Management

Obviously enough, the chief problem is that of haemorrhage at operation, but in view of the overall rarity of such tumours, the possibility of an intraosseous haemangioma is unlikely to be suspected from the clinical or radiographic appearances, if there has been no bleeding or superficial signs of a vascularity. Theoretically, haemangioma should be considered in the differential diagnosis of radiolucent lesions of the jaws, particularly those having the radiographic features described earlier. It is clearly not feasible to carry out angiography on every doubtful case, but it is probably the strongest argument for aspiration of cyst-like lesions of uncertain nature. However, an important warning

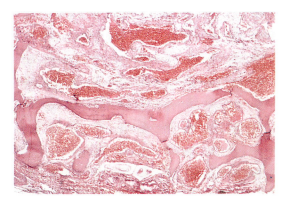

Figure 5.19   Intrabony haemangioma showing cavernous vascular channels within normal bony trabeculae

is the appearance of a bluish swelling when the periosteum is elevated at operation.

Opening a haemangioma or extracting a related tooth can give rise to torrential bleeding. Lamberg *et al.* (1979) reported a death and found reports of 10 earlier fatalities from this cause. Super-selective angiography indicates that haemangiomas can be venous (cavernous) capillary or arteriovenous. The last (fast-flow angiomas) have one or more large feeder arteries, tend to be the most rapidly expanding and are most likely to bleed severely, when opened. When there are identifiable feeder vessels, selective arterial embolization makes any subsequent resection very much easier and safer. Surgery should follow embolization as soon as possible, and certainly within 3 days as collateral vessels quickly open up. Wide en bloc resection, with the margins in normal bone, is the only practical method of dealing with high-flow haemangiomas, as recommended by Bunel and Sindet-Pedersen (1993) who also reviewed the variable clinical manifestations and treatment options. Following selective external carotid angiography, all feeder vessels should be tied off, if necessary including the ipsilateral external carotid artery. In the case of low-flow tumours, mucoperiosteal flaps are raised to expose the affected area, all related teeth are extracted and the haemangioma should be thoroughly curetted. The resulting cavity is then packed tightly with bone mush from the ilium. The mucoperiosteal flaps are then closed over the cavity. Healing can then progress without recurrence.

Should a tooth in the area of an unsuspected haemangioma be extracted, torrential haemorrhage can result. In such circumstances the tooth should be immediately reinserted into its socket and the patient told to bite hard pending transfer for definitive management of the tumour as already described.

Angiosarcoma of bone

Angiosarcoma is a particularly rare tumour, but in reviewing 133 reported cases, Barnes *et al.* (1985) identified 7 examples in the mandible.

Dull pain and swelling are typical symptoms and, as with other malignant tumours, teeth may become loosened. If neglected, the tumour can erode through the bone and spread into the soft tissues. The radiographic appearance is a poorly circumscribed area of radiolucency without any distinguishing features.

Microscopically, angiosarcomas range from those with capillary-like spaces lined by plump endothelial cells showing few mitoses (grade I), to those where vascular formation can only be recognized by reticulin staining to show malignant endothelial cells within its sheath (grade III). These cells are mitotically active, have prominent nucleoli and there are foci of necrosis. Lymphocytes and eosinophils can be so numerous in the stroma as sometimes to lead to misdiagnosis, if the biopsy is inadequate.

The treatment of choice appears to be wide surgical excision with radiotherapy for any inaccessible areas of tumour. The prognosis appears to depend greatly on the degree of differentiation, and well-differentiated examples (grade I; sometimes termed haemangioendotheliomas) are less likely to metastasize. Data on the prognosis of jaw tumours are limited.

Leiomyosarcoma of bone

Leiomyosarcoma is another rare tumour, but 40% of oral cases may arise in the maxilla or mandible where they form locally destructive lesions not clinically or radiographically distinguishable from many other malignant tumours.

The microscopic features are essentially the same as those of the soft tissue counterpart and described in Chapter 13.

The treatment is radical surgical excision, but the prognosis is poor.

Melanotic neuroectodermal tumour of infancy

This rare tumour was thought in the past to be odontogenic and termed *melanotic adamantinoma* because of its development in close proximity to the teeth. However it is widely accepted that its origin is from the neural crest.

Clinically, melanotic neuroectodermal tumours develop in the first year of life. Mosby *et al.* (1992) identified reports of 195 cases, of which 64% were in the maxilla, 11% in the mandible, 5% in the brain and isolated examples in almost any other site. In the maxilla it forms an expansile mass, stretching but not ulcerating through the overlying mucosa, which appears bluish because of the underlying pigmentation. Radiographs show an area of bone destruction with irregular margins and sometimes displacement of teeth.

Microscopy

The tumour consists of slit-like or larger spaces lined by cuboidal, melanin-containing cells in a fibrous stroma (Figure 5.20a). Small round cells, which are non-pigmented, form clusters in the stroma or lie in the alveolar spaces (Figure 5.20b). These round cells resemble those of a neuroblastoma and may be associated with neurofibrillary material resembling glia.

Ultrastructurally the pigmented cells show both epithelial and melanocytic features. The rounded, non-pigmented cells have a slender cell process and cytoplasmic neurofilamentous material that suggest a neuroblastic origin. Slootweg (1992) has reviewed the immunocytochemistry and confirmed that, unlike melanomas, none of the cells is S-100 positive.

Management

The radiographic, CT scans and MRI are not diagnostic in themselves, but the appearance of a

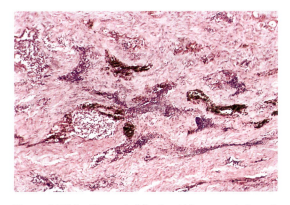

Figure 5.20(a) Pigmented (melanotic) neuroectodermal tumour of infancy showing deeply pigmented cells in a fibrous stroma surrounding non-pigmented cells

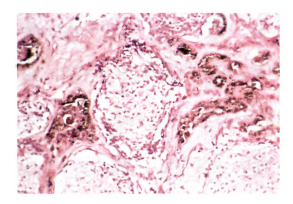

Figure 5.20(b) Pigmented (melanotic) neuroectodermal tumour of infancy showing non-pigmented cells lying in spaces and surrounding pigmented cells

destructive maxillary tumour in an infant, together with high levels of vanillylmandelic acid, is distinctive. Melanotic neuroectodermal tumour is widely thought to be benign, but up to 15% of cases may recur and a few have metastasized. Radical excision may be indicated, but where this was not feasible, radiotherapy and/or chemotherapy has been used.

Primary lymphoma of bone

Involvement of the jaws is typical of African Burkitt's lymphoma but, rarely, other primary lymphomas can arise in bone. Pileri *et al.* (1990) have reported 17 cases affecting the mandible in detail. There are no distinctive clinical features and radiographically the tumour forms a poorly demarcated area of bone destruction. The diagnosis depends purely on the microscopic findings.

Microscopy

Most lymphomas of bone appear to be large B cell lymphomas and earlier were frequently categorized as 'reticulum cell sarcomas' as the lymphocytes may resemble histiocytes. However, the nuclei are larger, with fine nuclear chromatin and more abundant cytoplasm. Fine reticulin fibres surround single or small groups of these lymphocytes.

Diagnosis and particularly differentiation from Ewing's sarcoma depend on immunostaining or gene product analysis which will indicate whether these large cells are B or T lymphocytes.

Management

It is necessary first to exclude disseminated lymphoma.

In the case of a true primary bone lymphoma, excision should be followed by multi-agent chemotherapy. Little data on the prognosis after modern treatment of these rare tumours is available, but they possibly have a better prognosis than most soft tissue non-Hodgkin lymphomas.

Multiple myeloma and solitary plasmacytoma

Multiple myeloma is a neoplasm of plasma cells which causes multifocal bone-destructive lesions. These are usually the main cause of symptoms, namely, bone pain and tenderness. However, a jaw lesion occasionally gives rise to the first symptoms. Alternatively, one of the major complications, in particular amyloidosis, may dominate the clinical picture.

Skeletal radiographs typically show multiple punched-out areas of radiolucency, particularly in the vault of the skull.

As a result of the proliferation of myeloma cells in the marrow, there is frequently anaemia and sometimes thrombocytopenia. Increased susceptibility to infection may result from depressed production of normal immunoglobulins.

The picture just described is that of advanced disease. However, myeloma can be detected early in its asymptomatic phase by the chance finding, in a routine blood examination, of a greatly raised ESR, as a result of the overproduction of immunoglobulin. The diagnosis is confirmed by electrophoresis showing a monoclonal immunoglobulin or fragment spike.

Microscopy

Myeloma appears as sheets of plasma cells which, when well differentiated, have an eccentric nucleus with peripheral clumping of the chromatin, giving a cartwheel appearance and a perinuclear halo (Figures 5.21 and 5.22). The area of cytoplasm is relatively large and baso- or amphophilic. With loss of differentiation, the nuclei become larger and lose their characteristic chromatin pattern, while the cytoplasm may form no more than a rim round the nucleus. Multiple nuclei and mitoses may be seen.

Investigation

Bone marrow biopsy is usually diagnostic, but recognition, by microscopy alone, of poorly differentiated myeloma may be difficult. Confirmation depends on the electrophoretic findings as well as the clinical features. Serological findings in multiple myeloma are a greatly raised ESR, rouleaux formation of red cells in a blood sample and raised plasma protein levels, all of which result from the increased immunoglobulin production. Serum electrophoresis shows a monoclonal spike of IgG in the majority of cases.

Immunocytochemical demonstration of monoclonal production of immunoglobulin or immunoglobulin fragments provides substantiation. Light chain overproduction, demonstrable by serum electrophoresis, is common and leads to Bence-Jones proteinuria.

Management

There is frequently an initial response to treatment with combination chemotherapy, but the median survival for multiple myeloma is about 2 years.

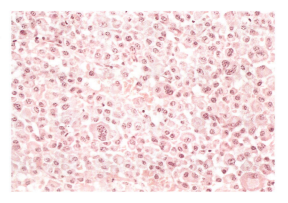

Figure 5.21 Multiple myeloma: well-differentiated tumour consisting of sheets of neoplastic plasma cells

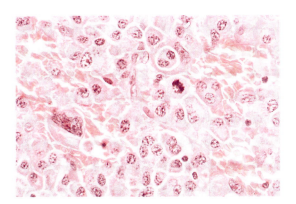

Figure 5.22 Multiple myeloma: moderately well-differentiated tumour with pleomorphic plasma cells and mitoses

Fewer than 20% of patients survive for 5 or more years.

Dental treatment may be complicated by anaemia, haemorrhagic tendencies or abnormal susceptibility to infection.

Solitary, soft tissue (extramedullary) plasmacytoma

These are rare tumours, but approximately 80% of them form in the head and neck, usually in the nasal cavity or nasopharynx rather than the mouth. Involvement of the antrum may, however, give rise to a maxillary tumour. Microscopically, extramedullary plasmacytoma does not differ from multiple myeloma and can be shown to be monoclonal by immunocytochemistry. Solitary extramedullary plasmacytoma is not associated with a monoclonal peak in the serum.

Irradiation is highly effective, but multiple myeloma develops in up to 50% of patients, usually within 2 years.

Solitary plasmacytoma of bone

This equally rare tumour occasionally develops in the jaws but has a significantly better prognosis than soft tissue plasmacytoma.

Clinically, bone pain, tenderness or a swelling and a sharply defined area of radiolucency or,

rarely, a soap-bubble appearance are typical features.

Microscopically, the cellular features are the same as those of multiple myeloma, which should be excluded as described earlier. A small rise in serum or urine monoclonal immunoglobulin is detectable in a minority of patients with solitary endosteal plasmacytoma. The monoclonal peak in the serum should disappear with treatment, but persistence indicates that treatment has been inadequate or that the disease has disseminated.

Treatment is by localized radiotherapy. Over 65% of patients survive for 10 or more years, but the majority eventually develop multiple myeloma, occasionally even after several decades.

Amyloidosis

Amyloidosis is the deposition in the tissues of an abnormal protein with characteristic staining properties and electron-microscopic appearances. It can be systemic or localized, and is classified according to the nature of the amyloid fibril and of the related serum protein. A fibrillary protein forms the essential structural element of amyloid, but a non-fibrillary glycoprotein (amyloid P component – AP) is present in virtually all types. In the case of myeloma and monoclonal gammopathies, amyloidosis results from overproduction of immunoglobulin light chains.

Amyloid deposition in the mouth, particularly the tongue, is most commonly a manifestation of a monoclonal gammopathy (non-neoplastic, plasma cell dyscrasias with overproduction of immunoglobulin) or of myeloma. In a survey of 225 patients, Kyle and Greip (1983) found macroglossia in 22% of cases of light chain associated amyloidosis (myeloma or monoclonal gammopathy). Reactionary (secondary) amyloidosis, resulting from rheumatoid arthritis or chronic infections, is more common overall, but rarely affects the mouth.

Clinically, deposits of amyloid can cause macroglossia or soft tissue tags or swellings, particularly on the gingivae. An enlarged tongue due to amyloid is frequently lobulated, particularly along the margins, and can be so large as to protrude from the mouth. Purpura and anaemia may also be associated and give the tongue a pale or purplish colour, or cause ecchymoses in the surrounding tissues.

Microscopy

Amyloid appears as weakly eosinophilic, hyaline homogeneous material which is often perivascular. It stains positively with Congo red, which also shows a characteristic apple green birefringence under polarized light (Figures 5.23 and 5.24). There is also positive fluorescence with thioflavine T and a characteristic fibrillary structure by electron microscopy.

If the underlying disease has not already been identified, a blood picture and plasma protein electrophoresis should be followed, if positive, by marrow biopsy and skeletal radiographs.

Management

The prognosis of myeloma-associated amyloidosis is poor, either from the tumour itself or from widespread amyloid deposition and, in particular, renal damage. So-called benign monoclonal gammopathy has a poor prognosis ultimately, either as a result of eventual development of myeloma or of widespread amyloid deposition and renal failure. However, progress of the disease may be delayed by chemotherapy with melphelan and prednisolone.

Tongue reduction, though desirable, should be avoided if possible, as the tissue is friable, bleeding can be difficult to control and any benefit is often only temporary.

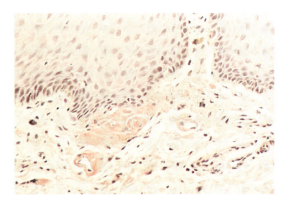

Figure 5.23 Amyloidosis: submucosal deposits stained with Congo red

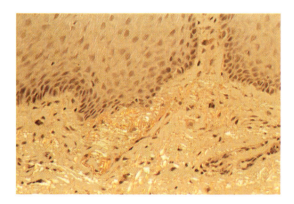

Figure 5.24 Amyloidosis: typical birefringence of Congo red stained specimen under polarized light

Langerhans cell histiocytosis (histiocytosis X, eosinophilic granuloma)

In this rare, predominantly osteolytic, tumour-like disease, there is a proliferation of histiocyte-like Langerhans cells. Both the surface markers of Langerhans cells and the characteristic Birbeck granules can be found in the tumour histiocytes. Three main forms, in order of severity, are usually recognized:

1. Solitary eosinophilic granuloma
2. Multifocal eosinophilic granuloma (including Hand–Schuller–Christian disease).
3. Letterer-Siwe disease.

Letterer-Siwe disease was thought to be a different entity such as a lymphoma, but Birbeck granules have also been demonstrated in the tumour cells and the bone lesions may not be distinguishable microscopically from those of the other variants. In a review of 1120 cases, Hartman (1980) found that there was oral involvement in 114 cases and that the mandible was affected in 73%.

Solitary eosinophilic granuloma

Solitary eosinophilic granuloma predominantly affects adults and, when involving the jaws, usually affects the mandible to produce a localized area of bone destruction with swelling and often pain. A typical radiographic appearance is a rounded area of radiolucency with margins somewhat less sharply defined than those of a cyst, and frequently extending into the alveolar ridge. Teeth which appear to be floating in air is a typical radiographic appearance. Dagenais *et al.* (1992), in reviewing the radiographic findings in 29 cases, found that they comprised solitary intraosseous lesions, multiple lesions of the alveolar ridge, saucerization or scooped-out lesions of the alveolar ridge, periosteal new bone formation and root resorption in 10 out of 15 cases. The radiolucent areas were well defined, but only those involving the alveolar ridge showed marginal sclerosis. The mandible alone was involved in 20 out of the 29 cases, and with the maxilla in 8 more. The maxilla was the sole site in only 1 case.

Occasionally, gross periodontal destruction with exposure of the roots of the teeth is a feature.

Microscopy

Histiocytes are associated with eosinophils, sometimes with other types of granulocytes. The histiocytes have pale, vesiculated and often lobulated nuclei, and weakly eosinophilic cytoplasm. Mitotic activity is typically absent. Eosinophils may be scattered among histiocytes or in conspicuous clusters. The matrix consists of unremarkable poorly fibrillar or granular material. These appearances may vary with the stage of the disease, with a high proportion of eosinophils at first (Figure 5.25), then growing numbers of histiocytes, and finally, in resolving cases, increasing fibrosis.

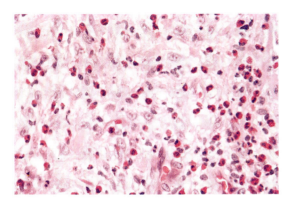

Figure 5.25 Eosinophilic granuloma showing sheets of histiocytes and eosinophils

The diagnosis may be confirmed by demonstration by electron microscopy of Birbeck granules but Fartarsch *et al.* (1990) have reported that positive staining of Langerhans cells for S-100 protein and peanut agglutinin is as reliable.

Multifocal eosinophilic granuloma

As well as the mandible, other sites of predilection are the skull, axial skeleton and femora. Almost any of the viscera (hepatosplenomegaly) or the skin (seborrhoeic dermatitis) may be involved in multifocal disease, but rarely without osseous lesions.

Such disease may be termed *Hand–Schuller–Christian disease*, but the classical triad of exophthalmos, diabetes insipidus and lytic skull lesions is present only in a minority.

Letterer–Siwe disease

Letterer–Siwe disease differs from the other types of Langerhans cell histiocytosis in that infants or, less often, young children are affected and the disease may be rapidly fatal. Though some believe that Letterer–Siwe disease is a separate entity, Birbeck granules have been seen and suggest that this disease is also a neoplasm of Langerhans cells. Both soft tissues and bone are commonly involved and rashes may be the earliest manifestation. Other features can include lymphadenopathy and splenomegaly, fever, anaemia and thrombocytopenia, and infections such as otitis media. Many organs can become involved and become enlarged as a result of histiocytic infiltration.

Radiographically, the bone lesions do not differ from those in other types of Langerhans cell histiocytosis.

Management

The natural history of Langerhans cell histiocytosis ranges from isolated lesions with spontaneous regression, to widespread disease and a rapidly fatal outcome despite treatment. Though the behaviour of this disease is unpredictable, the very young have the worst prognosis, and have a mortality rate of about 50%. In those over 2 years of age, the mortality is reported to be about 15%.

In general, the greater the number of organ systems affected, the poorer the prognosis. Monocytosis or thrombocytopenia are also associated with a high mortality.

In addition to biopsy of the oral lesions, physical examination, skeletal survey and blood picture will give an indication of any dissemination and its degree.

For a localized jaw lesion, curettage followed if necessary by corticosteroid or cytotoxic chemotherapy, or irradiation, usually suffices, but, as mentioned earlier, the course of the disease is so unpredictable that prolonged careful follow-up, and sometimes further treatment, is necessary. For multisystem disease, a combination of cytotoxic agents (often vinca alkaloids), corticosteroids and irradiation to active bone lesions is required.

Eosinophilic ulcer (atypical or traumatic eosinophilic granuloma)

Tumour-like, often ulcerated lesions with a microscopic picture resembling that of Langerhans cell histiocytosis may occasionally be seen in the oral soft tissues, particularly the tongue, but also the gingivae and, occasionally, other sites. In some cases there has been a history of trauma and, experimentally, crush injury to tongue muscle can induce a proliferative response with tissue eosinophilia. However, Doyle *et al.* (1989) found trauma to be a possible cause in only 5 out of 15 cases.

Clinically, the ulcerated mass may be mistaken for a carcinoma: almost any age can be affected.

Microscopy

The typical appearance is a dense aggregation of eosinophils and other cells which resemble histiocytes. The latter lack the ultrastructural features and surface markers of Langerhans cells, but there have been a few cases where these histiocytes were pleomorphic, and showed prominent nucleoli and mitotic activity. This cellular infiltrate may extend into the epithelium.

The differential diagnosis is from Langerhans cell histiocytosis, which can be excluded by investigations, as suggested above, and by the use of immunostaining to identify Langerhans cells. In practice, spontaneous resolution, usually within 3 to 8 weeks, is to be expected, and with an isolated soft tissue mass having these characteristics an expectant policy is usually justified.

Metastatic tumours

Most metastases in the jaws are carcinomas and the primary growth is usually in the bronchus, breast or prostate. These are common tumours and are the most common carcinomas to cause bony metastases. Other important sites of primary growths are the thyroid and kidney, but adenocarcinomas from almost any primary site can metastasize to the jaws.

Symptoms from a malignant deposit in the jaw can rarely provide the first sign of the disease and lead to diagnosis of the primary. In other cases the jaw is the first apparent site of secondary deposits from a growth treated a year or more previously. Though the jaw is much less frequently involved than other bones, secondary carcinoma is an important malignant tumour.

Patients are usually middle-aged or elderly. Typical symptoms are pain, which is often severe, or swelling of the jaw. Paraesthesia of the lip may be caused by involvement of a nerve trunk.

Radiography

Typically, there is an area of radiolucency with a hazy outline (Figures 5.26 and 5.27). It sometimes simulates an infected cyst or may be quite irregular and simulate osteomyelitis. Sometimes the entire mandible may have a moth-eaten appearance. Sclerotic areas may rarely be the main feature, particularly with metastases from the prostate.

Microscopy

Secondary deposits are usually adenocarcinomas or less frequently squamous cell carcinoma, according to the nature of the primary growth. Bone destruction by osteoclasts near the periphery of the deposit is the most common effect, but bone sclerosis can result particularly from metastases from the prostate. The latter are associated with raised prostate-specific antigen levels.

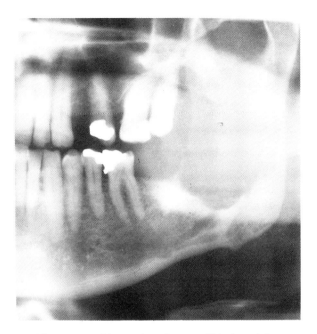

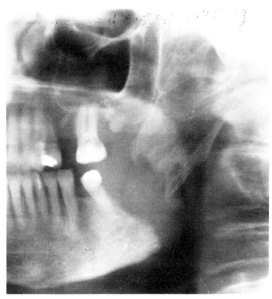

Figure 5.26   Metastatic melanoma. This deposit has filled the greater part of the left ramus but has relatively sharply defined margins despite its rapid growth

Figure 5.27   Metastasis from carcinoma of the breast causing a pathological fracture

References

Barnes, L., Peel, R.L., Verbin, R.S. *et al.* (1985) Diseases of the bones and joints. In *Surgical Pathology of the Head and Neck* (ed. L. Barnes), Marcel Dekker, New York, pp. 883–1044

Besly, W., Wiesenfeld, D., Kleid, S. *et al.* (1993) Malignant fibrous histiocytoma of the maxilla – a report of two cases. *British Journal of Oral and Maxillofacial Surgery*, **31**, 45–48

Block, M.S., Cade, J.E. and Rodriguez, F.H. (1986) Malignant fibrous histiocytoma of the maxilla. *Journal of Oral and Maxillofacial Surgery*, **44**, 404–412

Bunel, K. and Sindet-Pedersen, S. (1993) Central hemangioma of the mandible. *Oral Surgery, Oral Medicine and Oral Pathology*, **75**, 565–570

Clark, J.L., Unni, K.K., Dahlin, D.C. *et al.* (1983) Osteosarcoma of the jaw. *Cancer*, **51**, 2311–2316

Dagenais, M., Pharoah, M.J. and Sikorski, P.A. (1992) The radiographic characteristics of histiocytosis X. A study of 29 cases that involve the jaws. *Oral Surgery, Oral Medicine and Oral Pathology*, **74**, 230–236

Damm, D.D., White, D.K., Geissler, R.H. *et al.* (1985) Chondromyxoid fibroma of the maxilla. Electron microscopic findings and review of the literature. *Oral Surgery, Oral Medicine and Oral Pathology*, **59**, 176–183

Dehner, L.P. (1993) Primitive neuroectodermal tumor and Ewing's sarcoma. *American Journal of Surgical Pathology*, **17**, 1–13

Management

Biopsy of the mass in the jaw will usually indicate whether it is a metastasis. A detailed history, especially of previous operations, and general examination are necessary. Radiographs of the rest of the skeleton may show other deposits. Blood examination is necessary to exclude anaemia due to replacement of the marrow by metastases.

The primary tumour should be treated if this is still feasible, but bony metastases are a sign of bloodstream spread of the disease and only palliative treatment may be possible. However, in many cases of breast cancer, tamoxifen can dramatically prolong survival, sometimes with complete resolution of bony metastases for several years. In prostatic cancer, anti-androgenic treatment may cause secondary deposits to regress for a time. If all else fails, irradiation may make the patient more comfortable and cause the tumour to regress for a time. Should the deposit fungate into the oral cavity or face, cryosurgery may help to control pain and haemorrhage, and reduce bulk.

Some sarcomas, particularly Ewing's sarcoma, can metastasize to other bones and exceptionally rarely the jaws are involved.

Doyle, J.L., Geary, W. and Baden, E. (1989) Eosinophilic ulcer. *Journal of Oral and Maxillofacial Surgery*, **47**, 349–352

Fartarsch, M., Vigneswaran, N., Diepgen, T.L. *et al.* (1990) Immunohistochemical and ultrastructural study of histiocytosis X and non-X histiocytoses. *Journal of the American Academy of Dermatology*, **23**, 885–892

Flanagan, A.M., Tinkler, S., Horton, M.A. *et al.* (1988) The multinucleate cells in giant cell granulomas of the jaw are osteoclasts. *Cancer*, **62**, 1139–1145

Garrington, G.E. and Collett, W.K. (1988a) Chondrosarcoma. I. A selected literature review. *Journal of Oral Pathology*, **17**, 1–11

Garrington, G.E. and Collett, W.K. (1988b) II. Chondrosarcoma of the jaws: analysis of 37 cases. *Journal of Oral Pathology*, **17**, 12–20

Garrington, G.E., Scofield, H.H., Cornyn, J. *et al.* (1967) Osteosarcoma of the jaws. Analysis of 56 cases. *Cancer*, **20**, 377–391

Hackney, F.L., Aragon, S.B., Aufdemorte, T.B. *et al.* (1991) Chondrosarcoma of the jaws: clinical findings, histopathology, and treatment. *Oral Surgery, Oral Pathology and Oral Medicine*, **71**, 139–143

Hartman, K.S. (1980) Histiocytosis X. A review of 114 cases with oral involvement. *Oral Surgery, Oral Medicine and Oral Pathology*, **49**, 38–54

Hashimoto, K., Mase, N., Iwai, K. *et al.* (1991) Desmoplastic fibroma of the maxillary sinus. *Oral Surgery, Oral Medicine and Oral Pathology*, **72**, 126–132

Henry, C.H., Granite, E.L. and Rafetto, L.K. (1992) Osteochondroma of the mandibular condyle. Report of a case and review of the literature. *Journal of Oral and Maxillofacial Surgery*, **50**, 1102–1108

Kurt, A.-M., Unni, K.K., Sim, F.H. *et al.* (1989) Chondroblastoma of bone. *Human Pathology*, **20**, 965–976

Kyle, R.A. and Greipp, P.R. (1983) Subject review, amyloidosis (AL): clinical and laboratory features in 229 cases. *Proceedings of the Mayo Clinic*, **58**, 665–683

Lamberg, M.A., Tasanen, A. and Jääskelainen, J. (1979) Fatality from central hemangioma of the mandible. *Journal of Oral Surgery*, **37**, 578–584

Lustman, J., Gazit, D., Ulmansky, M. *et al.* (1986) Chrondromyxoid fibroma of the jaws: a clinicopathological study. *Journal of Oral Pathology and Medicine*, **15**, 343–346

Millar, B.G., Browne, R.M. and Flood, T.R. (1990) Juxtacortical osteosarcoma of the jaws. *British Journal of Oral and Maxillofacial Surgery*, **28**, 73–79

Mintz, G.A., Abrams, A.M., Carlsen, G.D. *et al.* (1981) Primary malignant giant cell tumor of the mandible. Report of a case. *Oral Surgery, Oral Medicine and Oral Pathology*, **51**, 164–171

Mosby, E.L., Lowe, M.W., Cobb, C.M. *et al.* (1992) Melanotic neuroectodermal tumor of infancy. Review of the literature and report of a case. *Journal of Oral and Maxillofacial Surgery*, **50**, 886–894

Pileri, S.A., Montanari, M., Falini, B. *et al.* (1990) Malignant lymphoma involving the mandible. Clinical, morphologic and immunohistochemical study of 17 cases. *American Journal of Surgical Pathology*, **14**, 652–659

Slootweg, P.J. (1992) Heterologous tissue elements in melanotic neuroectodermal tumor of infancy. *Journal of Oral Pathology and Medicine*, **21**, 90–92

Tran, L.M., Mark, R., Meier, R. *et al.* (1992) Sarcomas of the head and neck. Prognostic factors and treatment strategies. *Cancer*, **70**, 169–177

Whitaker, S.B. and Waldron, C.A. (1993) Central giant cell lesions of the jaws. A clinical, radiologic and histopathologic study. *Oral Surgery, Oral Medicine and Oral Pathology*, **75**, 199–208

White, V.A., Fanning, C.V., Ayala, A.G. *et al.* (1988) Osteosarcoma and the role of fine-needle aspiration biopsy. A study of 51 cases. *Cancer*, **62**, 1238–1246

Wood, R.E., Nortje, C.J., Hesseling, P. *et al.* (1990) Ewing's tumor of the jaw. *Oral Surgery, Oral Medicine and Oral Pathology*, **69**, 120–127

6

Genetic, metabolic and other non-neoplastic bone diseases

Craniofacial defects – surgical considerations

Many developmental defects such as cleft lip and palate, branchial arch defects, craniostenoses or supernumerary teeth are genetic traits. However, the family history is informative in relatively few of these patients. Most arise by new gene mutations and only then become potentially heritable. There are also chromosomal defects of which the most common is Down's syndrome (trisomy 21), which is not usually heritable.

Other conditions such as the Pierre Robin anomaly probably have an entirely environmental cause. Here, it appears that the developing fetus is unable to extend the neck due to deficiency of amniotic fluid. As a result the tongue does not descend from between the developing palatal shelves and prevents them from fusing in the midline. Failure of the fetal neck to extend also causes the developing chin to press on to the sternum. Gross mandibular hypoplasia with consequent obstruction of the airway are the results. However, it is important to note that, in such congenital defects, growth potential is normal. If early nursing difficulties can be overcome, mandibular growth will ultimately catch up and, as there is no intrinsic shortage of palatal tissue, anatomical repair of the cleft palate can often be achieved without detriment to subsequent maxillary growth.

For many of these conditions, any distinction between a genetic or environmental aetiology is academic. Once the condition has become established, management depends more on appreciation of the scope of the primary defect than on its aetiology. For example, in hemifacial microsomia the intrinsic defect is probably confined to structures arising from the mandibular arch. Early surgery to the young mandible should therefore encourage normal growth of the maxilla, thus avoiding developmental defects which are predominantly secondary to the mandibular asymmetry.

In many conditions, knowledge of the growth potential of various parts of the developing facial skeleton is incomplete, and clinical findings have often been distorted by the effects of earlier surgery. The best example is in the study of the growth of the maxilla in cleft lip and palate patients. It is only comparatively recently that sufficient sound evidence has accumulated to establish that the middle third of the face in unoperated clefts has a normal growth potential in all dimensions. Nevertheless, gross cosmetic defects should usually be repaired early in life, but the timing and nature of such surgery should be such as to minimize damage which lessens the intrinsic growth potential.

In this text, only the more common craniofacial defects can be considered as examples of what may be susceptible to surgical improvement.

Facial clefts and associated anomalies

Cleft lip with or without cleft palate

The overall incidence is about 1 per 1000 Caucasian live births, only 0.4 per 1000 births in Afro-

Americans, but in Japan reaches 1.7 per 1000 births. In general, males are more frequently affected. Isolated cleft lip may be unilateral or bilateral: when unilateral, 70% are on the left side. Eighty-five per cent of bilateral cleft lips and 70% of unilateral cleft lips are associated with complete clefts of the hard and soft palate.

Isolated cleft palate

This appears to be a separate entity with an incidence of approximately 1 per 2000 live births in Caucasians and Afro-Americans. There is a 2:1 female predominance for complete palatal clefts, but an equal sex incidence of clefts of the soft palate only. Bifid uvula (an incomplete form of cleft palate) is present in 1:80 Caucasians and may be associated with a submucous palatal cleft in which there is imperfect muscle union across the velum but an intact mucosal surface. Often there is an associated notch in the posterior hard palate.

Because of the different patterns and associations of cleft lip and palate, it has been difficult to analyse the patterns of inheritance. However, there clearly is a strong familial influence. The risk of having a cleft is much higher if a parent or sibling is affected (Table 6.1).

Associated anomalies   The association of congenital lower lip pits with cleft lip and palate is strong and due to an autosomal dominant gene showing 80% penetrance. Other rare associated anomalies are talipes equinovarus, syndactyly and various eye

defects, but there is a great variety of craniofacial syndromes where clefting is a feature, as Gorlin *et al.* (1971) have described.

The Pierre Robin anomaly (cleft palate, micrognathia and glossoptosis) is probably quite different from other clefting conditions in aetiology and management. As discussed earlier, there is no inherent lack of tissues in this condition; growth can catch up if early nursing difficulties can be overcome.

Surgical aspects of cleft lip and/or palate
Until relatively recently it was believed that maxillary hypoplasia in all three planes was an intrinsic feature of clefts. However, studies on unoperated clefts have shown that they have an almost normal growth potential (Ortiz-Monasterio *et al.*, 1959; Mars and Houston, 1990). Without early surgery, facial and dental development are normal. It seems, therefore, that postnatal surgery to close the cleft lip and palate defect inhibits subsequent growth. Two factors are important. First, in developing vomerine flaps to close the hard palate, the vomerine growth centre is irrevocably damaged, inhibiting downward and forward development of the maxilla. Secondly, the surgery itself results in extensive scar formation which also inhibits growth. von Langenbeck or Wardill-type flaps in the palate leave bare areas to granulate and scarring can restrict subsequent transverse growth. Dissection in the anterior floor of the nose for lip closure inhibits subsequent alveolar growth, often resulting in infra-occlusion. The timing and planning of procedures to limit these problems is therefore critical.

One approach has been to delay hard palate closure until 8 or 9 years of age when a considerable amount of maxillary growth has taken place. As a consequence, growth inhibition and distortion could be minimized. Hotz and Gnoinski (1979) adopted this regimen and used a modified Widmaier procedure for the anatomical closure of the soft palate only (Perko, 1979). The extensive hard palate fistula could be obturated with an appliance until hard palate closure was carried out at 8 years. Hotz and Gnoinski (1979) are among the few cleft teams who have kept meticulous records. They have followed up their patients carefully, and convincingly shown excellent results in terms of facial growth and dental occlusion. However, some controversy persists as to the ultimate quality of

Table 6.1   Risk levels for clefts for those with affected relatives (After Tolorava, 1972)

	Cleft lip and/or palate	Isolated cleft palate
Normal parents		
One affected sibling	4%	3.5%
One affected parent		
No affected siblings	4%	3.5%
One affected sibling	12%	10%
Both parents affected		
No affected siblings	35%	25%
One affected sibling	45%	40%

their patients' speech; this may be acceptable in the more guttural Germanic languages but is less acceptable for English.

Another approach has been adopted in Norway, where all cleft surgery for the entire country is undertaken by two small teams that have become, as a result, very experienced. A more traditional approach has been adopted and the hard and soft palates together are closed before 18 months, using conventional von Langenbeck-type procedures. Nevertheless, results have been excellent and osteotomy procedures to correct subsequent growth deficiencies have rarely been required. This suggests that extensive experience and very gentle handling of the tissues can minimize the secondary growth defects consequent on the primary surgery. However, the genetic pool may be different in Norway and palatal clefts there may be less severe than elsewhere in Europe and America.

Another approach has been developed by Precious and Delaire (1993) in France, where it is argued that for harmonious balanced growth in the cleft lip and palate subject it is necessary, at the time of lip repair and, later, at the time of palate repair, to mobilize widely all the associated muscles from their anomalous insertions and restore them to their normal anatomical arrangement. Only under the influence of normal muscle function can the face and jaws develop normally, as described by Markus *et al.* (1993).

Although there have been advances in the repair of palatal clefts since the days when it was performed without benefit of anaesthesia, it cannot be said that there is any consensus about the most satisfactory technique. Moreover, the evaluation of current techniques is by no means satisfactory, as Roberts *et al.* (1991) have confirmed. The only conclusion that can be drawn is that all surgery results in some scar tissue and that scar tissue does not grow. Therefore, all surgery in cleft lip and palate patients should be kept to a minimum, but a convincing case seems to have been made for Delaire's muscle mobilization technique and late closure of the hard palate.

Lateral facial clefts

An extensive variety of lateral facial clefts with associated anomalies of the ear, eyelids and malars have been described. Their association with other defects such as polydactyly, syndactyly or absence of digits has led to the suggestion that these deformities result from persistent amniotic bands. The most useful classification of these clefts is that of Tessier (1976).

Hemifacial microsomia (Goldenhar syndrome, oculo-auriculovertebral dysplasia, first and second branchial arch syndrome)

This group of conditions has not been shown to possess any significant familial predisposition. They appear once in approximately 3000 live births, with an equal sex ratio. In the majority (70%) the condition is unilateral but, when bilateral, is always asymmetrical. Seven per cent of cases are associated with a cleft lip and palate. The defects may vary from slight to severe when they extend well beyond the mandible and can include defects of the auricle, middle ear, malar, maxilla, squamous temporal bone and related soft tissues including muscles of mastication and parotid gland. Rarely, there are facial palsy, unilateral coloboma and epibulbar dermoids. Anomalies of the cervical spine and ribs are also seen. Poswillo (1973) has suggested, from animal and clinical studies, that rupture of the stapedial arterial system in the 35-day fetus results in focal necrosis of tissues in the vicinity of the developing mandibular ramus. The expanding haematoma is unselective in its effects, and clinical cases vary in severity according to the degree of primary destruction and the capacity of the tissues to effect compensatory repair.

Surgical aspects

The skeletal tissues are not only defective or absent, but the soft tissues which comprise the functional matrix are also affected. Thus treatment planning should take account of any lack of functioning muscle, as it will lead to atrophy of any bone grafts used to augment the facial skeleton. However, when some functional muscle is present, serial bone grafting may prevent the onset of secondary deformities. Indeed, costochondral bone grafts have sometimes been seen to grow under the influence of the functional matrix. When there is little functioning soft tissue, it is necessary to introduce new hard and soft tissue into the area to facilitate facial reconstruction. Currently, micro-vascular surgery is being used for this purpose.

Down's syndrome (mongolism; trisomy 21)

Down's syndrome is the most common autosomal chromosome abnormality and also the most common of the clinically recognizable categories of mental handicap. Down's syndrome has an incidence of approximately 1 in 700 live births and accounts for about one-third of severely mentally handicapped children. The trisomic mongol is usually born of an older mother and the risk rises to 1 in 100 at 45 years of age. The translocation type is born to a younger mother; in about 50% this defect is inherited from a parent, usually the mother. The risk to these mothers of having a further Down's syndrome baby is 1 in 3–6.

All Down's syndrome children are mentally subnormal to some degree, but usually amiable and cooperative. Congenital cardiac defects are found in up to 50%. The main types are atrial septal defect, mitral valve prolapse or, less often, atrio-ventricular canal and ventricular septal defect. About one-third die in the first few years of life from heart disease. There are typically also multiple immunological defects so that infections of the skin, gastrointestinal and respiratory tracts are common, especially in institutionalized patients. However, infective endocarditis does not appear to be unusually frequent. The risk of acute leukaemia (usually acute lymphoblastic) in Down's syndrome is 20 times greater than in the general population. Though life expectancy has been greatly extended by cardiac surgery and control of infections, premature ageing is characteristic and like those with Alzheimer's disease, there is reduplication of the amyloid gene in Down's syndrome.

There are many oral abnormalities: the most obvious is an open-mouth posture. The tongue is frequently abnormally large, protrusive and fissured. The circumvallate papillae enlarge, but filiform papillae may be absent. The lips tend to be thick, dry and fissured and there is a poor anterior oral seal. Anterior open bite, to which a strong tongue thrust contributes, posterior crossbite and other types of malocclusion are common. The maxillae and malars are small, the mandible is somewhat protrusive and class III malocclusion is common. The palate often appears high, with horizontal palatal shelves, but a short palate is more characteristic. About 0.5% have a cleft palate and there is also a high incidence of bifid uvula and cleft lip. Tooth formation and eruption are retarded. Up to 30% have morphological abnormalities of both dentitions, particularly short, small crowns and roots.

There is also severe early onset of periodontal disease, and lower anterior teeth, in particular, are usually lost early. By contrast, caries incidence is usually low in both dentitions.

Down's children are generally more easily managed than many other mentally handicapped patients. Dental treatment can usually be carried out under local anaesthesia with sedation if necessary.

General anaesthesia needs to be carried out by a specialist because of the frequency of cardiac defects and respiratory disease. Intubation may be difficult because of the hypoplastic midface; congenital respiratory tract anomalies may be associated and there is abnormal susceptibility to chest infections. Anaemia, a risk of atlanto-axial subluxation when extending the neck, and possible hepatitis B carriage are other hazards. Despite these difficulties, improvement in the facial appearance by maxillofacial reconstruction and plastic surgery may be considered.

Clefts of lip or palate should be treated as in any other child. When adolescence is reached, assessment in conjunction with parents or guardians, for orthognathic surgery should be carried out. Many have an anterior open bite with poor facial muscle tone and a large tongue. These require bimaxillary surgery with advancement and impaction of the posterior maxilla and reduction of the mandible. Frequently, tongue reduction is also needed and sometimes also reduction of the lower lip to improve lip posture and seal. In severe cases it is also possible to carry out canthal surgery to improve the mongoloid slant of the palpebral fissures.

Down's syndrome children accept such treatment with few difficulties and the benefits from the improvement in their appearance are very encouraging.

Psychological aspects of remedial surgery

Surgical reconstruction of many genetic or other developmental jaw defects is not a practical proposition because of the technical difficulties and stress on the child of multiple operations. In addition, associated mental defect has generally been considered to be a contraindication to surgery. However, there is now a move towards cosmetic surgery for those with mild mental defect. In the case of Down's syndrome, the most common of such disorders, it appears that removal of the facial stigma leads to a considerable improvement in the children's performance and in their ability to integrate with their normal peers. Absence of insight or self-awareness should not necessarily, therefore, be thought to be an essential concomitant of mental defect, and anything that can be done to enable these children to integrate into 'normal' society will optimize their subsequent development (Figure 6.1–6.3).

Osteogenesis imperfecta (brittle bone syndrome)

Osteogenesis imperfecta is characterized by abnormal fragility of bones and is usually inherited as an autosomal dominant trait. The underlying defect is in type I collagen formation, but at least five subtypes are recognized. In addition to those with positive family histories, sporadic cases due to new mutations are relatively common.

Typical features are that the bones are capable of growing to their normal length but are abnormally thin and weak. Multiple fractures follow minimal or unnoticed trauma and the most severe form (type II – autosomal recessive) is lethal as a result of multiple fractures *in utero* and almost complete failure of ossification of the skull.

About 80% of cases are type I. They suffer multiple fractures in childhood and usually therefore become grossly deformed. The thin sclerae appear blue and there is hearing loss due to overgrowth of soft spongy bone round the oval window or to fractures of the auditory ossicles. Joints are frequently also hypermobile and the aortic valves are thin. The teeth are abnormally translucent with weak attachment of the enamel to

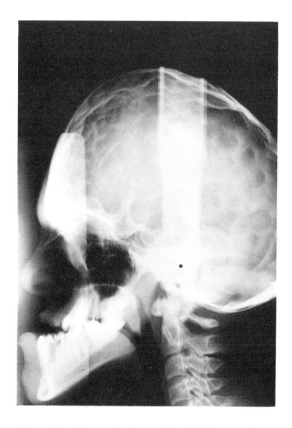

Figure 6.1 Crouzon's disease. The skull has a striking copper-beaten appearance and the maxillary hypoplasia is also typical

the dentine (dentinogenesis imperfecta), particularly in type IV.

The long bones typically have slender shafts but normal epiphyses, giving them a trumpet-like shape. Fracture healing is not delayed but usually leads to distortion of the bones and there is frequently excessive callus formation which can rarely undergo sarcomatous change.

Microscopy
Bone is both inadequate in amount and typically woven in character (Figure 6.4). Osteoblasts are sometimes excessively numerous.

Management
Though the long bones are fragile and care must be taken when carrying out extractions, fractures of

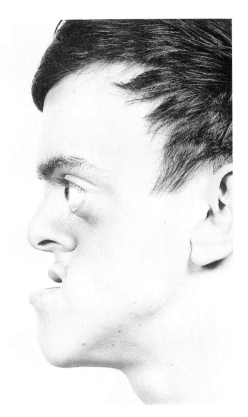

Figure 6.2   Crouzon's disease

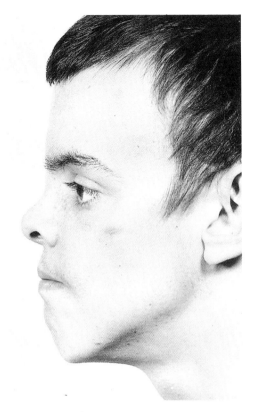

Figure 6.3   Crouzon's disease. The postoperative picture shows the enormous improvement in the patient's appearance and also the less dangerously prominent orbit

the jaws are uncommon. Management of dentinogenesis imperfecta, when present, depends on specialized restorative procedures.

Osteopetrosis (marble bone disease)

Osteopetrosis is a genetically heterogeneous group of disorders characterized by defective osteoclast function. As a consequence there is failure of normal bone modelling, formation of abnormally dense bone with loss of differentiation between cortical and cancellous types and complete or almost complete obliteration of medullary spaces. The two main forms are a milder, usually dominant type with bone defects as the main manifestations, and a severe, usually recessive, type with anaemia or pancytopenia, widespread extramedullary hae-

mopoiesis, and neurological complications of the bone disease. Blindness, deafness and facial palsy or trigeminal nerve pain result from cranial nerve compression by overgrowth of bone. There may also be multiple dental defects. The bones, though abnormally dense, are weak and fracture readily; osteomyelitis is a recognized complication as a result of the impaired blood supply. Craniofacial abnormalities in severe osteopetrosis include frontal bossing and exophthalmos.

Microscopy

In mild cases there may be an attempt to form normal lamellar bone, but the medullary cavity is replaced by bone containing minute marrow spaces and little or no haemopoietic tissue (Figure 6.5). Younai *et al.* (1988) have described three distinct

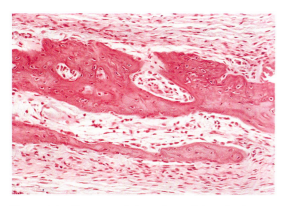

Figure 6.4 Osteogenesis imperfecta of the calvarium showing only cellular woven bone

patterns of bone abnormality in a severely affected mandible. These comprised a tortuous pattern of lamellar bone trabeculae, amorphous globular areas and an osteophytic pattern. Osteoclasts were numerous but appeared to be inactive.

Management

The dominant type is compatible with normal survival with only occasional effects such as those described. Symptoms may even be absent and the abnormalities discovered only by chance on routine radiography. Intermediate forms are characterized by rickets-like skeletal disease and renal tubular

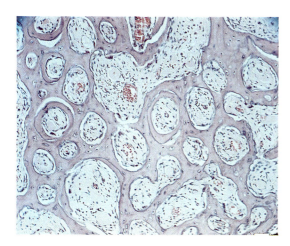

Figure 6.5 Osteopetrosis showing dense bony trabeculae penetrated by vascular channels and moderate numbers of osteoclasts

acidosis. In the most severe, recessive type, haemopoiesis is so much impaired that death in childhood from anaemia, haemorrhage or infections is usual, but bone marrow transplantation can be life-saving.

The chief risk from dental surgery and particularly extractions is that of osteomyelitis, which can also follow dental infections. Long-term antibiotic treatment, sequestrectomy and hyperbaric oxygen may be required.

Hypophosphatasia

Severe (infantile) hypophosphatasia is recessively inherited, but the milder adult form may be due to a dominant trait. The typical biochemical abnormalities are a low plasma alkaline phosphatase level and a high phosphoethanolamine level in the urine (Fallon *et al.*, 1984).

Infantile hypophosphatasia may be lethal due to hypercalcaemia and renal failure. In childhood hypophosphatasia, the main features are rickets-like skeletal disease leading to short-limbed dwarfism. Radiographically, the ends of the long bones are ragged or invisible and there is failure of mineralization of wide areas of the skull. Early synostosis of cranial sutures can lead to oxycephaly and exophthalmos. Adults with hypophosphatasia have frequent fractures and may have rickets-like deformities. However, premature exfoliation of deciduous teeth due to failure of cementum formation is sometimes the only clinical abnormality. These teeth may have abnormally large pulp chambers and hypoplastic enamel defects. Permanent teeth are less frequently shed spontaneously.

Cleidocranial dysplasia

This rare autosomal dominant disorder is characterized by defective formation of the clavicles, delayed closure of the fontanelles, but the presence of multiple Wormian bones, and retrusion of the maxilla. Partial or complete absence of clavicles may allow patients to bring the shoulders together in front of the chest.

Cleidocranial dysplasia is a cause of delayed or, often, failure of eruption of permanent teeth. The latter frequently remain embedded in the jaw and are associated with multiple supernumerary teeth. Cyst formation round these embedded teeth is common, but unless this happens there is no justification for wholesale removal of buried teeth as this leads to gross atrophy of the jaws. However, surgery is required when teeth erupt late in life under a denture.

Marfan's syndrome

Marfan's syndrome is a relatively common defect of collagen formation inherited as an autosomal dominant trait. Typical features are a tall, slender body habitus with arachnodactyly, dislocation of the lens and cardiovascular defects. The underlying defects include unstable crosslinkage and increased solubility of the collagen molecule or other defects in type I collagen. This leads to weakness of many important connective tissue structure such as joint capsules or the media of arteries.

Clinically, there is wide variation in expression of Marfan's syndrome. In addition to the typical body habitus, about 50% of patients have mild to severe ectopia lentis and up to 90% of patients have mitral valve prolapse and regurgitation, and an enhanced susceptibility to infective endocarditis. Aortic dilatation and regurgitation are less common but more serious, and the main cause of shortened expectation of life is aortic dissection. Aortic and mitral valve dysfunction may be associated with hypermobile joints in some of these patients.

The palatal vault is high and hypermobility can lead to recurrent subluxation of the temporomandibular joint. Cleft palate or bifid uvula may be associated in some cases. Prognathism and malocclusion are common. Cardiovascular disease can affect the management of the patient when surgery is required.

Sickle cell disease and the thalassaemias

Sickle cell disease and the thalassaemias are genetically determined haemolytic diseases in which bone abnormalities can result from bone marrow hyperplasia or, in sickle cell anaemia, from bone infarction.

Sickle cell anaemia

Sickle cell anaemia mainly affects people of African, Afro-Caribbean, Indian, Mediterranean or Middle Eastern origin. There are estimated to be about 5000 persons in Britain who have sickle cell anaemia (homozygotes), but many more with sickle cell trait (heterozygotes).

In homozygotes, formation of abnormal haemoglobin (HbS) brings the risk of haemolysis, anaemia and other effects. In heterozygotes, sufficient normal haemoglobin (HbA) is formed to allow normal life with only rare complications.

The complications arise from the polymerization of deoxygenated HbS which is less soluble than HbA, and forms long fibres. These deform the red cells into the characteristic sickle shapes and cause them to be readily haemolysed. Haemolysis causes chronic anaemia with a haemoglobin level around 8 g/dl. Nevertheless patients, under normal circumstances, typically feel well, as HbS releases its oxygen content to the tissues more readily than HbA, and are in a steady state which does not require treatment.

Exacerbation of sickling causes increased blood viscosity and blocking of capillaries. Factors which precipitate sickling include (a) hypoxia from poorly conducted anaesthesia or chest infections, (b) dehydration, and (c) infection, acidosis and fever. Infections (occasionally dental) can not merely precipitate painful crises, but these patients are also abnormally susceptible to infection, particularly pneumococcal or meningococcal.

Sickle cell crises are of three main types:

1. Painful crises caused by blockage of blood vessels and bone marrow infarcts.
2. Anaemic crises due to marrow aplasia. They require immediate transfusion.
3. Sequestration crises probably due to extensive sickling, particularly in the viscera. An acute chest syndrome, characterized by pain, fever and leucocytosis, is the most common cause of death.

Painful crises can affect the jaws, particularly the mandible, and mimic acute osteomyelitis. Bone infarcts form foci susceptible to infection and salmonella osteomyelitis is a recognized hazard in these patients. Infarcts in the jaws may mimic toothache or osteomyelitis. Rarely, the true nature of a crisis with jaw infarction may not be recognized and biopsy has to be carried out. The oral mucosa may also be pale or yellowish due to haemolytic jaundice.

Radiography
Abnormalities result from expansion of the haemopoietic marrow causing thickening but apparent osteoporosis of the bones of the skull. In severe cases, the changes resemble those of thalassaemia. Bone infarcts may appear relatively radiolucent at first, but become sclerotic. Rarely, jaw lesions can be the sole radiographic manifestation of the disease. Sclerotic areas in the skull or jaws may be seen in radiographs as a result of earlier infarcts.

Microscopy
Biopsy is only likely to be carried out under unusual circumstances such as unexplained jaw pain or radiographic changes. Typical-features of a bone infarct are erythrocytic haemopoiesis, sickled erythrocytes and haemosiderin-filled macrophages.

Management
Tests for the sickling trait should be carried out particularly in those of Afro-Caribbean origin, if general anaesthesia is anticipated. If the haemoglobin is less than 10 g/dl, then the patient is probably a homozygote with sickle cell disease.

In those with sickle cell trait, the main precaution is that general anaesthesia, if unavoidable, should be carried out with full oxygenation. Occasionally, crises may be precipitated by dental infections such as acute pericoronitis. Regular dental care and prompt antibiotic treatment of infections are therefore necessary for these patients.

Painful bone infarcts should be treated with non-steroidal anti-inflammatory analgesics and fluid intake should be increased (at least 3 litres/day for adults). Admission to hospital is required for severe painful crises not responsive to simple analgesics.

Rigorous routine dental care is necessary because of the susceptibility to infection. General anaesthesia, if utterly unavoidable, should be carried out

in hospital where precautions include exchange transfusions to raise the HbA level, rehydration and avoidance of hypoxia and acidosis if anaesthesia has to be given.

The thalassaemias

Bone disease in the thalassaemias is also due to bone marrow hyperplasia. The alpha-thalassaemias mainly affect Asians, Africans and Afro-Caribbeans, while the beta-thalassaemias mainly affect the Mediterranean littoral, such as Greece (thalassaemia: literally, sea in the blood). Alpha- and beta-thalassaemias result from inadequate synthesis of the alpha and beta globin chains of haemoglobin. The imbalance between the production of the globin chains means that the normal chains are present in the red cells in relative excess and tend to precipitate out. In homozygous thalassaemia, haemolysis can therefore result.

The severity of the disease depends on the numbers of alpha or beta globin genes affected, but in simplified terms the diseases are thalassaemia minor in heterozygotes and thalassaemia major in homozygotes.

Thalassaemia minor is characterized by mild but persistent microcytic anaemia (Hb over 9 g/dl), but is otherwise asymptomatic, apart sometimes from splenomegaly.

Thalassaemia major (usually homozygous beta-thalassaemia) is characterized by severe hypochromic, microcytic anaemia, great enlargement of liver and spleen and skeletal abnormalities due to marrow hyperplasia. The results are failure to thrive and early death if repeated blood transfusions are not given.

Radiography
The diploic spaces of the skull are enlarged and there is thinning of the cortex with a 'hair on end' appearance. The maxillae may also be expanded, causing severe malocclusion. The zygomatic bones are pushed outwards and the nasal bridge depressed in severe cases.

Management
Regular transfusions prevent the development of bony deformities, but lead to progressive

deposition of iron in the tissues. In those that survive, therefore, haemosiderosis can lead to dysfunction of glands and other organs. Typical complications include diabetes mellitus, hepatic cirrhosis and cardiac failure in early life. A Sjögren-like syndrome can result from iron deposition in the salivary glands.

Desferrioxamine, a chelating agent, may lessen the effects of the iron overload and folic acid treatment may ameliorate the haemolytic anaemia.

Other genetic disorders affecting the jaws

Gardner's syndrome is discussed in Chapter 5, the Gorlin–Goltz syndrome in Chapter 3 and cherubism below.

Fibro-osseous lesions

Fibro-osseous lesions range from fibrous dysplasia to the well-circumscribed lesions of ossifying or cementifying fibroma. Apparently, intermediate variants have features of both types of lesions, but this is a controversial area where the diagnosis must take into account clinical and radiographic as well as the microscopic findings.

Fibrous dysplasia

Typical monostotic fibrous dysplasia is characterized by focal but poorly circumscribed fibro-osseous replacement of an area of bone to form a swelling that starts in childhood but is likely to undergo arrest with maturation of the skeleton. The jaws are the most frequently affected site in the head and neck region, but overall these represent only 20–25% of cases, as the ribs and femur are considerably more frequently involved. Males and females are almost equally often affected.

Polyostotic fibrous dysplasia is relatively rare and is characterized by histologically similar lesions affecting several or many bones. Females are affected in the ratio of 3 to 1 male, and some show precocious puberty.

Albright's syndrome comprises polyostotic fibrous dysplasia, skin pigmentation and sexual precocity. Lesions are typically unilateral or segmental in distribution.

The aetiology of fibrous dysplasia is unknown. Unlike cherubism, which frequently has a similar natural history, there is no evidence of any genetic component.

Clinically, monostotic fibrous dysplasia is mainly seen in young adults, usually in their 20s, while polyostotic fibrous dysplasia is more frequently seen in childhood. The lesion typically forms a painless, smoothly rounded swelling in the maxilla more often than the mandible. The mass may be large enough to cause disturbance of function in some sites; malocclusion, for example, can result from displacement of teeth. Though the fibro-osseous mass weakens the bone, pathological fracture of the jaws is rare but relatively common in long bones.

Polyostotic fibrous dysplasia involves the head and neck region in up to 50% of cases. A jaw lesion may be the most conspicuous feature and the patient may appear to have monostotic disease. In a young girl, in particular, a search for other skeletal lesions and pigmentation may be appropriate. Skin pigmentation consists of tan to brown macules, 1 cm or more across, with an irregular outline. Pigmentation frequently overlies affected bones but has a predilection for the back of the neck, trunk, buttocks or thighs. Though any skin area can be affected, pigmentation of the oral mucosa is very rare.

Radiography
Most characteristic is an area of lessened radiopacity, with a fine orange-peel texture which merges imperceptibly with the surrounding normal bone. The outer surface may have an eggshell thin cortex of expanded normal bone. However, a variety of appearances can be seen and depend on the state of ossification of the lesion. Predominantly fibrous lesions may mimic cysts or cystic tumours. More heavily ossified lesions may have a pagetoid pattern or a patchily sclerotic appearance (Figure 6.6).

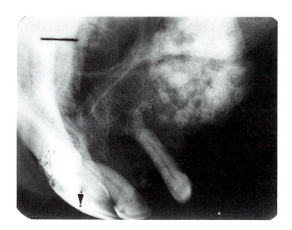

Figure 6.6 Fibrous dysplasia. Patchy sclerosis has produced the mottled appearance of this ill-defined maxillary lesion

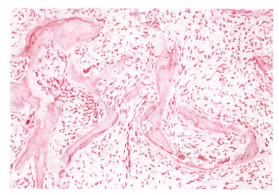

Figure 6.8 Fibrous dysplasia showing lamellar bone with little osteoblastic rimming, in a cellular fibroblastic stroma

Microscopy

The typical appearance is of loose cellular fibrous tissue in which there are evenly distributed trabeculae of woven bone (Figure 6.7). The trabeculae tend to be slender and arcuate or branched but very variable in shape. Osteoblasts are scattered throughout the substance of the trabeculae. This may contrast with the more conspicuous osteoblastic rimming seen in ossifying fibroma, where, in addition, the bone is typically lamellar rather than woven. However, lamellar bone or calcified spherules can also be seen in fibrous dysplasia (Figure 6.8). The types and amount of bone vary considerably from case to

case, but more important is the lack of definable borders where the trabeculae of fibrous dysplasia merge imperceptibly into the surrounding normal bone.

In addition to the mainly trabecular pattern of fibrous dysplasia, there may be myxoid areas or small foci of giant cells scattered in the fibrous stroma. These giant cells are not in such compact masses as those of giant cell lesions.

Management

There is nothing as yet to suggest that different patterns of bone formation are of any value in predicting the behaviour of the lesion or its response to treatment. The natural history is of steady progression until (very approximately) skeletal maturity is reached, when most lesions become static. Though the time of arrest is variable and doubt has been expressed as to whether this happens in all cases, there are undoubtedly numerous cases which have been followed up for sufficient periods to confirm spontaneous arrest. Moreover, unlike some benign tumours, there appear to have been no cases of untreated elderly patients with actively proliferating fibrous dysplasia.

The chief concern is usually therefore largely cosmetic or to ameliorate serious interference with function. There is also a small possibility of sarcomatous change which is more frequent in polyostotic disease and typically develops in early adult life. Ebata *et al.* (1992) were able to identify

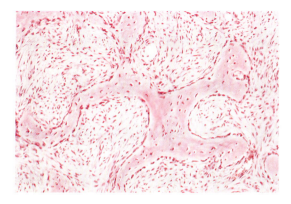

Figure 6.7 Fibrous dysplasia. Thin trabeculae of woven bone bordered by osteoblasts lie in a fibroblastic stroma

89 reported cases: the majority (61%) were osteo-sarcomas. The tendency to malignant change in fibrous dysplasia appears to be related to the disease itself, as only a minority (approximately 30%) of the reported cases had received radiation treatment.

Treatment for fibrous dysplasia, when indicated, should be resection. However, this is only justifiable for disfiguring lesions or those which seriously interfere with function. Recurrence usually within two or three years may be expected in up to 30% of cases, largely because of the difficulty of defining the extent of and completely eradicating the disease. Occasionally, fibrous dysplasia involves the orbital region and can cause proptosis and, rarely, blindness. In such cases, early radical excision and reconstruction is required. This may be undertaken via a transcranial approach planned on three-dimensional CT reconstructions of the region.

If sarcomatous change develops, wide radical excision is indicated, as for other sarcomas.

Cherubism

Cherubism is an autosomal dominant disease (formerly known as *familial fibrous dysplasia*) with variable expressivity. Due to weaker penetrance of the trait in females, the disorder is approximately twice as common in males. Like other genetic diseases, many non-familial cases appear as a result of new mutations.

The characteristic abnormalities are multiple, symmetrical pseudocystic masses in the jaws. These form in infancy or childhood and give the face an excessively chubby or, less frequently, a so-called cherubic appearance. Partial or complete resolution of the lesions with skeletal maturation is the general rule.

Clinically, the onset is typically between the ages of 6 months and 7 years and symmetrical mandibular swelling is the characteristic manifestation. Radiographic changes may be seen considerably earlier than the swelling of the jaws. The time of the onset of clinically evident disease and the rapidity of progress of the lesions are both variable.

Frequently, only the mandible, particularly the region of the angles, is involved. Maxillary involvement is usually associated with widespread mandibular disease and is seen in about 65% of cases. Extensive maxillary lesions cause the eyes to appear to be turned heavenward; this together with the plumpness of the face, is the cause of these patients being likened to cherubs. The appearance of the eyes is due to such factors as the maxillary masses pushing the floors of the orbits and eyes upwards, with the result that the sclera below the pupils becomes exposed. Expansion of the maxillae may also cause stretching of the skin and some retraction of the lower lids; rarely, the infra-orbital ridges may be destroyed and support for the lower lid is weakened.

The alveolar ridges are expanded and the mandibular swelling may sometimes be so gross lingually as to interfere with speech, swallowing or even breathing. Maxillary involvement can cause the palate to become an inverted V shape. Teeth are frequently displaced and may be loosened.

Despite the lack of inflammation, there is frequently cervical lymphadenopathy, due to reactive hyperplasia and fibrosis.

Radiography

The defects are usually more extensive than is clinically apparent. The angles of the mandible are bilaterally involved and the process extends towards the coronoid notch and sometimes also forwards along a considerable part of the body of the mandible. The appearances resemble multilocular cysts as a result of fine bony septa extending into the soft tissue masses. Progressive expansion of the latter reduces the bony cortices to eggshell thickness.

Maxillary involvement is shown by diffuse rarefaction of the bone, but spread of the soft tissue' masses can cause opacity of the sinuses. A distinctive radiographic sign described by Cornelius and McClendon (1969) is exposure of the posterior part of the hard palate in lateral skull films, as a result of forward displacement of the teeth. In severe cases, upward bulging of the orbital floor and destruction of part of the infra-orbital ridges may be seen. Even after complete clinical resolution of the facial swelling, bone defects may be evident radiographically.

Microscopy

The soft tissue masses consist of highly cellular and vascular fibrous tissue containing many giant cells (Figure 6.9). The fibrous tissue may be loose and relatively delicate in some areas but dense in others. Blood vessels are numerous and are typically surrounded by a cuff of eosinophilic fibrin-like material (Figure 6.10).

The giant cells have variable numbers of nuclei and may be in compact foci or scattered. There may also be small irregular bone trabeculae of which some are probably metaplastic, but others are remnants of normal bone undergoing resorption. Occasionally, epithelial remnants of teeth whose development has been aborted by the disease may be seen.

A limited biopsy of cherubism tissue may be indistinguishable microscopically from some areas of fibrous dysplasia, but overall the many giant cells and scanty bone of cherubism are in contrast with the pattern of bone trabeculae but scanty giant cells which are typical of fibrous dysplasia. More important are the clinical presentation and distinctive radiographic features. In particular, the early onset and symmetrical distribution of the lesions distinguish cherubism from fibrous dysplasia and from other giant cell lesions. A positive family history helps to confirm the diagnosis.

Management

Most cases can be allowed to progress to spontaneous resolution and the parents reassured accordingly. Exceptionally, treatment may be

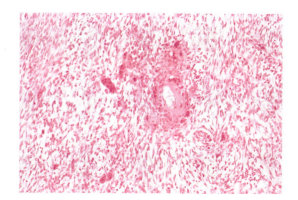

Figure 6.10 Cherubism. There are scanty giant cells in this field but the perivascular hyaline cuffing is prominent

necessary for extensive lesions which interfere with function or are disfiguring. Surgery is the only feasible method of treatment, as the possible complications of radiotherapy in a child preclude its use. Treatment, ranging from conservative curettage, repeated as necessary, to more aggressive resection and filling the void with autogenous bone chips, has been advocated from time to time. Nevertheless, radical or conservative surgery are equally likely to be followed by recurrence and further bone destruction if carried out while the disease is still active. Any surgery should be delayed, if possible until the disease is becoming quiescent in adolescence. However, by this time, treatment may be less necessary. Moreover, residual bone lesions persisting after clinical resolution of the disease should not be interfered with as this may provoke renewed activity. Though it has been suggested that extraction of related teeth may halt jaw expansion, extractions in a case reported by Ireland and Eveson (1988) led to fungation of the giant cell tissue through the socket, despite complete clinical regression of the disease. Control of the soft tissue proliferation could be achieved only by covering it with a mucoperiosteal flap.

Paget's disease of bone

The clinical and pathological features of Paget's disease of bone (osteitis deformans) were first described in detail by Sir James Paget in 1877 (Paget, 1877).

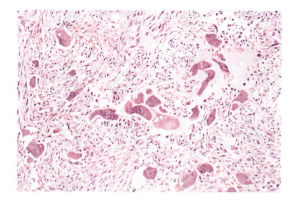

Figure 6.9 Cherubism showing scattered multinucleated giant cells in a fibroblastic stroma and characteristic hyaline material

Paget's disease is characterized by the onset in later life of anarchic osteoclastic and osteoblastic activity leading to distortion and weakening of bones. One or many bones may be affected, but though the cranium is a relatively common site, the maxillofacial skeleton is infrequently and the mandible very rarely involved.

Paget's disease is common, particularly if asymptomatic cases are included. The detection rate rises with the age of the population sample and on radiographic rather than clinical signs of the disease. In a survey of over 13 000 persons, Barker *et al.* (1977) found radiographic signs of the disease in 7–8% in people aged over 55 years in several adjacent towns in Lancashire, and an average prevalence of 5% in other counties. There was a considerably higher prevalence in men (6.2%) than women (3.9%). Smith (1992), from reported data, suggested that 0.75 million people have Paget's disease in Britain and that 5% (150 000) of them have substantial disability.

Barker (1984) noted that in the USA the prevalence of Paget's disease ranged from 1.2% to 2.6% for black and 0.9% to 3.9% for white persons over 55 years of age, and that the prevalence was low in many European countries, notably Sweden where it was only 0.4%. These variations appear to be compatible with an environmental influence such as a slow virus, superimposed on a genetic factor conferring susceptibility. A genetic component has been confirmed by Sofaer *et al.* (1983), who found that in 13.8% of 463 patients there was a family history of the disease and in them the mean age of onset was earlier (approximately 54 years) than in sporadic cases (57 years).

In addition to a possible genetic factor, intranuclear inclusions are visible by electron microscopy in bone and other cells of Paget's disease. Immunofluorescence and *in situ* hybridization studies show these inclusions to be compatible with a paramyxovirus, such as the measles or respiratory syncytial virus which can be shown in both osteoblasts and osteoclasts. The most recently proposed candidate is the canine distemper virus, but the evidence for Paget's disease being due to a slow virus remains incomplete.

Clinical features

As noted earlier, Paget's disease is a disease of old age. It is polyostotic in approximately 90% of cases, though frequently localized to a single site initially.

The bones chiefly affected (in declining order of frequency) are the lumbar vertebrae, sacrum, skull, femur, tibia, clavicle, humerus and ribs. When the skull is involved, the cranial bones, particularly the calvarium, are considerably more frequently affected than the facial skeleton and the mandible is exceptionally rarely involved.

The effects depend on the bones affected but, in general, they become thickened and larger but weaker. As a result, long bones become distorted by the stresses put on them. Increased vascularity of diseased bones may cause the overlying skin to feel warm and bone pain can be severe.

In the case of Paget's disease of the vault of the skull, the bone becomes thickened and enlarged until it may bulge forward over the face. Differentiation of the inner and outer plates is progressively lost and the diploic space becomes obliterated until ultimately a section of the skull appears grossly uniform but porous. Involvement of the temporal bone can cause deafness. Other neurological effects are compression of the VIIIth and occasionally of the optic nerve.

Involvement of the maxilla causes bulging of the central third of the face. Gross thickening of the alveolar ridges causes them to become enlarged, broad and rounded and the teeth may become spaced. Similar effects can rarely be seen in the mandible.

Paget's disease usually remains active for 3–5 years and then may become virtually static. Bone pain is often the most troublesome feature, but widespread disease can cause high-output heart failure due to the excessive vascularity of many bones producing, in effect, an arteriovenous shunt.

Radiography

Paget's disease of the vault of the skull shows well-defined, irregular areas of abnormal radiolucency ('osteoporosis circumscripta') in the early stages. This is followed by sclerosis which is patchy at first but spreads to produce the typical cottonwool appearance.

In the jaws, the normal trabecular pattern is lost and, as in the calvarium, areas of radiolucency are followed by the development of cottonwool opacities. In the early stages, loss of the lamina dura and resorption of periapical bone may mimic infection. Later there is typically gross craggy hypercementosis and bony ankylosis.

Microscopy

The characteristic features are anarchic, apparently uncontrolled, alternating resorptive and appositional activity of bone cells with osteoclastic activity predominating at first (Figure 6.11). The result is a pattern of scalloped areas of resorption, replaced in turn by irregular, basophilic reversal lines giving a jigsaw puzzle-like ('mosaic') pattern, when apposition follows. In the active stages, rimming of the bone by numerous osteoclasts and osteoblasts is conspicuous. The osteoclasts are frequently abnormally large with an excessive number of nuclei. Later, these cells become scanty but the jigsaw puzzle pattern of reversal lines persists (Figure 6.12). In addition, the bone marrow is replaced by highly vascular, loose connective tissue and in widespread disease extramedullary haemopoiesis may result.

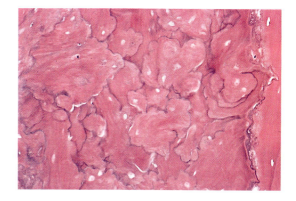

Figure 6.12   Paget's disease: late stage showing dense mass of bone with distinct basophilic resting and reversal lines

Biochemistry

Blood calcium and phosphate levels are typically normal, but the alkaline phosphatase levels are higher than in any other disease and can be as high as 700 u/l. Hypercalcaemia can result from the patient having become immobile or bedridden. Urinary hydroxyproline levels are raised during active, resorptive phases.

Management

Treatment is not indicated for asymptomatic cases. Aspirin or other anti-inflammatory analgesics may be effective for pain. In more severe cases, calcitonin can be given particularly for bone pain, to lessen any neurological complications or for hypercalcaemia. Though effective for these purposes, calcitonin is unlikely to improve the skeletal lesions and formation of neutralizing antibodies may limit its benefits. Salcatonin is less immunogenic, but does not remove the risk. Bisphosphonates, particularly disodium etidronate, are adsorbed on to hydroxyapatite crystals to slow their growth and resorption. The rate of bone turnover is slowed as a consequence and the biochemical abnormalities usually return to normal. Toxic effects of bisphosphonates include nausea and diarrhoea: in high doses they may worsen bone pain and increase the risk of fractures.

Giant cell tumours in areas of Paget's disease occasionally develop in the skull or facial skeleton. Their behaviour is similar to that of central giant cell granulomas and they also respond to conservative curettage. Sarcoma in Paget's disease is well recognized, with an estimated incidence of 0.1–1%, but there are few authenticated cases involving the jaws. Both giant cell lesions and sarcomas develop much later in life than in otherwise normal persons.

Oral complications include difficulty with dentures and bleeding or infection of the bone, particularly as a result of attempted extraction of grossly hypercementosed teeth.

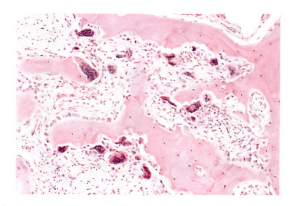

Figure 6.11   Paget's disease showing active irregular bone resorption by large osteoclastic giant cells and concomitant osteoblastic activity

Hyperparathyroidism

Hyperparathyroidism can be primary or secondary and results from overproduction of parathyroid hormone. This raises the blood calcium level, partly by bone resorption, but there is also increased calcium absorption from the gut and renal re-absorption. Bone resorption may not therefore be seen in early cases and significant bone lesions are now rarely seen in hyperparathyroidism.

Approximately 80% of cases of primary disease are due to a parathyroid adenoma, while the remainder are due to hyperplasia or, more rarely, carcinoma of the gland. Even more rarely, hyperparathyroidism can be a manifestation of the multiple endocrine neoplasia syndromes, either type I or II.

Secondary hyperparathyroidism is a reaction to a persistent hypocalcaemia due to chronic renal failure or prolonged renal dialysis, or rarely to malabsorption.

Clinically, the diagnosis is made in the majority of patients from biochemical screening, either as a chance finding or for the investigation of gastro-intestinal symptoms, renal stones, hypertension, fluid retention, stiffness or other musculoskeletal symptoms or psychiatric disorders. In the elderly, symptoms of hypercalcaemia are more common and cause dehydration, with thirst and nocturia, anorexia, vomiting or constipation, and confusion or depression. In secondary hyperparathyroidism, bone disease is common but renal stones relatively uncommon.

Localized bone lesions ('osteitis fibrosa cystica') can cause pain, deformity or pathological fractures. However jaw lesions, a well-recognized feature in the past, can be painless or cause localized swellings. Rarely, jaw lesions have been the first sign of the disease. Even more rarely, hyperparathyroidism can give rise to a soft tissue lesion similar both clinically and microscopically to a giant cell epulis.

Hyperparathyroidism can cause lethal renal damage. Accurate diagnosis of a giant cell lesion of the jaw is therefore essential. Hyperparathyroidism should particularly be suspected in a patient of a middle age or over. In such patients, blood biochemistry and possibly parathormone assay must be carried out. In doubtful cases, this may be supplemented by a skeletal survey, starting with the fingers.

In patients with carcinoma of the breast or lung there may be bone metastases which can mimic Paget's disease radiographically. However, in carcinoma of the lung the biochemical findings can also be similar to those of primary hyperparathyroidism. A chest radiograph may therefore be required.

Secondary hyperparathyroidism may be seen in a child: in such a case the history of renal disease will suggest the diagnosis. Rarely, a jaw lesion due to secondary hyperparathyroidism may be an early sign of rejection of a kidney graft.

Radiography
The most characteristic change is generalized osteoporosis. Localized bone lesions appear as moderately well-defined, cyst-like areas often with a multiloculated pattern. These may be associated with other bone lesions such as resorption and tufting of the terminal phalanges, or cyst-like areas of bone resorption in the cranial vault or long bones. Disappearance of the lamina dura of the teeth is inconstant and an unreliable sign. The nature of the jaw lesions is unlikely to be recognized until after microscopy.

Microscopy
The bone lesions appear grossly as soft, livid masses which are typically brown due to altered blood (brown tumours). Microscopically, they are non-specific giant cell lesions (Figure 6.13) which can be distinguished from giant cell granulomas of the jaws only by blood chemistry. Some lesions consist predominantly of fibrous tissue (Figures 6.14 and 6.15).

Management
Blood for calcium levels must be taken from a fasting patient and, to avoid venous stasis, without a tourniquet. The level should be related to the serum albumin level and venepuncture may need to be repeated several times as elevation of serum calcium may only be intermittent. The reference range for albumin-adjusted serum calcium is 2.20–2.65 mmol/l, but 2.20–2.70 mmol/l for women aged over 69 years. Hypophosphataemia is frequently but inconstantly associated. Alkaline phosphatase levels are raised in proportion to the extent of the bone disease. Immunoassay of

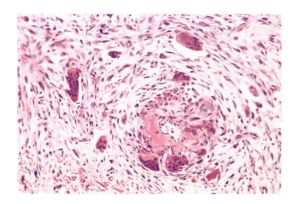

Figure 6.13   Hyperparathyroidism. Typical giant cells lie in a vascular fibroblastic stroma

parathormone is sometimes necessary, but the levels in hyperparathyroidism overlap with the normal range and the level is also raised in renal failure.

Other causes of hypercalcaemia must be excluded, particularly the considerably more common hypercalcaemia secondary to tumours of the lungs, breast and other sites, or myeloma. The biochemical findings are the same of those of hyperparathyroidism, but the hypercalcaemia usually responds to corticosteroids. Other possible causes of hypercalcaemia include sarcoidosis, thyrotoxicosis, immobility and milk-alkali syndrome. However, these should not cause confusion in a patient with a giant cell lesion of the jaw.

In primary hyperparathyroidism, removal of the parathyroid adenoma is curative, though the

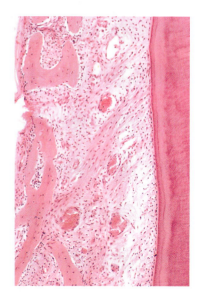

Figure 6.15   Hyperparathyroidism showing grossly widened periodontal ligament due to resorption of the lamina dura

tumour may be difficult to find. This is the required treatment for .those with bone lesions and particularly for those with renal complications of the disease. For those without symptoms, where hypercalcaemia has been a chance finding, prolonged follow up shows an unexpectedly favourable outcome without surgery.

For those with secondary hyperparathyroidism, treatment of the underlying renal disease, and if possible a renal transplant, is necessary.

Idiopathic osteosclerosis (solitary bone islands)

These foci of abnormal bone density have been thought in the past to result from chronic inflammation (Chapter 2).

Massive osteolysis (phantom bone disease)

Massive osteolysis is a rare disease which sometimes affects the maxillofacial bones. Frederiksen *et*

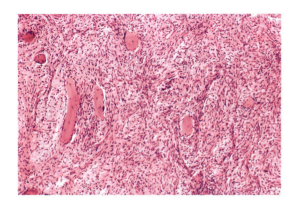

Figure 6.14   Hyperparathyroidism showing replacement of bone by cellular fibroblastic tissue with only occasional multinucleated giant cells

al. (1983) reviewed 14 cases and added another. The cause is unknown and no genetic or biochemical abnormalities have been found.

The onset can be at any age, but appears to be most frequent in young adults. When the maxillofacial bones are affected, the mandible appears to be first and most severely affected and the first symptoms are usually loosening and exfoliation of teeth or there may be spontaneous fracture of the mandible.

Radiography

Early signs may be subcortical foci of radiolucency with indistinct margins. These coalesce and involve the cortex. The mandible can be progressively resorbed along its whole length from the alveolar ridge downwards, until only the lower border and the ramus remains, but even these may disappear. Heffez *et al.* (1983) reviewed 43 earlier cases and reported, in a 13-year-old boy, resorption of the mandible from condyle to symphysis, the posterior zygomatic arch, the hyoid bone, the lower thirds of the pterygoid plates, the mastoid tip, the occipital bone and the lateral aspect of the middle cranial fossa. Nine months later the maxilla and other bones, including the cervical vertebrae, were affected.

Microscopy

The main features are dilated vascular channels, active osteoclastic resorption at the interface with normal bone and fibrous tissue proliferation.

Management

Massive osteolysis may have to be distinguished from haemangioma of the jaws or the osteolysis that occasionally complicates systemic sclerosis. No reliably effective treatment for idiopathic osteolysis is known, but the disease may be self-limiting. Frederiksen *et al.* (1983) replaced the lost mandibular tissue with a rib graft, but this too was almost completely resorbed and had to be removed. Two years later the disease was still active. By contrast, in the patient reported by Heffez *et al.* (1983) with more extensive disease, a CT scan taken a year after presentation showed stabilization and partial recalcification of osteolytic foci in the mandible and vertebrae. A short course

of radiotherapy had been given, but it is not clear whether it was of any benefit.

Management is therefore essentially palliative with regular CT scanning to check progress and treatment of complications as they arise.

References

Barker, D.J.P. (1984) The epidemiology of Paget's disease of bone. *British Medical Bulletin*, **40**, 396–400

Barker, D.J.P., Clough, P.W.L., Guyer, P.B. *et al.* (1977) Paget's disease of bone in 14 British towns. *British Medical Journal*, **1**, 1181–1183

Cornelius, E.A. and McClendon, J.L. (1969) Cherubism – hereditary fibrous dysplasia of the jaws. Roentgenographic features. *American Journal of Roentgenology*, **106**, 136–143

Ebata, K., Usami, T., Tohnai, K. *et al.* (1992) Chondrosarcoma and osteosarcoma arising in polyostotic fibrous dysplasia. *Journal of Oral and Maxillofacial Surgery*, **50**, 761–764

Fallon, M.D., Teitelbaum, S.L., Weinstein, R.S. *et al.* (1984) Hypophosphatasia: clinicopathologic comparison of the infantile, childhood and adult forms. *Medicine*, **63**, 12–24

Frederiksen, N.L., Wesley, R.K., Sciubba, J.J. *et al.* (1983) Massive osteolysis of the maxillofacial skeleton. A clinical, radiographic, histologic and ultrastructural study. *Oral Surgery, Oral Medicine and Oral Pathology*, **55**, 470–480

Gorlin, R.J., Cervenka, J. and Pruzansky, S. (1971) Facial clefting and its syndromes. *Birth Defects*, **7**, 3–49

Heffez, L., Doku, H.C., Carter, B.L. *et al.* (1983) Perspectives on massive osteolysis. Report of a case and review of the literature. *Oral Surgery, Oral Medicine and Oral Pathology*, **55**, 331–343

Hotz, M.M. and Gnoinski, W.M. (1979) Effects of early maxillary orthopaedics in coordination with delayed surgery for cleft lip and palate. *Journal of Maxillofacial Surgery*, **7**, 201–210

Ireland, A.J. and Eveson, J.W. (1988) Cherubism: a report of a case with unusual post-extraction complication. *British Dental Journal*, **164**, 116–117

Markus, A.F., Smith, W.P. and Delaire, J. (1993) Primary closure of cleft palate: a functional approach. *British Journal of Oral and Maxillofacial Surgery*, **31**, 71–77

Mars, M. and Houston, W.J. (1990) A preliminary study of facial growth and morphology in unoperated male unilateral cleft lip and palate subjects over 13 years of age. *Cleft Palate Journal*, **27**, 7–10

Ortiz-Monasterio, F., Rebeil, A.S., Valderrama, M. *et al.* (1959) Cephalometric measurements on adult patients with nonoperated cleft palates. *Plastic and Reconstructive Surgery*, **24**, 53–61

Paget, J. (1877) On a form of chronic inflammation of bones (osteitis deformans). *Medical Chirurgical Transactions,* **60,** 37–64

Perko, M.A. (1979) Two stage closure of cleft palate (Progress report). *Journal of Maxillofacial Surgery,* **7,** 76–80

Poswillo, D. (1973) Pathogenesis of the first and second branchial arch syndrome. *Oral Medicine and Oral Pathology,* **35,** 302–308

Precious, D.S. and Delaire, J. (1993) Clinical observations of cleft lip and palate. *Oral Surgery, Oral Medicine and Oral Pathology,* **75,** 141–151

Roberts, C.T., Semb, G. and Shaw, W.C. (1991) Strategies for the advancement of surgical methods in cleft lip and palate. *Cleft Palate and Craniofacial Journal,* **28,** 141–149

Smith, R. (1992) Paget's disease of bone (editorial). *British Medical Journal,* **305,** 1379–1380

Sofaer, J.A., Holloway, S.M. and Emery, A.E. (1983) A family study of Paget's disease of bone. *Journal of Epidemiology and Community Health,* **37,** 226–231

Tessier, P. (1976) Anatomical classification of facial, craniofacial and latero-facial clefts. *Journal of Maxillofacial Surgery,* **4,** 69–92

Tolorava, M. (1972) Empirical recurrence risk factors for genetic counselling of clefts. *Acta Chirurgiae plasticae,* **14,** 234–235

Younai, F., Eisenbud, L. and Sciubba, J.J. (1988) Osteopetrosis: a case report including gross and microscopic findings in the mandible at autopsy. *Oral Surgery, Oral Medicine and Oral Pathology,* **65,** 214–221

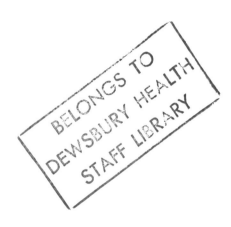

7

Disorders of the temporomandibular joints and periarticular tissues

Disorders of the temporomandibular joint can cause various combinations of limitation of movement of the jaw, pain, locking or clicking sounds. Pain, in particular, is a frequent cause of limitation of movement. Few of these complaints are due to organic disease of the joint and many are due to trauma. However, these functional disorders must be considered in the differential diagnosis.

Limitation of movement (trismus)

Trismus may be defined as inability to open the mouth due to muscle spasm, but the term is usually used for limited movement of the jaw from any cause. Inability to open the mouth fully is usually temporary and causes include the following:

Infection and inflammation in or near the joint The main cause is acute pericoronitis with associated muscle spasm. Mumps can also cause temporary limitation of movement. Rare causes include suppurative arthritis, osteomyelitis, cellulitis and suppurative parotitis. Submasseteric abscess results in profound trismus (Chapter 2), but infection in the pterygoid, lateral pharyngeal or submandibular spaces may also cause varying degrees of trismus.

Mandibular block injections may cause inflammation of the muscles around the joint and oedema, either because of irritation by the local anaesthetic or by introduction of infection. Occasionally, limitation of movement may be more persistent, possibly due to organization of haematoma after the passage of the needle through the medial pterygoid muscle during the injection. If voluntary jaw exercises fail to achieve opening, forced manipulation under general anaesthesia may be necessary. Often the scar tissue can be felt to tear during the forced opening.

Injuries Unilateral condylar neck fracture usually only produces mild limitation of opening with deviation of the jaw to the affected side, but closing into centric occlusion may be difficult. Bilateral displaced condylar fractures cause an anterior open bite with limited movement. Rarely, a fall on the chin can result in unilateral or bilateral dislocation of the condylar head into the middle cranial fossa and severe restriction of all movements. Less severe injuries frequently result in an effusion into the temporomandibular joint; both wide opening and complete closure are then prevented.

Any unstable mandibular fracture causes protective muscle spasm with limitation of movement. Patients suffering from displaced Le Fort II or III fractures often complain of limited opening, whereas in reality they are fully open with the jaws wedged apart by the displaced middle third. Reduction of the fracture allows closure.

Tetanus and tetany These are rare causes of masticatory muscle spasm. Trismus (lockjaw) is a classical early sign of tetanus which, though rare, must be excluded because of its high mortality. This possibility should be considered whenever a patient develops acute severe limitation of movement of the jaw without local cause but has had a penetrating wound, even if small, elsewhere.

Tetany is most likely to be seen as a result of anxiety and hyperventilation syndrome.

Temporomandibular pain dysfunction syndrome Pain dysfunction syndrome is one of the most common causes of temporary limitation of movement of the temporomandibular joint, as discussed later.

Hysterical trismus Inability to open the mouth is occasionally the main symptom in disturbed patients.

Drugs Phenothiazine neuroleptics can cause tardive dyskinesia with uncontrollable, involuntary grimacing or chewing movements. Tardive dyskinesia is typically a result of long-term treatment: unlike drug-related Parkinsonism, there is little response to treatment. Metoclopramide, which has phenothiazine-like properties, can cause limitation of movement of the jaw.

Management
In all these conditions the essential measure is to relieve the underlying complaint.

Permanent limitation of movement (ankylosis)

Management of ankylosis depends on its aetiology and can be classified for surgical purposes as follows:

1. Pseudo-ankylosis (mechanical interference with opening, well away from the joint).
2. False ankylosis (extracapsular limitation of opening).
3. True ankylosis (intracapsular fixation).

Pseudo-ankylosis

Causes include:

- *trauma:* depressed fracture of the zygomatic bone or arch
- *hyperplasia:* developmental overgrowth of the coronoid process

- *neoplasms:* osteochondroma, osteoma, osteosarcoma of the coronoid process
- *miscellaneous:* myositis ossificans, congenital anomalies.

Extracapsular ankylosis

Causes include:

- *trauma:* periarticular fibrosis (wounds/burns); posterior or superior dislocation; long-standing anterior dislocation
- *infection:* chronic periarticular suppuration
- *neoplasia:* fibrosarcoma of the capsule; chondroma or chondrosarcoma
- *periarticular fibrosis:* irradiation; oral submucous fibrosis; progressive systemic sclerosis.

Irradiation

The penetrating power of modern sources such as cobalt 60 or linear accelerators are such that high doses can damage deep tissues without a superficial burn. Radiation involving the region of the masticatory muscles, for the treatment of a maxillary tumour for instance, can lead to fibrosis of muscle and fibrous adhesions to the surrounding fascial layers, producing a fixed mass bound to the jaw. When this happens there is severe limitation of opening the mouth or complete ankylosis.

Treatment is difficult and may involve division of muscle attachments from the jaw or section of the angle or body of the mandible to produce a false joint. Bone surgery is complicated by the risk of osteoradionecrosis and infection (Chapter 2).

In children, irradiation can result in inhibition of condylar cellular activity with subsequent inhibition of mandibular growth.

Oral submucous fibrosis

Oral submucous fibrosis is a disease which produces changes similar to those of scleroderma but limited to the oral tissues. The disease is virtually only seen in those from the Indian subcontinent.

In their review, Pillai *et al.* (1992) conclude that the aetiology is unknown, but suggested factors have been irritants (chillis) in the diet, betel (areca nut) chewing, genetic factors or a questionable relationship to progressive systemic sclerosis. However, there are no immunological findings to suggest any relationship between oral submucous fibrosis and systemic sclerosis.

The main contributor is thought by Jayanthi *et al.* (1992) to be the chewing of a preparation (*pan*) which typically consists of areca nut, tobacco and lime wrapped in betel leaf. While tobacco may possibly contribute to the premalignant potential of this disease, similar changes are not seen in the oral mucosa from long-term use of oral tobacco in other countries where the typical response is keratosis (Chapter 9).

Experimentally, an alkaloid component of the areca nut, arecoline, can induce fibroblast proliferation and collagen synthesis and it may penetrate the oral mucosa to cause progressive crosslinking of collagen fibres. Susceptibility to submucous fibrosis also appears to be related to specific HLA types. The fact that oral submucous fibrosis is an almost specifically Indian disease also strongly suggests a genetic factor, and the use of areca nut is mainly restricted to that subcontinent. It is probably the tobacco content of the betel quid, rather than an areca nut, which induces epithelial atypia and any tendency to malignant change (Chapter 10). Pillai *et al.* (1992) conclude, therefore, that the aetiology of this disease is multifactorial.

Clinically, symmetrical fibrosis of such sites as the buccal mucosa, soft palate or inner aspects of the lips is characteristic. The overlying mucosa may be normal or there may be a vesiculating stomatitis. Fibrosis causes extreme pallor of the affected area which becomes so hard that it cannot be indented with the finger. Ultimately, opening the mouth may become so limited that eating and dental treatment become increasingly difficult and tube feeding may become necessary.

Microscopy
The subepithelial connective tissue becomes thickened, hyaline and avascular, and there may be infiltration by modest numbers of chronic inflammatory cells. The epithelium usually becomes thinned and may show atypia. Underlying muscle fibres undergo progressive atrophy.

Investigation
In patients from the Indian subcontinent, with these lesions and especially with the characteristic histological changes on biopsy, the diagnosis can rarely be in doubt. Scleroderma should be readily differentiated by the dermal and visceral involvement, the less severe oral changes and the autoantibodies.

Management
Treatment is unsatisfactory. Patients must stop the habit of betel chewing and intralesional injections of corticosteroids may be tried in association with muscle-stretching exercises to prevent further limitation of opening, but the benefit is not great. Wide surgical excision of the affected tissues including the underlying buccinator muscle, together with skin grafting, can be carried out, but is likely to be followed by relapse. Borle and Borle (1991), in comparing treatments in 326 patients, concluded that injections could be hazardous and conservative treatment by topical applications of such preparations as corticosteroids or vitamin A derivatives, and oral iron, were as effective. However, no form of treatment is more than palliative and in some cases operative treatment may become unavoidable. Jayanthi *et al.* (1992) suggest that the most important measure is prevention and that use of pan should be forbidden in patients. This may be initially effective, but fibrosis often recurs even though the patient complies. Regular follow-up is important because of the premalignant potential of this disease.

Progressive systemic sclerosis (scleroderma)

Systemic sclerosis is an uncommon connective tissue disease characterized by widespread subcutaneous and submucous fibrosis. Though the most obvious feature is the progressive stiffening of the skin, the gastrointestinal tract, lungs, heart and kidneys can also be affected. Unlike oral submucous fibrosis, the prognosis is poor as a result.

Systemic sclerosis is a connective tissue (collagen vascular) disease. There are circulating antinuclear antibodies in about 50% of patients, antinucleolar antibodies or antibodies to RNA. An antinuclear antibody Scl 70 appears to be restricted to this disease, but is found in only about 20% of patients. Other laboratory findings are a normochromic anaemia and a raised ESR.

Clinically, women between the ages of 30 and 50 years are predominantly affected. Raynaud's phenomenon is the most common early manifestation, often associated with arthralgia. A hallmark of the disease is involvement of the hands, causing such changes as atrophy of or ischaemic damage to the tips of the fingers and contractures preventing straightening of the fingers.

The skin becomes thinned, stiff, tethered, pigmented and marked by telangiectases. The head and. neck region is involved in over 75% of patients and, in a minority, symptoms start there. Narrowing of the eyes and taut, mask-like limitation of facial movement (Mona Lisa face) can give rise to a characteristic facial appearance. The lips may be constricted (fish mouth) or become pursed with radiating furrows. Occasionally, involvement of the periarticular tissues of the temporomandibular joint, together with the microstomia, may greatly limit opening of the mouth. Involvement of the oral submucosa may cause the tongue to become stiff and narrowed (chicken tongue), but the clinical effects on the oral soft tissues are typically relatively minor compared with those seen in oral submucous fibrosis. Widening of the periodontal membrane space is another abnormality characteristic of systemic sclerosis, but seen in fewer than 10% of cases. The mandibular angle may be resorbed or rarely there is gross extensive resorption of the jaw. Sjögren's syndrome also develops in a significant minority.

Microscopy

There is great thickening of the subepithelial connective tissue, degeneration of muscle fibres and atrophy of minor glands (Figure 7.1). The collagen fibres are swollen and eosinophilic. There are scattered infiltrates of chronic inflammatory cells which are frequently perivascular, and arterioles typically show fibro-intimal thickening of their walls.

Complications and prognosis

The main disabilities caused by systemic sclerosis are dysphagia and pulmonary, cardiac or renal involvement. Visceral disease, particularly dysphagia and reflux oesophagitis, are common and

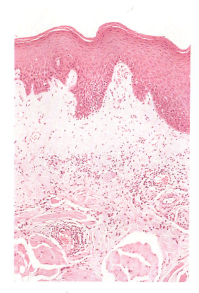

Figure 7.1 Systemic sclerosis (scleroderma). The thickened and hyalinized subepithelial connective tissue overlies atrophic muscle fibres and vessels with a perivascular infiltrate

are sometimes the initial symptoms. Pulmonary involvement leads to impaired respiratory exchange and, eventually, dyspnoea and pulmonary hypertension. Cardiac disease can result from the latter or myocardial fibrosis and these are potential contraindications to general anaesthesia. Renal disease secondary to vascular disease is typically a late effect; it leads to hypertension and is an important cause of death. The overall 5-year survival rate is approximately 70%.

No specific treatment is available. Immunosuppressive drugs are ineffective. Penicillamine may be given to depress fibrous proliferation but can cause loss of taste, oral ulceration, lichenoid reactions and other complications. Symptomatic measures such as those described for oral submucous fibrosis can be used to prevent undue limitation of jaw movement. Complications such as renal failure are managed by conventional means.

Localized scleroderma (morphoea)

Morphoea is characterized by similar tissue changes to systemic sclerosis, but limited to a single area of skin and without visceral disease or systemic effects. A typical manifestation is involvement of the side of the face causing an area of scar-like contraction like a sword wound (*coup de sabre*) and there may be atrophy of the underlying bone. Facial hemiatrophy may be the result from morphoea starting in childhood.

Intracapsular ankylosis

Important causes include:

- *Trauma:*
  Intracapsular comminuted fracture. Intracapsular fracture of the condyle disorganizes the joint. Bleeding may be followed by organization and bone formation. Early mobilization of such injuries should prevent bony ankylosis.
  Penetrating wounds.
  Forceps delivery at birth.
- *Infection:*
  Otitis media/mastoiditis.
  Osteomyelitis of the jaws.
  Haematogenous pyogenic arthritis.
  Acute pyogenic arthritis is exceedingly rare but, if treated inadequately, ankylosis follows.
- *Systemic:*
  Juvenile arthritis.
  Psoriatic arthropathy.
  Osteoarthritis (rarely).
  Rheumatoid arthritis (rarely).
- *Neoplasms:*
  Chondroma, osteochondroma, osteoma, sarcoma, fibrosarcoma, synovial sarcoma.
  Metastases to the condyle.
- *Miscellaneous:*
  Synovial chondromatosis.

Management
These conditions are described in previous or subsequent sections. If ankylosis cannot be prevented, the objectives of surgery are to establish joint movement and function, to prevent relapse, to restore appearance and occlusion in the adult and to achieve normal growth and occlusion in the child by interceptive surgery and orthodontics.

Simple division of bone and fibrous tissue at the articular surface (osteoarthrotomy) is seldom indicated and results in early relapse. Osteoarthrectomy, in which a block of bone is removed either as a condylectomy or gap arthroplasty, is more effective and is the usual technique employed in adults. Relapse is prevented by interposition of a temporalis muscle flap, silicone rubber or metal. In the growing patient, joint reconstruction using a free costochondral bone graft gives better results as in many cases the graft will grow with the patient, preventing subsequent facial deformity.

Other techniques sometimes used are ramus osteotomies (Ward's technique) in which a false joint is created in the ramus. Relapse is prevented by interposition of a cobalt–chrome cap or angle ostectomies (Esmarch's technique) in which a section of bone is removed at the angle and bony union prevented by the interposition of masseter and medial pterygoid muscles. Occasionally, the joint is reconstructed with a cobalt–chrome or titanium prosthesis articulating in a silicone rubber articular fossa. However, long-term results with such prostheses have been disappointing and have resulted in much litigation.

Arthritis and other causes of pain in or around the joint

The main causes are as follows:

- *Injury.* Dislocation, joint effusion or fractures of the neck of the condyle can cause pain of varying severity, but surprisingly often, fractures in this region pass unnoticed.
- *Infection and inflammation.* Acute pyogenic arthritis and osteomyelitis are rare but exceedingly painful.
- *Rheumatoid and other arthritides.* The temporomandibular joints tend to be much less severely affected than other small joints, although if specifically asked, many patients with rheumatoid arthritis admit to temporomandibular joint symptoms, but overall, pain is not conspicuous. Pain associated with osteoarthritis of this joint is even more uncommon.
- *Vascular disease.* Cranial arteritis is an important cause of ischaemia and pain in the masticatory muscles while chewing.

- *Muscle spasm.* Probably the most common causes of pain in the region of the temporomandibular joint is the so-called pain dysfunction syndrome, as discussed later.
- *Salivary gland disease.* Painful conditions of the parotids (inflammatory or neoplastic) can cause pain in this region.
- *Ear disease.* Otitis externa, otitis media and mastoiditis are potent causes of pain referred to the temporomandibular joint.

Rheumatoid arthritis

The main feature of this common multi-system disease is chronic inflammation of many joints, pain, progressive limitation of movement, varying degrees of constitutional upset and immunological abnormalities.

Rheumatoid arthritis is the only important inflammatory disease of the temporomandibular joints, but is nevertheless an infrequent cause of significant symptoms there.

Clinical features
Women are affected, particularly in the third and fourth decades. Loss of weight, malaise and depression are common. The smaller joints are mainly affected (particularly those of the hands), and the distribution tends to be symmetrical.

The main symptoms of temporomandibular joint involvement are crepitus and limitation of movement, but severe pain is surprisingly uncommon. The temporomandibular joints are never involved alone and the other affected joints usually dominate the picture. Among 100 patients with rheumatoid arthritis sufficiently severe for them to attend a large rheumatology centre, Chalmers and Blair (1973) found 71% to have clinical abnormalities of the temporomandibular joints (compared with 41% for controls), while 79% showed radiographic abnormalities compared with 34% for controls. In spite of the fact that these were middle-aged patients with long-standing disease, pain was *not* significantly more common than in control patients. The main clinical abnormalities were limitation of opening or crepitus, both of which were considerably more common than in other patients.

Radiography
Flattening of the condyles with loss of contour and irregularity of the articular surface are typical findings. The joint space may be widened by exudate in the acute phases, but later narrowed. The underlying bone may be osteoporotic and the margins of the condyles may be irregular. There may be limitation of condylar movement.

Microscopy
There is proliferation and hypertrophy of the synovial lining cells and infiltration of the synovium by dense collections of lymphocytes and plasma cells (Figure 7.2). The inflammatory cells are often arranged as focal aggregates with germinal centres. There is effusion into the synovial fluid which contains neutrophils and fibrinous exudation from the hyperaemic vessels on to the surface of the synovial membrane. A vascular, inflamed mass of granulation tissue (pannus) spreads over the surfaces of the articular cartilages from their margins (Figure 7.3) and is followed by death of chondrocytes and loss of intercellular matrix. Fibrous adhesions form between the joint surfaces and the meniscus. The meniscus may eventually be destroyed and inflammatory changes in the ligaments and tendons can lead to fibrous ankylosis or loss of stability of the joint.

Management
Diagnosis is based on the clinical, radiographic and autoantibody findings. Serum IgG is usually raised

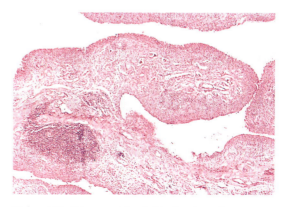

Figure 7.2 Rheumatoid arthritis showing villous hypertrophy of the synovium and focal areas of dense lymphoplasmacytic inflammatory infiltration

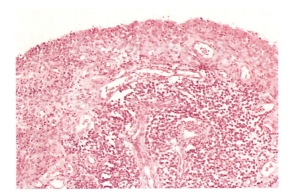

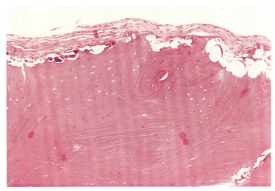

Figure 7.3   Rheumatoid arthritis. Vascular granulation tissue (pannus) is growing over the articular surface

Figure 7.4   Osteoarthritis. Subarticular erosion and underlying dense bone

and a variety of autoantibodies particularly rheumatoid factor and antinuclear antibodies may be detected.

Generally speaking, though rheumatoid arthritis is a common disease, it is not a major cause of temporomandibular joint pain, and radiographic changes appear to be more severe than the symptoms. The mainstay of treatment is the use of non-steroidal anti-inflammatory drugs, but any gross abnormalities of occlusion, such as overclosure, should be corrected to reduce stress on the temporomandibular joints.

Osteoarthritis

Osteoarthritis has long been thought to be a degenerative (wear-and-tear) phenomenon, particularly affecting chronically overstressed joints such as the hips and knees in elderly patients. However, it is now clear that osteoarthritis is a systemic disease: trauma is only a contributory factor, but heavy stress on affected joints is the cause of pain.

Osteoarthritis of the temporomandibular joint is a post mortem finding in many elderly patients, is occasionally seen by chance in radiographs, but is not a cause of significant symptoms (Figures 7.4 and 7.5). Nevertheless, the conviction that osteoarthritis is a significant cause of temporomandibular joint pain, even in young persons, is widely held in the USA, to justify surgical interference.

However, the argument that the temporomandibular joint is prone to osteoarthritis because of the heavy stresses it has to bear is hardly consistent with the types of operation that are used. It would be unlikely, for example, that excision of the head of the femur would be appropriate treatment for osteoarthritis of the hip.

In the rare event that a patient has pain associated with osteoarthritis of the temporomandibular joint, any factor contributing to stress on the joint should be relieved. Non-steroidal anti-inflammatory analgesics in generous doses are the main line of treatment. A high condylar shave is also effective in reducing symptoms either by denervating the joint or by decompressing the condylar head.

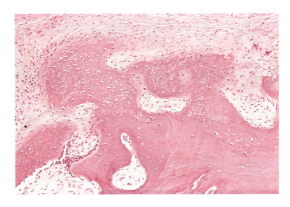

Figure 7.5   Osteoarthritis. Bony repair at the periphery of the damaged joint surfaces

The concept of temporomandibular joint 'internal derangement' is also open to a variety of interpretations. Some regard it as an underlying cause of pain dysfunction syndrome, others that it is a contributory cause of temporomandibular joint osteoarthritis. After an International Conference on Temporomandibular Joint Surgery, Goss (1993) commented disarmingly that 'it was noted that facts are commonly not allowed to interfere in discussions of TMJ problems'. Although some degree of consensus was reached at this conference it was apparent that neither the pathogenesis nor the effectiveness of surgical treatment of this condition were firmly established. It therefore remains too controversial a subject to discuss here.

Other types of arthritis

Many other types of arthritis can affect the temporomandibular joints but rarely do so. They include psoriatic arthritis, the juvenile arthritides, gout, ankylosing spondylitis, Lyme disease and Reiter's disease (Könönen, 1992). Psoriatic arthropathy can cause ankylosis of temporomandibular joint (Miles and Kaugars, 1991; Koorbusch *et al.*, 1991). Some of the variants of juvenile arthritis such as Still's disease are severe and disabling. Destruction of the condylar head, severely limited opening and secondary micrognathia have been reported by Larheim and Haanaes (1981). Management is essentially that of the underlying disease.

Cranial (giant cell) arteritis

Cranial arteritis occasionally causes ischaemic pain in the masticatory muscles in elderly patients and should be considered in patients over middle age who complain of headache and pain on mastication.

Clinically, women, usually after the age of 55, are predominantly affected. The disease may start with malaise, weakness, low-grade fever and loss of weight. Severe throbbing headache is the most common symptom. The temporal artery frequently becomes red, tender, firm, swollen and tortuous.

In 20% of patients, there is ischaemic pain in the masticatory muscles, comparable to and often misnamed jaw claudication (claudication is, literally, *limping*). More important is involve-ment of the ophthalmic artery causing disturbances of vision or sudden blindness. Polymyalgia rheumatica may be associated. There is then weakness and pain of the shoulder or pelvic girdles associated with the febrile symptoms. The erythrocyte sedimentation rate is usually greatly raised.

Microscopy

Inflammation involves the arterial media and intima. The infiltration by mononuclear cells is typically associated with multinucleate cells (Figures 7.6 and 7.7). Intimal damage leads to formation of thrombi, which usually become organized, and there may be severe damage to the internal elastic lamina, sometimes going on to complete destruction. Healing is by fibrosis, particularly of the media, thickening of the intima and partial recanalization of the thrombus. Lesions skip short lengths of an artery and a biopsy should be at least 3 cm long.

Management

The possibility of complications, particularly blindness which develops in up to 50% of untreated patients, makes it essential to start treatment early. Systemic prednisolone (starting with 60 mg/day) should be given on the basis of inflamed scalp

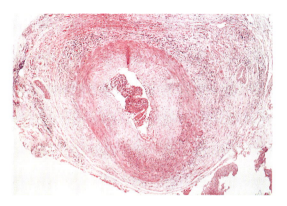

Figure 7.6   Giant cell arteritis (low power). There is intimal proliferation and a medial fibroblastic reaction

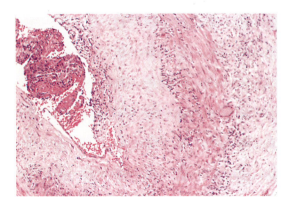

Figure 7.7   Giant cell arteritis. Higher power view shows disruption of the elastic lamina and closely associated multinucleated giant cells

vessels and a high (>70 mm/h) ESR. Corticosteroids are usually quickly effective and should be continued until the ESR falls to normal.

Pain dysfunction syndrome

Pain dysfunction syndrome is probably the most common cause of pain in the temporomandibular joint region. It predominantly affects young women and typical features, in varying combinations, are pain, clicking sounds from the joint and limitation of movement. Despite intensive investigation over several decades and a voluminous literature, no organic disease of the temporomandibular joints has been convincingly demonstrated. However, a significant number of patients have been noted by Buckingham *et al.* (1991) to have hypermobility syndrome.

Aetiology
The female to male predominance is nearly 4 to 1. Most patients are aged between 20 and 40 years. Older persons are rarely affected. There is no evidence that the disease is progressive and goes on to produce permanent changes, or that there is disease of the joint itself. Symptoms may be sufficiently troublesome to justify treatment, but in the majority of patients symptoms resolve after two or three years, even without treatment.

Malocclusions have been held responsible, but the evidence is unconvincing. Lack of posterior occlusal support sometimes appears to be a contributory factor. Trauma, particularly from minor injuries, is a possible factor, but the evidence is anecdotal. However, some abnormal habits seem to contribute. An obvious one is habitual grinding, particularly at night time. The habit of holding a telephone receiver between the shoulder and chin for prolonged periods, to free the hands for writing, and the lateral deviation of the chin to grip the telephone can result in instability of the meniscus on the opposite side. Violinists occasionally have similar trouble. Woodwind and brass players sometimes develop temporomandibular joint symptoms when their embouchure involves abnormal posturing of the mandible. Other patients aggravate their symptoms by habitually and forcefully biting into hard food; in the susceptible patient this too can lead to instability of the meniscus, particularly in patients with a deep overbite. Modification of these habits can lead to relief of symptoms.

Electromyographic and arthrographic studies suggest that incoordination of the upper fibres of the lateral pterygoid muscle attached to the anterior margin of the joint meniscus results in inappropriate movements of the meniscus during opening and closing. This incoordination results in the characteristic clicking and locking.

Patients with pain dysfunction syndrome tested by means of standard psychological scoring methods also appear to have significantly higher scores for neuroticism, anxiety and related factors affecting muscle tension, and significantly lower pain thresholds than controls. Psychiatric factors probably underlie pain dysfunction syndrome in many cases and, in older patients especially, more serious underlying psychopathology has been reported (Kaban and Belfer, 1981).

To summarize, pain dysfunction syndrome typically affects only a restricted group of the population. It has little organic basis, is self-limiting and does not cause permanent damage or degenerative arthritis later in life. Defective neuromuscular coordination and areas of fatigue or spasm in the masticatory muscles appear to be the main cause of the symptoms.

Clinical features
The onset is usually gradual, but a few patients ascribe the onset to violent yawning, laughing or

some similar incident. Pain is usually one-sided and typically a poorly localized dull ache made worse by mastication. The condylar region is the main site. Pain is typically felt in front of the ear, but sometimes felt lower down the ramus, occasionally at the angle of the jaw and, more rarely still, in the neck or occiput.

Limitation of opening or 'locking' of the jaw in the partially open or closed position is frequently associated. A clicking sound associated with deviation, when the mouth is opened or closed, is common. Defects of occlusion can often be found, as they can in asymptomatic patients.

Management

In view of the absence of objective signs, diagnosis is largely by exclusion. Rheumatoid or other arthritis should be excluded by appropriate investigation. Tenderness or swelling of the joint suggests organic disease. Trigeminal neuralgia should be suspected in patients of middle age or over with severe pain, since it can occasionally be triggered by movement of the jaw and is also unassociated with any detectable abnormalities. Trigeminal neuralgia is subject to spontaneous remissions and if remission follows the fitting of an appliance then the wrong conclusions can be drawn. However, the pain of trigeminal neuralgia is far more acute than that of pain dysfunction syndrome and stabbing in character.

Movements of the head of the condyle can be felt through the overlying skin or with a finger in the external auditory meatus. With practice, abnormal excursions or asymmetrical movement of the condyles or crepitus may be detected.

Lateral radiographs of the joints should be taken with the jaw in the open and closed positions, to make sure that movements are equal and not excessive in either direction. The main value of radiographs is to exclude organic disease shown by increased size of the joint space or damage to or deformity of the joint surfaces. Signs of hypermobility should also be sought.

Arthrography, magnetic resonance imaging or direct arthroscopy via a fine endoscope can all be used to demonstrate an unstable meniscus which is often displaced anteriorly. These investigations are invasive or costly or both, but merely serve to confirm the clinical findings. They should be reserved for patients resistant to conservative management or when there is real doubt about diagnosis.

Treatment options may be considered under six main headings:

- reassurance
- use of appliances
- muscle training and modification of habits
- occlusal equilibration
- antidepressive treatment
- surgery.

Many other forms of treatment (sufficient in fact to fill large textbooks) have been recommended, but this is merely another reflection of how little is known about this disorder.

Reassurance Once the diagnosis has been established, reassurance alone is sometimes effective. A benzodiazepine may be helpful for its anxiolytic and muscle relaxant action, but should only be used for a limited period. However, there is wide individual variation in patients' response and the risk of dependence should be borne in mind.

Overlay appliances In many cases an acrylic overlay appliance covering the occlusal surfaces of the teeth is effective. This allows free occlusion without cuspal interference and tends to relieve abnormal grinding habits. It is not uncommon for these patients to be over-closed with a deep anterior overbite and locked occlusion. This also can be managed by means of an appliance, using an anterior bite plane, but full occlusal cover is essential to prevent over-eruption of the posterior teeth.

Overlay appliances should be worn day and night in severe cases and may have to be replaced or built up as necessary, as they wear down during use. The appliances should be firmly fitting and retained by means of cribs. Patients usually accommodate quickly to these appliances which, after a day or so, interfere little with speech or mastication. In many cases, the relief of pain or other symptoms is a strong impetus to continue wearing the appliance.

Overall, the use of these types of appliances is probably the most satisfactory form of treatment. They are usually effective and are much less time-consuming than other methods.

Muscle exercises and modification of habits There is no firm evidence that this time-consuming method of treatment produces any more satisfactory results than the use of overlay appliances.

Antidepressive treatment Pain dysfunction syndrome may sometimes be part of the spectrum of atypical facial pain. Psychiatric assessment and antidepressive treatment is appropriate and successful in such cases.

Occlusal equilibration Objective evidence of the value, other than a placebo effect, of detailed occlusal analysis and equilibration has yet to be established.

Surgery In the USA in particular, surgery is widely used. Over the years many techniques – closed condylotomy, open condylotomy, high condylar shave, condylectomy, capsular rearrangement and reattachment of the joint meniscus – have been advocated. In the short term most of these procedures provide symptomatic relief. This may be due to a placebo effect, surgical denervation of the joint or perhaps modification of some defect such as a dislocated meniscus. However, in the long term the relapse rate is high, and surgery should therefore be reserved for those patients with objective organic joint disease who have failed to respond to more conservative management.

To summarize, pain dysfunction syndrome frequently responds to a relatively simple type of occlusal appliance, and in some patients this may be usefully combined with antidepressive treatment. Harris *et al.* (1993) have reviewed the prosthetic and psychiatric aspects of management of this complaint, and possible medicolegal problems. Surgical interference should generally be avoided.

'Costen's syndrome'

This syndrome was said to comprise headache, ear symptoms (tinnitus or deafness) and burning pain in the tongue and throat and was ascribed to over-closure causing excessive backward movement of the head of the condyle.

This syndrome does not exist, but the term 'Costen's syndrome' persists in medicine and is often thought to be synonymous with pain dysfunction syndrome.

Condylar hyperplasia

Condylar hyperplasia is a rare, usually unilateral, overgrowth of the mandibular condyle. It causes facial asymmetry, deviation of the jaw to the unaffected side on opening, and a crossbite. The condition usually manifests after puberty and is slowly progressive. Pain in the affected joint is variable. Serial models and radiographs are used to monitor the condition. An isotope bone scan confirms the diagnosis by showing greatly increased bone activity in the affected condyle. If the condition is still active at the time of diagnosis, an intracapsular condylectomy should be performed to destroy the active growth centre. If the disease has stabilized – usually at the end of puberty or shortly afterwards – corrective osteotomies should restore the occlusion and facial symmetry.

Neoplasms

Tumours of the temporomandibular joint are rare, but may arise from the condyle   either the bone or articular cartilage – or from the joint capsule. Metastatic tumours such as those from the breast, prostate and thyroid occasionally metastasize to the condylar head (Chapter 6).

Though otherwise rare in the facial skeleton, osteochondroma (Chapter 5) is probably the most common tumour of the condyle or coronoid process, as reviewed by Kerscher *et al.* (1993) who found 30 reports of coronoid osteochondromas, while Forssell *et al.* (1985) were able to find 26 examples of condylar osteochondromas up till then. Osteoma and chondroma and their malignant counterparts may develop, but apart from their interference with joint function and disturbance of occlusion, their behaviour and management are the same as when they arise elsewhere in the jaws. Condylectomy may be required for a neoplasm such as an osteochondroma and an external approach may be used.

Synovial sarcoma is an exceptionally rare tumour and, paradoxically, arises more frequently in the soft tissues adjacent to joints, such as tendons or tendon sheaths, rather than in joint cavities, or in soft tissues unrelated to joints (Chapter 13). White *et al.* (1992), in reporting a synovial sarcoma of the temporomandibular joint, could find only two earlier reports.

Loose bodies in the temporomandibular joints

Loose bodies are rare in the temporomandibular joints compared with other joints. The following types of loose bodies are recognized:

- *Fibrinous:*
  tuberculosis or haemorrhage
  pyogenic arthritis
- *Fibrous:* tuberculosis, syphilis or haemorrhage
- *Cartilaginous:* fragments of meniscus (1–3 bodies)
- *Osteocartilaginous:*
  osteochondritis dissecans (1–3 bodies)
  intracapsular fractures (1–3 bodies)
  osteoarthritis (1–10 bodies)
  synovial chondromatosis (50–500 bodies)
  rheumatoid arthritis
  tuberculosis or syphilis
- *Foreign bodies:* following trauma or surgery.

Osteochondritis dissecans

This is the main cause of loose bodies in joints, most commonly in the knee. It is believed to result from trauma causing an area of subchondral bone to undergo avascular necrosis with subsequent degenerative changes in the overlying articular cartilage. This area subsequently separates to produce one or several loose bodies. In the temporomandibular joint, the patient has discomfort and episodes of locking. The loose body may be seen on tomography, arthrography or arthroscopy. Surgical removal of the loose body, which is always in the lower joint compartment, relieves the symptoms.

Synovial chondromatosis

In this disease, foci of cartilage develop in the synovial membrane; it is thought to be a benign neoplasm. Synovial chondromatosis rarely affects the temporomandibular joint, but can cause swelling and limitation of movement, with deviation to the affected side on opening. Conventional radiographs may show radiopaque masses in the region of the joint capsule, but if no abnormality may be seen, MRI should reveal multiple cartilaginous nodules and distension of the capsule. Both upper and lower joint compartments are involved and exceptionally rarely the process may extend into the cranial cavity (Sun *et al.*, 1990).

Microscopically, there is proliferation and atypia of chondrocytes in the subsynovial connective tissue, with formation of microscopic or larger nodules of cartilage (Figures 7.8 and 7.9). These nodules enlarge, and may calcify and escape into the joint cavity. The appearance of the chondrocytes is such that it is possible to mistake the lesion for a chondrosarcoma if the pathologist is not made aware of the clinical history and operative findings. Fujita *et al.* (1991) demonstrated immunohistochemically that most of the nuclei of the chondrocytes were inactive and that malignancy could be excluded.

Removal of the loose bodies and the whole of the affected synovium are curative. Incomplete excision can be followed by recurrence.

Dislocation

The temporomandibular joint may become fixed in the open position by anterior dislocation; this is due

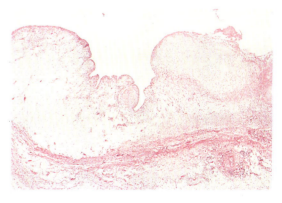

Figure 7.8 Synovial chondromatosis showing chondodroblastic proliferation within the synovial tissue

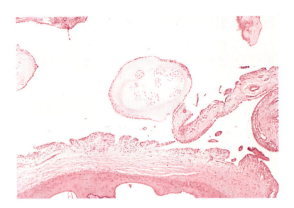

Figure 7.9 Synovial chondromatosis showing exophytic and free cartilaginous islands in the joint space

to forcible opening of the mouth by a blow on the jaw, or during dental extractions under general anaesthesia. In the latter case, the condition should be noticed immediately. It must be corrected before the patient recovers consciousness, by pressing downwards and backwards on the lower posterior teeth. Occasionally a patient will dislocate spontaneously while yawning. Epileptic patients sometimes also dislocate during a fit.

Occasionally the dislocation remains unnoticed and, surprisingly, a patient may tolerate the disability and discomfort for weeks or even months. In these cases, effusion into the joint, following injury, becomes organized to form fibrous adhesions. When this happens, manual reduction may be impossible and open reduction, with division of adhesions, must be carried out.

Recurrent dislocation

Recurrent dislocation of the temporomandibular joint is more common and is typically seen in adolescent girls and young adults. It is a typical feature of floppy joint syndromes, notably Ehlers–Danlos and Marfan's syndromes or the benign type with no underlying systemic disorder.

Techniques advocated for the management of recurrent dislocation have included surgical reduction of the articular eminence (eminectomy), augmentation of the eminence (by bone grafting or by down-fracture of the malar arch using the Dautrey procedure or down-fracture of the eminence with interpositional grafting) and capsular plication to limit condylar movement. Augmentation of the eminence by bone graft or down-fracture of the eminence are overall the most successful procedures.

References

Borle, R.M. and Borle, S.R. (1991) Management of oral submucous fibrosis: a conservative approach. *Journal of Oral and Maxillofacial Surgery,* **49,** 788–791

Buckingham, R.B., Braun, T., Harinstein, D.A. *et al.* (1991) Temporomandibular joint dysfunction: a close association with systemic joint laxity (the hypermobile joint syndrome). *Oral Surgery, Oral Medicine and Oral Pathology,* **72,** 514–519

Chalmers, I.M. and Blair, G.S. (1973) Rheumatoid arthritis of the temporomandibular joint. A clinical and radiological study using circular tomography. *Quarterly Journal of Medicine,* **42,** 369–386

Forssell, H., Happonen, R.-P., Forssell, K. *et al.* (1985) Osteochondroma of the mandibular condyle, report of a case and review of the literature. *British Journal of Oral and Maxillofacial Surgery,* **23,** 183–189

Fujita, S., Iizuka, T., Tuboi, Y. *et al.* (1991) Synovial chondromatosis of the temporomandibular joint with immunohistochemical findings. *Journal of Oral and Maxillofacial Surgery,* **49,** 880–883

Goss, A.N. (1993) Toward an international consensus on temporomandibular joint surgery. Report of the Second International Consensus Meeting, April 1992, Buenos Aires, Argentina. *International Journal of Oral and Maxillofacial Surgery,* **22,** 78–81

Harris, M., Feinmann, C., Wise, M. *et al.* (1993) Temporomandibular joint and orofacial pain: clinical and medicolegal management problems. *British Dental Journal,* **174,** 129–136

Holmlund, A., Reinholt, F. and Bergstedt, H. (1992) Synovial chondromatosis of the temporomandibular joint. Report of a case. *Oral Surgery, Oral Medicine and Oral Pathology,* **73,** 266–268

Jayanthi, V., Probert, C.S.J., Sher, K.S. *et al.* (1992) Oral submucosal fibrosis – a preventable disease. *Gut,* **33,** 4–6

Kaban, L.B. and Belfer, M.L. (1981) Temporomandibular joint dysfunction: an occasional manifestation of serious psychopathology. *Journal of Oral Surgery,* **39,** 742–746

Kerscher, A., Piette, E., Tideman, H. *et al.* (1993) Osteochondroma of the coronoid process of the mandible. *Oral Surgery, Oral Medicine and Oral Pathology,* **75,** 559–564

Könönen, M. (1992) Signs and symptoms of craniomandibular disorders in men with Reiter's disease. *Journal of Craniomandibular Disorders and Facial Pain,* **6,** 247–253

Koorbusch, G.F., Zeitler, D.L., Fotos, P.G. *et al.* (1991) Psoriatic arthritis of the temporomandibular joints with ankylosis. *Oral Surgery, Oral Medicine and Oral Pathology,* **71,** 267–274

Larheim, T.A. and Haanaes, H.R. (1981) Micrognathia, temporomandibular joint changes and dental occlusion in juvenile rheumatoid arthritis of adolescents and adults. *Scandinavian Journal of Dental Research,* **89,** 329–338

Lustmann, J. and Zeltser, R. (1989) Synovial chondromatosis of the temporomandibular joint. Review of the literature and case report. *International Journal of Oral and Maxillofacial Surgery,* **18,** 90–94

Miles, D.A. and Kaugars, G.A. (1991) Psoriatic involvement of the temporomandibular joint. Literature review and report of two cases. *Oral Surgery, Oral Medicine and Oral Pathology,* **71,** 770–774

Pillai, R., Balaram, P. and Reddiar, K.S. (1992) Pathogenesis of oral submucous fibrosis. Relationship to risk factors associated with oral cancer. *Cancer,* **69,** 2011–2020

Rosati, L.A. and Stevens, C. (1990) Synovial chondromatosis of the temporomandibular joint presenting as an intracranial mass. *Archives of Otolaryngology and Head and Neck Surgery,* **116,** 1334–1337

Sun, S., Helmy, E. and Bays, R. (1990) Synovial chondromatosis with intracranial extension. *Oral Surgery, Oral Medicine and Oral Pathology,* **70,** 5–9

White, R.D., Makar, J. and Steckler, R.M. (1992) Synovial sarcoma of the temporomandibular joint. *Journal of Oral and Maxillofacial Surgery,* **50,** 1227–1230

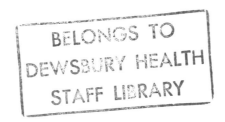

8

Diseases of the oral mucous membranes

Mucosal, particularly ulcerative, diseases include both surgically treatable conditions and non-surgical conditions, though they are not always easy to differentiate. Nevertheless, some of them, such as lupus erythematosus, are important indicators of severe underlying systemic disease. Of current concern is the prevalence of HIV infection, in which any of a great variety of oral mucosal lesions may be seen. If, therefore, stomatitis has unusual features, a resolute attempt should be made to make a firm diagnosis from the history, clinical features, biopsy and, if necessary, other laboratory investigations. Particular attention should be given to the medical and drug history, and whether other mucous membranes or the skin are affected.

Biopsy is mandatory, particularly in the bullous diseases. In such cases, the diagnosis can frequently only be confirmed by microscopy. In other cases, microscopic findings can be less definite, but often (as in the cases of major aphthae, for example) serve to exclude more serious diseases.

Frequently, a critical factor is the adequacy of the specimen and it has never ceased to be a source of wonder to the authors that some surgeons, who may have carried out commando operations leaving little remaining between the eyes and larynx, sometimes produce soft tissue biopsies so small as often (without exaggeration) to be difficult to find in the specimen bottle.

Though the subject of biopsies has been discussed earlier, it must be emphasized again that a mucosal specimen must be at least 1 cm long. In many mucosal diseases, such as lichen planus, the specimen needs to be no more than 5 mm deep, but in others such as Crohn's disease it should be as deep as can safely be made.

Infections

Primary herpetic stomatitis

Primary infection is caused by the herpes simplex virus, usually type 1, which, in the non-immune, results in an acute vesiculating stomatitis. Thereafter, recurrent (reactivation) infections usually take the form of *herpes labialis* (cold sores or fever blisters).

Transmission of herpes is by close contact and where there are large, poor, urban communities, up to 90% develop antibodies to herpesvirus during early childhood. In more affluent countries, the incidence of herpetic stomatitis has declined and it is seen in adolescents or adults, rather than children, and is more common in the immuno-compromised such as in HIV infection. In many British and US cities, by contrast, approximately 70% of 20 year olds may be non-immune, as a result of lack of exposure to the virus.

Clinical features
The early lesions are vesicles which can affect any part of the oral mucosa, but the hard palate and dorsum of the tongue are characteristic sites. The vesicles are dome shaped and usually 2–3 mm in diameter. Recently ruptured vesicles leave flat, yellowish, disc-shaped lesions which progress to circular, sharply defined, shallow ulcers with yellowish or greyish floors and red margins. The ulcers are painful and may interfere with eating.

The gingival margins are frequently swollen and red, particularly in children, and the regional lymph nodes are enlarged and tender. There is often fever and systemic upset, sometimes severe, particularly in adults.

Oral lesions usually resolve within a week to 10 days, but malaise can persist so that an adult may not recover fully for several weeks.

Microscopy

The vesicle is sharply defined and forms in the upper epithelium; the roof is several cells thick and is therefore sufficiently strong that intact vesicles are often seen. Viral-damaged epithelial cells are seen in the floor of the vesicle (Figures 8.1 and 8.2). Direct smears from an early lesion show viral-damaged cells with ballooning degeneration of the nuclei or multinucleate cells. Later, the full thickness of the epithelium is replaced by viral-damaged cells and is destroyed to produce a sharply delimited ulcer.

A rising titre of antibodies, reaching a peak after 2–3 weeks, provides absolute but retrospective confirmation of the diagnosis.

Differential diagnosis

Teething An infant who develops an acutely sore mouth usually has herpetic stomatitis. Acute generalized soreness of the mouth, especially with lymphadenopathy, does not result from teething.

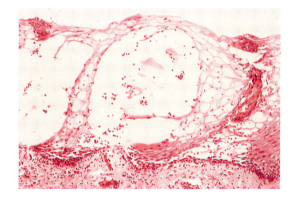

Figure 8.1 Herpes simplex: intraepithelial vesicle showing ballooning degeneration of keratinocytes

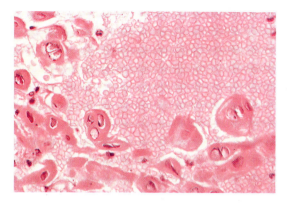

Figure 8.2 Herpes simplex. Multinucleate epithelial giant cells are present in the depths of the vesicle

Acute ulcerative gingivitis (AUG) Herpetic ulcers can sometimes affect the tips of the interdental papillae and adjacent gingiva and be mistaken for acute ulcerative gingivitis. However, vesicles and ulcers elsewhere in the mouth, and the lymphadenopathy or fever of herpes, readily distinguish the conditions. Acute gingival ulceration in children in the Western world is usually herpetic, but acute ulcerative gingivitis may be seen if they are immunocompromised.

Herpes zoster The first symptom is usually pain which may resemble toothache. The lesions have a characteristic distribution on one side of the skin of the face and mucosa supplied by the trigeminal nerve, as discussed below.

Recurrent aphthae Individual ulcers may resemble those of herpetic infection. However, there is usually a history of recurrences, no systemic upset and the regional lymph nodes are rarely enlarged. Usually only two or three aphthae appear in any one crop, are not preceded by vesicles and also, unlike herpes, do not affect the hard palate or gingival margins and rarely the dorsum of the tongue.

Hand-foot-and-mouth disease The infection is usually very much milder than herpetic stomatitis with only one or two small scattered oral ulcers. Intact vesicles are rarely seen, regional lymph nodes are not involved and there is no associated gingivitis. The vesicles on the extremities are distinctive and frequently there is a cluster of cases.

Treatment

Acyclovir is a potent antiherpetic drug. It is of low toxicity and is effective even for potentially lethal herpetic encephalitis or disseminated infection. Acyclovir suspension used as a rinse and then swallowed should accelerate healing of severe herpetic stomatitis if used sufficiently early. In AIDS or other immunodeficient patients, systemic acyclovir (tablets or intravenous injection) may be required.

In mild cases, topical tetracycline suspension, rinsed round the mouth several times a day, relieves soreness and may hasten healing by controlling secondary infection.

Patients who are unwell should preferably be kept in bed and given a soft diet. Young infants readily become dehydrated during the painful stomatitis and may rarely require intravenous rehydration.

Unusually prolonged or severe infections or failure to respond to acyclovir (200–400 mg five times daily by mouth for 7 days) suggest HIV infection. Herpetic ulceration persisting for more than a month is an AIDS-defining illness (Centers for Disease Control, 1987).

Herpes labialis

After the primary infection, the latent virus can be reactivated in 20–30% of patients to cause cold sores (fever blisters). Triggering factors include the common cold and other febrile infections, exposure to strong sunshine, menstruation or occasionally, emotional upsets or local irritation, such as dental treatment. Neutralizing antibodies produced in response to the primary infection are not protective.

Clinically, changes follow a consistent course with prodromal paraesthesia or burning sensations, then erythema at the site of the attack. Vesicles form after an hour or two, usually in clusters along the mucocutaneous junction of the lips, but can extend onto the adjacent skin.

The vesicles enlarge, coalesce and weep exudate. After 2 or 3 days they rupture, the raw area crusts over but new vesicles frequently appear for a day or two only to scab over and finally heal, usually without scarring. The whole cycle may take up to 10 days. Secondary bacterial infection may induce an impetiginous lesion which sometimes leaves scars.

Treatment

In view of the rapidity of the viral damage to the tissues, treatment must start as soon as the premonitory sensations are felt. Acyclovir cream may be effective if applied sufficiently early.

Herpetic cross-infections

Both primary and secondary herpetic infections are contagious. Herpetic whitlow is therefore a recognized though surprisingly uncommon hazard to dental surgeons and their assistants. Herpetic whitlows, in turn, can infect patients and have led to outbreaks of infection in hospitals and among patients in dental practice. In immunodeficient patients such infections can be dangerous, but acyclovir has dramatically improved the prognosis in such cases and is frequently given on suspicion.

Herpes zoster of the trigeminal area

Zoster (shingles) is characterized by pain, a vesicular rash and stomatitis in the related dermatome. The varicella zoster virus (VZV) causes chickenpox in the non-immune (mainly children), while reactivation of the latent virus causes zoster, mainly in the elderly. Unlike herpes labialis, repeated recurrences of zoster are very rare. Occasionally there is an underlying immunodeficiency. Herpes zoster is a hazard in organ transplant patients and can be an early complication of some tumours, particularly Hodgkin's disease or, increasingly, of AIDS where it is five times more common than in HIV-negative persons and potentially lethal.

Clinical features

Herpes zoster usually affects adults of middle age or over, but occasionally attacks even children. The first signs are pain and irritation or tenderness in the dermatome corresponding to the affected ganglion. The pain can be severe and may be felt by the patient as toothache. Prodromal toothache which led to extensive, unjustified dental treatment has been described by Goon and Jacobsen (1988) among others. Malaise and fever are usually associated.

Vesicles form on one side of the face and in the mouth up to the midline. The regional lymph nodes are enlarged and tender. The acute phase usually lasts about a week. Pain continues until the lesions crust over and start to heal, but secondary infection may cause suppuration and scarring of the skin.

The fact that patients are sometimes unable to distinguish the pain of trigeminal zoster from severe toothache has sometimes led to a demand for a tooth to be extracted. When this is done, the rash follows as a normal course of events, and this has given rise to the myth that dental extractions can precipitate facial zoster. Alternatively, the rash may be misinterpreted as an allergic reaction to a local anaesthetic.

Microscopically, the varicella zoster virus produces similar epithelial lesions to those of herpes simplex, but also inflammation of the related posterior root ganglion.

Management

Herpes zoster is an uncommon cause of stomatitis, but readily recognizable. It is distinguished from herpes simplex and other types of stomatitis by:

● pain (usually severe) preceding the rash
● facial rash accompanying the stomatitis
● localization of the lesions to one side, within the distribution of the second and third divisions of the trigeminal nerve.

According to the severity of the attack, oral acyclovir (200–800 mg, 5 times daily, usually for 7 days) should be given at the earliest possible moment, together with analgesics. In immunodeficient patients, intravenous acyclovir is required and may also be justified for this debilitating infection in the elderly.

Complications

Post-herpetic neuralgia mainly affects the elderly. The pain can resemble trigeminal neuralgia but is persistent rather than paroxysmal and unresponsive to carbamazepine. Analgesics may be of some help, but though antidepressants or other drugs

such as amantadine have been tried, there is no consistently reliable treatment. However, transcutaneous electrical stimulation is sometimes effective. Whether very early and vigorous treatment with acyclovir reduces the risk of post-herpetic neuralgia developing remains unconfirmed.

A rare complication is maxillary osteomyelitis and spontaneous tooth exfoliation. Mintz and Anavi (1992), in reporting a case and reviewing earlier reports, managed the bone necrosis by closed nasal-vestibular drainage.

Hand-foot-and-mouth disease

This common, mild viral infection, which often causes minor epidemics among schoolchildren, is characterized by ulceration of the mouth and a vesicular rash on the extremities.

Hand-foot-and-mouth disease is usually caused by strains of Coxsackie A virus. It is highly infectious, frequently spreads through a classroom in schools and may infect a teacher or parent. The incubation period is probably between 3 and 10 days. It should not be confused with foot and mouth disease of cattle, a rhinovirus infection, which rarely affects humans.

Clinical features

The small, scattered oral ulcers usually cause little pain. Intact vesicles are rarely seen, and the gingivae are not affected. Regional lymph nodes are not enlarged except in unusually severe cases, and systemic upset is mild or absent.

The rash consists of vesicles, which are sometimes deep seated, or occasionally bullae. It is mainly seen around the base of fingers or toes, but any part of the limbs may be affected. The rash is often the main feature and such patients are unlikely to be seen by a dentist. In some outbreaks, either the mouth or the extremities alone may be affected. Serological confirmation of the diagnosis is possible but rarely required, as the history, especially of other cases, and clinical features are usually adequate. The disease usually resolves within a week. No specific treatment is available or needed, but myocarditis or encephalitis are rare complications.

Cytomegalovirus infection

Shallow, painful oral ulcers showing typical owl-eye inclusion bodies in the base have been seen in immunodeficient patients, particularly those with AIDS. Though it is not certain whether cytomegalovirus is the cause of the ulcers in these patients, the response of the ulcers to ganciclovir in 3 cases reported by French *et al.* (1991) suggests that it was responsible.

The acute specific fevers

Fevers which cause oral lesions are rarely seen in dentistry. Those which cause vesicular rashes (smallpox and chickenpox) produce the same lesions in the mouth.

In the prodromal stage of measles, Koplik's spots may be seen on the buccal mucosa and soft palate and are pathognomonic. Palatal petechiae or ulceration, involving the fauces especially, are seen in glandular fever and are accompanied by the characteristic, usually widespread, lymphadenopathy.

Kawasaki's disease (mucocutaneous lymph node syndrome)

Kawasaki's disease is endemic in Japan, but though uncommon in Britain it is frequently unrecognized and the cause of a significant mortality.

Clinical features
Children are affected and have persistent fever, oral mucositis, ocular and cutaneous lesions, and acute cervical lymphadenopathy. Oral lesions consist of widespread mucosal erythema with swelling of the lingual papillae (strawberry tongue), but are of minor significance compared with the serious cardiac effects. Other features are discussed in Chapter 14.

Tuberculosis

The recrudescence of tuberculosis in the West is partly a consequence of the AIDS epidemic, and multiply-resistant mycobacteria are becoming widespread. Oral tuberculosis is rare as yet, but is a complication of open pulmonary disease with infected sputum. Elderly men or those with HIV infection are the main victims. The typical lesion is an ulcer on the mid-dorsum of the tongue; the lip or other parts of the mouth are less often affected. The ulcer is typically angular or stellate, with overhanging edges and a pale floor, but can be ragged and irregular. It is painless in its early stages and the regional lymph nodes are usually unaffected.

The diagnosis is rarely suspected until biopsy has shown tubercle follicles in the floor of the ulcer (Figure 8.3). *Mycobacteria* can be demonstrated in the sputum (but rarely in the oral lesion) and chest radiographs show advanced infection.

Tuberculosis or non-tuberculous mycobacterial infection must be considered in patients with AIDS who develop oral ulceration with granuloma formation, microscopically.

No local treatment is needed; oral lesions clear up rapidly if there is effective chemotherapy for the pulmonary infection.

Tuberculous cervical lymphadenopathy (see Chapter 14)

Syphilis

Oral lesions in each stage of syphilis are clinically quite different from each other. Oral lesions are rarely seen or may pass unrecognized.

Primary syphilis

An oral chancre appears 3–4 weeks after infection and may form on the lip, tip of the tongue or, rarely, other oral sites. It consists initially of a firm nodule about 6 or 7 millimetres across. The surface breaks down after a few days, leaving a rounded

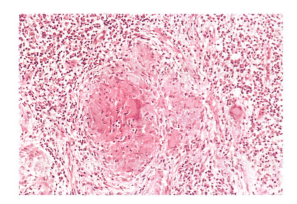

Figure 8.3 Tuberculosis. Tubercle follicle with Langhans multinucleate giant cells in the floor of an ulcer

ulcer with raised indurated edges, which may resemble a carcinoma, if on the lip. However, the appearances are variable. In the absence of secondary infection, the lesion is painless. The regional lymph nodes are enlarged, rubbery and discrete. A biopsy may only show non-specific inflammation but sometimes there is a conspicuous perivascular infiltrate (Figure 8.4).

Serological reactions are negative at first. Diagnosis therefore depends on finding *Treponema pallidum* which can be seen by dark-ground illumination of a smear from the chancre, but must be distinguished from other oral spirochaetes. Clinical recognition of oral chancres is difficult but important. They are highly infective, and treatment is most effective at this stage.

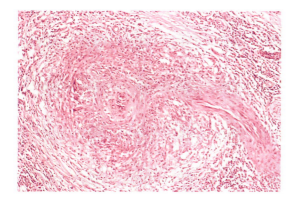

Figure 8.4 Primary syphilis showing conspicuous perivascular inflammatory infiltration

After 8 or 9 weeks the chancre heals, often without scarring.

Secondary syphilis

The secondary stage develops 1–4 months after infection. It typically causes mild fever with malaise, headache, sore throat and generalized lymphadenopathy, soon followed by a rash and stomatitis.

The rash is variable, but typically consists of pinkish (coppery) macules, symmetrically distributed and starting on the trunk. It is not irritating or painful and may last for a few hours or for a few weeks. The presence or history of such a rash is a useful aid to diagnosis. Oral lesions are rarely seen without the rash. The tonsils, lateral borders of the tongue and lips are the main sites, and the usual findings are flat ulcers covered by greyish membrane. The lesions may be irregularly linear (snail's track ulcers) or may coalesce to form well-defined rounded areas (mucous patches).

The discharge from the ulcers contains many spirochaetes and saliva is highly infective. Serological reactions (see below) are positive and diagnostic at this stage, but biopsy is unlikely to be helpful.

Tertiary syphilis

The late stage of syphilis develops in many patients about 3 years of more after infection. The onset is insidious and during the latent period the patient may appear well. A characteristic lesion is the gumma.

Clinically, a gumma, which may affect the palate, tongue or tonsils, can vary from two to several centimetres in diameter. It begins as a swelling, sometimes with a yellowish centre which undergoes necrosis leaving a painless indolent deep ulcer. The ulcer is rounded, with soft, punched-out edges. The floor is depressed and pale (washleather) in appearance. It eventually heals with severe scarring which may distort the soft palate or tongue, or perforate the hard palate or destroy the uvula.

Microscopically, there may be no more than a predominance of plasma cells in the inflammatory infiltrate (a common finding in oral lesions) but associated with peri- or endarteritis. Granuloma

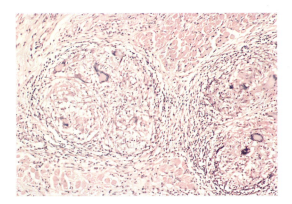

Figure 8.5   Tertiary syphilis – epithelioid granuloma formation

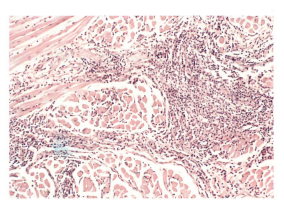

Figure 8.6   Tertiary syphilis – chronic interstitial glossitis. Diffuse chronic inflammatory infiltration of the lingual muscles can be seen

formation (Figure 8.5) may be seen but is rare; also rarely, there may be diffuse chronic inflammatory infiltration of the lingual muscles (Figure 8.6) or coagulative necrosis mimicking caseation. However, even arteritis may be absent and the appearances can be completely non-specific. Diagnosis therefore depends on the serological findings.

Leucoplakia of the tongue may also develop during this late stage (Chapter 9), and other effects of syphilis such as aortitis, tabes or general paresis of the insane may be associated.

Serological diagnosis of syphilis

Tests are either specific, such as the FTA-ABS, or non-specific, such as the VDRL (Table 8.1). The VDRL becomes positive 4–6 weeks after infection, and becomes negative only after effective treatment, but false positives can result from a variety of other causes. The FTA-ABS test acts as a check against false-positive or false-negative results, but remains positive despite effective treatment for the life of the individual.

Table 8.1   Interpretation of serological tests for syphilis

VDRL	FTA-ABS	Usual interpretation
+	–	False-positive
+	+	Active syphilis
–	+	Treated syphilis

Treatment

Antibiotics, particularly penicillin, are the mainstay, but tetracycline and erythromycin are also effective. Treatment must be continued until non-specific serological reactions (VDRL) are persistently negative.

Candidosis

Candidal infection can cause the formation of whitish plaques or areas of erythema. These are discussed in Chapter 9.

Non-infective ulceration

Traumatic ulcers

Traumatic ulcers are usually caused by a denture and often in the buccal or lingual sulcus. They are tender, and have a yellowish floor and red margins; there is no induration. A similar ulcer, caused by the sharp edge of a broken-down tooth, is usually on the tongue or buccal mucosa.

A traumatic ulcer heals a few days after elimination of the cause, and thus confirms the diagnosis. If it persists for more than 7–10 days, or there is any other cause for suspicion, biopsy must be carried out.

Aphthous stomatitis (recurrent aphthae)

Recurrent aphthae are the most common disease of the oral mucosa and may affect 10–20% or more of the population. The distinctive feature is painful shallow ulcers which recur at more or less regular intervals. Ulcers resembling major aphthae can also be a feature of AIDS.

Aetiological aspects
Suggested factors have been extensively reviewed by Scully and Porter (1989) and include the following:

Infection   There is no evidence that herpes simplex or any other virus is the cause. *Streptococcus sanguis* and L-forms have been implicated in the past, but though microorganisms may secondarily infect aphthae there is no evidence that they are a direct cause or that cross-reacting microbial antigens play a significant role.

Immunological aspects   It has been fashionable to regard recurrent aphthae as an autoimmune disease. However, the enormous variety of immunological abnormalities reported over the years have been by no means consistently found. No convincing case for an immunopathogenesis has been made and Jonsson *et al*. (1990), for example, do not include recurrent aphthae in their review of immunologically mediated oral diseases. The facts that the majority of patients are otherwise healthy and that there is no association with, or any other features of, any of the better substantiated autoimmune diseases make it difficult to sustain an autoimmune hypothesis. The microscopic features are also not suggestive of an immunologically mediated reaction and, unlike autoimmune disease, recurrent aphthae are self-limiting in most cases.

Haematological and gastrointestinal disease   Between 10% and 15% of patients with recurrent aphthae may have haematological abnormalities, particularly iron or, less often, folate or vitamin B_{12} deficiency. Folate deficiency itself, though uncommon, is probably one of the few diagnosable and reliably treatable causes of aphthous stomatitis. Typical aphthous stomatitis is occasionally the first overt manifestation of folate deficiency and resolves when folate is given. However, Porter *et al*. (1988), in an investigation into the haematological status of 69 patients with recurrent aphthae, express doubts about the contribution to the oral ulceration of the deficiency states found in over 12% of them.

In the case of a possible association between ulcerative colitis, Crohn's disease or coeliac disease, it is difficult to exclude coincidence, since recurrent aphthae are very common in healthy persons. Nevertheless, intestinal disorders can cause folate or vitamin B_{12} deficiency and may promote aphthae indirectly.

In a minority of women, aphthae are worse premenstrually and may improve during pregnancy.

Clinical features
Patients with recurrent aphthae frequently show mild anxiety or obsessional traits. Extensive surveys, particularly that by Sircus *et al*. (1957), have shown that they come almost exclusively from clerical, semi-professional or professional social groups, and the vast majority are non-smokers. Occasionally, the onset of a severe exacerbation of aphthous stomatitis follows cessation of smoking. Most patients with aphthous stomatitis have mouths that are well cared for and this suggests that local factors may be less important than has been suggested.

Recurrent aphthae often start in childhood or adolescence, peak in early adult life, then wane spontaneously. They usually resolve entirely before middle age and often much earlier.

The frequency, number and size of ulcers is very variable. Many patients have had sporadic small solitary ulcers for many years, but seek treatment because of increasing severity. Most such patients have ulcers at intervals of 2–4 weeks but, in severe cases, ulcers are continuously present – as some heal, others form. Quite commonly, there are remissions of a month or two and this makes the assessment of treatment difficult.

Aphthae appear singly, in crops of two or three or occasionally in much greater numbers. The first symptom is often a pricking sensation as if a toothbrush bristle had stabbed the mucous membrane. The ulcers soon become painful and tender and, in severe cases, may cause difficulties with eating or talking.

The ulcers are usually shallow, circular or elliptical and about 2–4 mm in diameter. The floor of an ulcer is yellowish, with a sharply defined red margin which is sometimes raised by oedema to make the ulcer crater shaped. Pain usually persists for three or four days. Healing follows without scarring in about a week.

Recurrent aphthae have a characteristic distribution which is a useful guide to the diagnosis. Unlike those of herpetic stomatitis, for example, aphthae affect only non-keratinized areas and not the masticatory mucosa of the hard palate or gingival margins. Only patients with severe aphthous stomatitis occasionally have ulcers on the dorsum of the tongue. If ulcers are seen in the vault of the palate, they are unlikely to be aphthae.

Clinical variants

- *Minor aphthae (Mikulicz type)* are by far the most common and have the features already described.
- *Herpetiform aphthae* comprise only a small minority. They are small (2–3 mm) ulcers which may be innumerable and become confluent. There is widespread erythema of the mucous membrane. The term 'herpetiform' applies only to the appearance, not the aetiology. Unlike herpetic ulcers, herpetiform aphthae lack preceding vesicles, are much less sharply defined and are more irregular in size and shape.
- *Major aphthae* also form a minority but are a very severe type, with ulcers one to several centimetres in diameter. They can persist for at least 3 months but sometimes much longer. Healing may be followed by scarring.

Among HIV-positive patients, any of the variants of recurrent aphthae may be seen, but MacPhail *et al.* (1991) report that herpetiform and major aphthae were more common in this group than in HIV-negative persons and also seemed to have coincided with development of immunodeficiency. Patients with major aphthae in particular tended to be more severely immunodeficient and to have lower CD4 counts.

Microscopically, aphthae show non-specific inflammation. Ulceration appears to start with infiltration of the epithelium by leucocytes associated with beads of exudate. A typical ulcer shows a mixed inflammatory infiltrate. In the early lesion, lymphocytes are said to predominate and neutrophils to replace them later, but such descriptions are based on arbitrary estimates of the duration of the lesion. Perivascular cuffing is also said to be characteristic, but in practice is rarely seen.

The main microscopic feature which may possibly distinguish aphthae from traumatic ulcers is that the inflammatory infiltrate may be more intense and extend more deeply.

Diagnosis

The most important feature is the history, often prolonged, of recurrence of ulcers at more or less regular intervals. Differentiation from herpetic stomatitis has been discussed earlier. However, the possibility should also be borne in mind of Behçet's syndrome, of which oral aphthae may be the first sign.

Exceptionally, major aphthae may mimic carcinoma. The history is an important guide, but patients with aphthous stomatitis are just as susceptible to cancer as anyone else. A clinical feature which helps to differentiate cancer from a major aphtha is that carcinomas of this size (one or more cm in diameter) are indurated, whereas a major aphtha remains relatively soft. Nevertheless, biopsy should be carried out where there is any doubt.

Management

Haematological investigation is important mainly in patients whose aphthae start or worsen late in life. Routine blood indices sometimes need to be supplemented with serum iron or ferritin, folic acid or vitamin B_{12} levels. In most cases, deficiency states are latent, and the haemoglobin is within normal limits. A depressed serum ferritin level (sideropenia) is the most common finding.

Any haematinic deficiency should be investigated and treated. However, as already mentioned, such treatment other than for folate deficiency may not improve aphthae significantly. Treatment is there-fore largely empirical and often unsatisfactory. Possible measures include the following:

Corticosteroids Some patients gain relief from Corlan (hydrocortisone sodium succinate 2.5 mg) pellets, allowed to dissolve in the mouth 3 times a day. Others favour the use of soluble betametha-sone (Betnesol) tablets as a mouthwash. Alterna-tively, beclomethasone (Becotide) aerosol can be used to spray more potent corticosteroids on to the ulcers.

Corticosteroids are unlikely to hasten healing of an ulcer, hence patients should preferably take pellets continuously (whether or not ulcers are present) to allow the corticosteroid to act in the earliest stages of ulcer formation, before symptoms develop. This is only feasible for those who have frequent ulcers, that is to say at two- or three-week intervals. Such a regimen should be tried for 2 months, then stopped for a month to assess whether there has been any improvement and whether there is any deterioration without treatment.

There is no evidence that currently available topical oral corticosteroids cause any significant adrenal suppression. Even continuous use of Corlan pellets appears to be harmless, but inter-ruption to assess the effect of treatment can also be regarded as a safety measure.

Tetracycline mouth rinses Despite the absence of any obvious rationale, controlled trials both in Britain and the USA have shown that tetracycline rinses significantly reduce both the frequency and severity of aphthae. Tetracycline may be used in conjunction with an antifungal drug. Tetracycline mixture (250 mg of tetracycline in 10 ml of fluid) can be held in the mouth for 2–3 min, 3 times daily. This should be done as soon as the patient feels that ulcers are starting to develop, but some find it helpful to use this mouth bath regularly for 3 days each week if they have frequent ulcers.

Chlorhexidine A 0.2% solution held in the mouth 3 times daily for at least 1 min after meals may sometimese lessen the duration and discomfort of aphthae to some degree. Zinc sulphate or zinc chloride solutions may also have some beneficial effect.

Topical salicylate preparations Salicylates have an anti-inflammatory action, and choline salicylate in a gel can be applied to aphthae. These prepar-ations, available over the counter, may help some patients with mild aphthae.

Cyclosporin Eisen and Ellis (1990) have reported successful treatment of recurrent aphthae with cyclosporin, but not all cases responded.

Major aphthae remain a difficult therapeutic problem. Systemic corticosteroids may give short-lived relief, then lose their effectiveness. Thalido-mide appears to be the drug most likely to give relief. Dapsone and azathioprine have also been claimed to be effective in some patients. Relief of major aphthae in patients with AIDS may follow treatment with zidovudine. All of these drugs have significant toxic effects, but their use may be justified for so severe a complaint. Scully and Porter (1989) have reviewed the agents used in the management of recurrent aphthae as well as the aetiology and pathogenesis.

Ultimately, topical local analgesics, such as lignocaine gel, are often the only preparations that allow the patient to eat in relative comfort.

In view of the lack of reliably effective treatment of aphthae, it is important to point out to patients, first, that there is no certain cure; second, that it is probable that the condition can be palliated and made at least tolerable and, third, that the disease is self-limiting, and that sooner or later it will clear up spontaneously.

Behçet's syndrome

This disease, which is rare in Britain, is character-ized by oral aphthae of any of the types described above, associated with eye lesions (particularly iridocyclitis), genital ulceration, thrombophlebitis, pyoderma, sometimes arthritis and other more or less severe systemic lesions. Young adult males aged between 20 and 40 years are chiefly affected. Diagnosis depends on recognizing the concurrence of the multi-site lesions: there are no definitive laboratory tests, so that, as Wechsler and Piette

(1992) have pointed out, confirmation of the diagnosis is sometimes difficult. The aetiology is still speculative and treatment is largely symptomatic. When major oral aphthae are troublesome, thalidomide may be the most effective treatment.

Lichen planus

Lichen planus, a common chronic inflammatory mucocutaneous disease, can give rise to white lesions, atrophic areas or erosions.

Aetiology
In spite of histological changes, which can be highly characteristic and specific, the aetiology of lichen planus remains obscure.

The predominantly T-lymphocyte infiltrate suggests the possibility of cell-mediated immunological damage to the epithelium. Nevertheless, tests of cellular immune responses to extracts of skin lesions of lichen planus have produced inconclusive results so far, and it has not been possible to demonstrate humoral or lymphocytotoxic mechanisms.

The fact that a disease indistinguishable from lichen planus can be induced by various drugs also suggests involvement of an immunopathogenesis. Lichen planus is also a characteristic feature of graft-versus-host disease, but nevertheless is not causally associated with any of the recognized autoimmune diseases. Lichen planus responds to immunosuppressive drugs (though not when associated with graft-versus-host-disease), but the nature of any immunological mechanism remains unclear.

The belief that lichen planus may be associated with an unusually high incidence of glucose intolerance or diabetes mellitus or, alternatively, with rheumatoid arthritis has not been confirmed. The so-called Grinspan syndrome of lichen planus, diabetes mellitus and hypertension appears to be no more than a chance association of these common disorders or related to the drugs used.

The traditional view that lichen planus is associated with emotional stress is difficult to evaluate or substantiate.

Clinical features
The white lesions are frequently asymptomatic. Nevertheless, lichen planus is probably the only disease which, if untreated, can cause unrelieved soreness of the mouth for many years. Middle-aged or older people are predominantly affected and the disease is rarely seen before the age of 30 years. Women account for at least 65% of patients.

The lesions have characteristic clinical appearances and distribution. Both features should be taken into account in making the diagnosis.

Striae are sharply defined and form lacy, starry or annular patterns. They may occasionally be interspersed with minute, white papules: rarely, papules may predominate. Striae may be impalpable or felt to have a stringy texture. Less common types of white lesions are confluent plaques. The latter are more likely to be seen on the dorsum of the tongue or in other sites in long-standing disease.

Atrophic areas, with redness and thinning but not ulceration of the mucosa, are often combined with striae.

Erosions are widespread, shallow irregular areas of epithelial destruction, usually covered by a slightly raised yellowish layer of fibrin. This appearance often gives rise to the idea that they are intact or recently ruptured bullae. However, bullous lichen planus is a rarity that is hardly ever authenticated.

The margins of erosions may be slightly sunken due to fibrosis and gradual healing at the periphery. Patterns of striae radiating from the margins of erosions may also be seen.

These three types of lesion have corresponding microscopic features.

Distribution
By far the most frequently affected sites are the buccal mucosa, particularly posteriorly, but the lesions may spread forward almost to the commissures. The next most common site is the tongue, either the edges or the lateral margins of the dorsum or less frequently the centre of the dorsum. Atrophic lichen planus often involves the gingivae, but striae are rare there. The lips are sometimes involved, but the palate is rarely, and the floor of the mouth hardly ever affected.

Lesions are very often symmetrical, often strikingly so, but may be more prominent on one side than another. Rarely, erosions may be the only sign or may precede the appearance of striae.

On the tongue, the lesions frequently form a narrow whitish band of depapillation along each side of the dorsum, sometimes with elongated erosions in the centre of each band. Occasionally, a dense snowy white (leucoplakia-like) plaque with irregular margins forms in the centre of the dorsum.

Gingival lichen planus

Gingival involvement may be the predominant feature, and needs to be distinguished from other types of gingivitis. Atrophic lesions are most common, the epithelium is then thin and appears almost transparent, shiny, red and smooth. Unlike marginal gingivitis, the inflammation can extend to the reflection of the mucosa, but may spare the gingival margin. Gingival lichen planus is often also patchily distributed and may involve the gingiva of only three or four teeth in one quadrant of the mouth. Also, it only affects the lingual and palatal gingivae uncommonly. Striae are rare on the gingivae, but may be present elsewhere in the mouth.

The soreness caused by these atrophic changes – often in the past labelled non-specifically as 'desquamative gingivitis' – makes toothbrushing difficult. Accumulation of plaque and associated inflammation seem to aggravate lichen planus, and a vicious circle is set up. The contribution of local irritation to gingival lichen planus is suggested by the fact that it disappears when the teeth are extracted. Lichen planus under a denture is virtually unknown.

Symptoms are variable. Striae may only be noticed by chance by a dentist. In others, striae may cause a sensation of roughness or slight stiffness of the mucous membrane. Atrophic lesions are sore and erosions may make eating difficult.

Skin lesions

Lichen planus is a common skin disease and 25–35% of patients with oral lichen planus may also have skin involvement. The skin lesions characteristically form purplish, 2–3 mm papules. They have a glistening surface marked by fine (Wickham's) striae which may only be visible with a magnifying glass. The rash is usually irritating and its appearance may be changed by scratching. Skin lesions should be looked for on the flexor surface of the forearms, especially on the wrists.

Microscopy

The classical features can be summarized as follows:

● a saw-tooth profile of the rete ridges
● liquefaction degeneration of the basal cell layer
● a band-like lymphohistiocytic infiltrate which hugs the epitheliomesenchymal junction.

Striae show parakeratosis or hyperorthokeratosis, sometimes with a prominent granular cell layer. The rete ridges tend to be pointed and saw-tooth in shape (Figure 8.7). Along the junction between the epithelium and connective tissue there may be degeneration and liquefaction, with beads of fluid accumulating along the basement membrane. The basal cell layer is not usually identifiable as such but colloid (Civatte) bodies (prematurely keratinized basal keratinocytes) may be present in the depths of the epithelium or extruded into the immediately underlying connective tissue (Figure 8.8). Fibrinogen deposition along the basement membrane zone may be conspicuous and there is often pigmentary incontinence (Figure 8.9).

In the corium, the infiltrate consists mainly of T lymphocytes, packed beneath the epithelium in a band-like distribution. These inflammatory cells form a compact zone which hugs the epitheliomesenchymal junction and has a well-defined lower border.

Atrophic lesions show severe thinning and flattening of the epithelium, but the inflammatory infiltrate often retains its characteristic distribution and may be more dense.

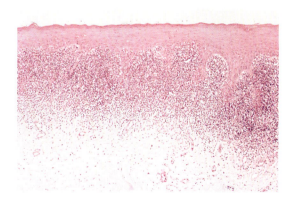

Figure 8.7 Lichen planus. Low-power view shows parakeratosis, saw-tooth rete ridges and dense, band-like chronic inflammatory infiltration of the superficial corium

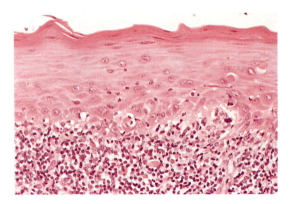

Figure 8.8 Lichen planus. Higher power view shows basal cell liquefaction degeneration with loss of clear delineation of the basal keratinocytes from the underlying dense lymphohistiocytic infiltrate. Eosinophilic colloid (Civatte) bodies are present in the epithelium and within the inflammatory infiltrate

In erosions, destruction of the epithelium leaves only the granulating connective tissue floor of the lesion, so that the appearances are non-specific. The diagnosis must be confirmed by finding typical lesions elsewhere in the mouth.

In many cases the microscopic features are not absolutely distinctive and no more than 'consistent with' lichen planus or difficult to distinguish from lupus erythematosus. The diagnosis must then be made in conjunction with the clinical features and laboratory investigation to exclude lupus erythematosus.

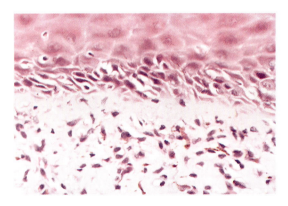

Figure 8.9 Lichen planus. Basal cell liquefaction degeneration, a sparse inflammatory infiltrate and pigmentary incontinence with melanin taken up by macrophages (melanophages) are shown

Management

The diagnosis of lichen planus can usually be made on the history, appearance and distribution of the lesions. If there is any doubt, a biopsy should be taken, particularly when striae are ill-defined. A streaky appearance is occasionally produced by dysplastic leucoplakias.

Tetracycline mouth baths (used as described for recurrent aphthae) seem sometimes to encourage erosions to heal. Hydrocortisone pellets or betamethasone mouth rinses are sometimes useful, but more potent anti-inflammatory corticosteroids such as beclomethasone aerosols sprayed into the mouth 4–6 times a day are probably more effective.

Thrush can be a side effect of the more potent topical corticosteroids, so that an antifungal drug such as miconazole may have to be given concurrently.

Gingival lichen planus is the most difficult to treat. The first essential is to maintain rigorous oral hygiene. If this cannot be maintained, the chances of improvement are small. Corticosteroids should be used in addition, as described above. In this site, triamcinalone dental paste may be relatively easy to apply.

In exceptionally severe cases and if topical oral treatment fails, systemic corticosteroids are effective. Alternatively, intralesional corticosteroids may be tried. Eisen *et al.* (1990) reported cyclosporin mouth rinses to be effective in a small group of patients.

Prognosis

As indicated earlier, lichen planus can be remarkably persistent, if untreated. In the past, patients have been known to have the disease for 20 or even 30 years. However, current treatment with potent corticosteroids is likely to be effective and patients with such long-standing disease are rarely seen.

The potential of lichen planus for malignant change has for long been controversial. A study by Holmstrup *et al.* (1988) involved 611 patients followed for a mean period of 7.5 years and, in this group, malignant change developed in 9 patients (1.5%). All the latter, except one, were women and malignant change followed the initial diagnosis after a mean period of 10 years (range 5–24 years). Compared with the estimated cancer risk in the population of Denmark, lichen planus would thus appear to increase it approximately 50-fold. Voute *et al.* (1992), in their follow-up study of

113 patients, concluded that the 3 cases of oral cancer found after an average period of 7 years provided 'some but not very strong support' for the belief that lichen planus was premalignant, because of doubt about the original diagnosis. However, Holmstrup (1992), on the basis of five previous studies reported since 1985, felt that there was no longer any doubt about this risk and that its magnitude was between 0.5% and 2.5%, but was unable to identify any predictive factors.

Drug-associated lichen planus

A great variety of drugs, notably methyldopa, gold and antimalarial agents, and contact with amalgam restorations, have been reported to cause disease indistinguishable from lichen planus. The treatment is, wherever possible, to change the drug or restoration for an appropriate alternative.

Lupus erythematosus

Lupus erythematosus is an uncommon connective tissue disease which has two main forms, namely systemic and discoid. Either can give rise to oral lesions which may appear similar to those of oral lichen planus. Systemic lupus erythematosus has protean effects. Arthralgias and rashes are most common, but virtually any organ system or serous surface can be affected. The most serious consequences are from renal or cerebral involvement. A great variety of autoantibodies is produced and, of these, antinuclear antibodies are the most characteristic and regularly detectable.

Discoid lupus is essentially a skin disease with mucocutaneous lesions indistinguishable clinically from those of systemic lupus. These may be associated with arthralgia but, rarely, significant autoantibody production.

Clinically, oral lesions are found in about 20% of cases of systemic lupus, in an unknown number of patients with discoid disease and can rarely be the presenting signs of this disease. Typical lesions are white, often striate, areas with irregular atrophic areas or shallow erosions, but the patterns, particularly those of the striae, are typically far less sharply defined than in lichen planus and in

discoid disease in particular. They often involve only a small area of one side of the mouth and may be in the vault of the palate – an unlikely site for lichen planus.

Lesions can be widespread and form variable patterns of white and red areas. There may also be small slit-like ulcers just short of the gingival margins. In about 30% of cases, Sjögren's syndrome develops and, rarely, cervical lymphadenopathy (Chapter 14) is the first clinical sign.

Microscopically, the oral lesions of discoid and systemic lupus show an irregular pattern of epithelial atrophy and acanthosis. The downgrowths of the latter may be flame-like in contour or long and slender, extending deeply into the corium (Figure 8.10). There may be surface keratinization which may rarely appear to be invaginating the epithelium (keratotic plugging) (Figure 8.11), liquefaction degeneration of the basal cell layer and thickening of the basement membrane zone by deposition of antigen/antibody complexes, which also appear in blood vessel walls, as shown by PAS staining. In the corium there is oedema and often a hyaline appearance. The inflammatory infiltrate is highly variable in density, typically extends deeply into the connective tissue and may have a perivascular distribution, but is frequently scanty in the lamina propria.

Though the appearances can sometimes be suggestive of either lichen planus or lupus erythematosus, the latter is unlikely to show the regular

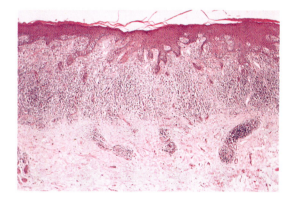

Figure 8.10 Lupus erythematosus. Low power shows hyperkeratosis, irregular acanthosis with flame-like downgrowths of the rete ridges and a dense inflammatory infiltrate both in the superficial corium and having a perivascular distribution more deeply

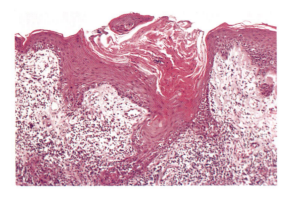

Figure 8.11 Lupus erythematosus. There is irregular epithelial hyperplasia and conspicuous keratotic plugging

patterns of acanthosis or, more particularly, the band-like distribution of lymphocytes in the papillary corium. Karjalainen and Tomich (1989), in a statistical analysis of a range of microscopic features seen in lichen planus and lupus erythematosus, found that distinguishing features of the latter were vacuolization of keratinocytes, thick patchy PAS-positive sub-epithelial deposits, oedema of the upper lamina propria, PAS-positive thickening of blood vessel walls and dense, deep or perivascular inflammatory infiltrate.

Using frozen sections, a band of immunoglobulins and complement (C3) with a granular texture deposited along the line of the basement membrane may be shown by immunofluorescence. This deposit underlies the lesions alone in discoid disease, but also underlies normal epithelium in systemic disease. In paraffin sections, immunoglobulin deposits may be detectable using immunoperoxidase staining. The only other feature that distinguishes systemic from discoid lupus microscopically is the characteristic, but rare, finding of frank vasculitis in the former.

Diagnosis of discoid lupus depends on the clinical features and particularly, rashes, often of a photosensitivity type. The autoantibody findings are of little importance except to distinguish discoid from systemic disease.

Mild systemic lupus can be difficult to distinguish clinically from discoid disease, and rarely there can be transition from discoid to systemic disease. However, systemic lupus should be recognizable by the pattern of autoantibody production. The most specific is that to double-stranded (native) DNA (dsDNA, nDNA).

Haematological findings in active SLE include a raised ESR, anaemia and, often, leucopenia or thrombocytopenia. Renal involvement is indicated by haematuria, proteinuria and red and white cell casts.

Oral lesions of discoid and systemic lupus respond in some degree to topical corticosteroids. Mild systemic lupus may be treated with anti-inflammatory agents alone, but more severe disease requires systemic corticosteroid or other immunosuppressive treatment. However, oral lesions frequently do not respond to doses of corticosteroids adequate to control systemic effects of the disease. Under such circumstances, palliative treatment is needed until disease activity abates.

Prognosis

Systemic lupus was thought at one time to have a high mortality and though uncommon, cerebral disease or, to a lesser degree, renal disease can be life-threatening. However, very many cases are relatively mild and ultimately self-limiting. Under such circumstances, over-enthusiastic immunosuppressive treatment can cause more trouble than the disease. As with other connective tissue diseases, there is an increased risk of cancer, especially lymphomas.

Pemphigus vulgaris

Pemphigus is a rare disease characterized by formation of vesicles or bullae on skin and mucous membranes and is usually fatal if untreated.

Aetiology

An immunopathogenesis can more readily be demonstrated in pemphigus than in any other oral disease. The two main findings are, first, a raised titre of antibodies (predominantly IgG) to the intercellular substances of the epithelium and, second, antibodies demonstrable by immunofluorescence along the intercellular junctions of the epithelium. The antibodies are tissue-specific and react only to the intercellular substance of squamous epithelium.

Clinical features

Women usually in the fourth or fifth decade are predominantly affected. Lesions may be seen first in the mouth but later involve the skin, particularly the trunk.

The vesicles are fragile and rarely seen intact in the mouth. A common appearance is therefore that of several small irregular erosions. These often have ragged edges and are superficial, painful and tender. When the mucous membrane is gently stroked, a vesicle or bulla may appear (Nikolsky's sign). Fluid taken from a recently ruptured vesicle should show characteristic rounded acantholytic epithelial (Tzanck) cells in a stained smear.

The rate of progress of the disease is very variable. It may be fulminating, with rapid development of widespread ulceration of the mouth and spread to other sites such as the eye within a few days and very soon afterwards to the skin. Occasionally, lesions may remain localized to the mouth for months or longer before they involve the skin.

The cutaneous vesicles or bullae vary from a few millimetres to several centimetres across. They at first contain clear fluid which may then become purulent or haemorrhagic. Rupture of the vesicles leaves painful erosions, with ragged margins of loose epithelium, which gradually crust over.

Microscopy

The essential feature is the loss of attachment of epithelial cells to each other (acantholysis). The changes are intra-epithelial and first seen as clefts just superficial to the basal cell layer (Figures 8.12 and 8.13). These splits widen until clinically visible vesicles or bullae form and finally rupture. The separated (acantholytic) epithelial cells become rounded, with their cytoplasm contracted round the nucleus (Figure 8.14), and can often be seen in small groups within a vesicle. Direct immuno-fluorescence, showing binding of immunoglobu-lins to the intercellular substance of the epithelium (Figure 8.15), is confirmatory. Electron microscopy has confirmed that this is the antibody-binding site.

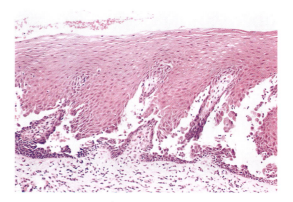

Figure 8.12   Pemphigus vulgaris. Suprabasal acantholysis has caused intra-epithelial vesiculation

Management

The severity of the disease may sometimes be such that the diagnosis must be confirmed as quickly as possible. As lesions spread over the body, loss of protein, fluid and electrolytes from the raw areas becomes severe and they readily become second-arily infected. Without treatment, death usually follows from septicaemia, but immunosuppressive drugs are usually life-saving. However, some cases pursue an indolent course.

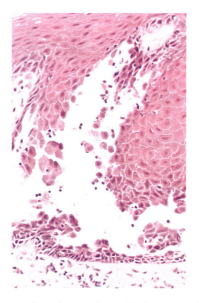

Figure 8.13   Pemphigus vulgaris. Higher power shows the rounded, acantholytic cells

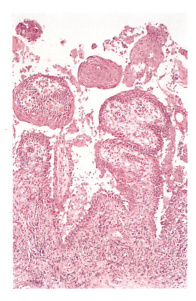

Figure 8.14 Pemphigus vulgaris. The roof of the blister has been lost during biopsy and the floor shows villous proliferation with the connective tissue processes still covered by epithelial basal cells

Biopsy is essential and the changes are usually sufficiently characteristic to make a diagnosis. Once the diagnosis has been confirmed, adequate immunosuppressive treatment is required. Systemic corticosteroids are the main standby but, to keep the dose within acceptable limits, azathioprine is usually also given. Treatment may have to be lifelong and withdrawal of treatment

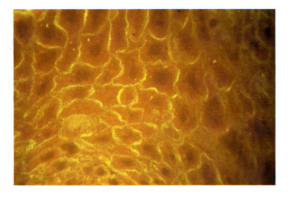

Figure 8.15 Pemphigus vulgaris. Immunofluorescent staining with anti-IgG shows deposits of immunoglobulin in the intercellular area

typically leads to relapse. However, immunosuppressive treatment can cause severe, even fatal, complications. Rarely, a patient may have non-progressive disease, as described by Lamey *et al.* (1992) who reviewed the response and alternative treatments for pemphigus.

Darier's disease (keratosis follicularis)

Darier's disease is a rare dominantly inherited genodermatosis characterized by acantholysis but, unlike pemphigus vulgaris, does not cause intraoral vesiculobullous lesions.

Clinically, the cutaneous lesions of Darier's disease include keratotic papules mainly of the upper parts of the body, palmar pits and dystrophy of the nails. The frequency of oral lesions ranges from 15% to 50% of patients. The palate is predominantly affected; it appears pebbly or may resemble smoker's keratosis. Recurrent salivary gland swelling due to duct obstruction was seen in 30% of 24 patients reported by Macleod and Munro (1991). Isolated oral lesions in the absence of skin disease have been termed *warty dyskeratoma*.

Microscopically, there is localized hyperkeratosis, acantholysis with suprabasal cleft formation and dyskeratosis. The last gives rise to large cells with eosinophilic cytoplasm (*corps ronds*) and pyknotic elongated nuclei (*grains*). Acantholysis appears to result from a defect of the tonofilament–desmosome complex.

Current treatment is with retinoids. Toxic effects limit their long-term tolerance, but even in the absence of treatment the disease is not disabling.

Epidermolysis bullosa

Epidermolysis bullosa (EB) is characterized by skin fragility and bulla formation. There are three main heritable types (dystrophic, junctional and simplex – each with several subtypes and different modes of inheritance), categorized according to the level of tissue cleavage. There is also an acquired type which appears to be immunologically mediated.

Wright *et al.* (1991), in an analysis of the variants of hereditary EB in 216 patients, found oral lesions in up to 100% of the recessive and 81% of the dominant dystrophic types, respectively. Oral lesions were present in up to 92% of the junctional types and in up to 59% of the simplex types, and were more frequent in association with generalized disease.

Clinically, oral lesions range from intermittent blistering in simplex-type disease to almost continuous blistering in response to minimal trauma and severe scarring in the generalized recessive dystrophic type. Scarring can be such as to obliterate the sulci, tie down the tongue and lead to microstomia. Intra-oral bulla formation can be severe in the junctional type, but disabling scarring is rare. In addition to blistering, intra-oral milia (small intra-epithelial cysts) may be seen particularly in dominant dystrophic EB, and appear as small papular swellings.

Microscopically, the different types of epidermolysis bullosa are distinguished by the level of cleavage. Cleavage can be intra-epithelial (epidermolytic, simplex type), through the lamina lucida (junctional type) or sub-epithelial (dermolytic, dystrophic type). In the simplex type, the mechanism is unusual in that cleavage is through the cytoplasm of basal cells and may be the result of a defect in keratin filaments, causing them to be fragile. As described earlier, the dystrophic type most frequently affects the oral mucosa and leads to the most severe scarring. In the dominant dystrophic type, intra-oral milia may form, probably as the result of epithelial cells becoming entrapped during blister formation.

Management

If seen sufficiently early, rigorous preventive dentistry needs to be enforced in all patients with a tendency to intra-oral scarring. Extreme gentleness during dental treatment is necessary to minimize trauma and prevent further damage to the oral mucosa, particularly in recessive dystrophic disease. It is essential to preserve the natural dentition, as distortion of normal oral morphology by scarring can make the retention of dentures impossible even if they could be tolerated. Patients with junctional type EB may be able to tolerate normal dental procedures once the potential for scarring has been assessed. In some patients, phenytoin lessens the frequency of cutaneous blistering and is worth giving prophylactically for dental treatment in any patients with a tendency to intra-oral scarring. Wright (1990) has described the dental care and anaesthetic management of patients with hereditary EB.

In generalized recessive dystrophic EB there is an enhanced risk of malignant change, either extra- or intra-oral in the scarred tissue. In those who survive into their thirties, regular oral examination is necessary to detect any carcinomatous change as early as possible.

Mucous membrane pemphigoid

Mucous membrane pemphigoid is an uncommon chronic disease causing bullae, painful erosions and sometimes scarring, particularly of mucous membranes. There can be serious complications such as blindness, but the disease is not lethal.

Clinical features

Women are mainly affected, and are usually aged over 50 years. The oral mucosa is often first affected and frequently the only site. Other sites are the eyes or the mucous membranes of the nose, larynx or oesophagus. The skin is rarely affected or to only a minor degree. Lesions are rarely widespread and progress is typically indolent.

In the mouth, bullae can often be seen intact but are sometimes filled with blood. Rupture of bullae leaves raw areas with a well-defined margin. Individual erosions can persist for weeks or months before healing. Further erosions may develop nearby and the process can persist for years. Other mucous membranes may eventually be involved. Nevertheless, in many patients lesions may remain localized to the mouth for very long periods.

Microscopy

Bulla formation results from loss of attachment of the epithelium to the connective tissue and is in the region of the basal lamina. In contrast to pemphigus, there is no acantholysis, but sub-epithelial bulla formation with separation of the full thickness of the epithelium from the connective tissue (Figure 8.16). Epithelium forms the roof of a bulla while the floor is formed by the corium, infiltrated with inflammatory cells which may also be seen in the bulla cavity.

The disease appears to be immunologically mediated, but linear deposition of immunoglobulin along the basement membrane zone is less readily demonstrable than complement components (Figure 8.17). Circulating autoantibodies against basement membrane zone proteins are detectable in low titre if sufficiently sensitive techniques are used.

Bullous pemphigoid is a similar disease but affects the skin, rarely involves the mouth and circulating autoantibodies are more readily and frequently detectable. It is also more frequent in males.

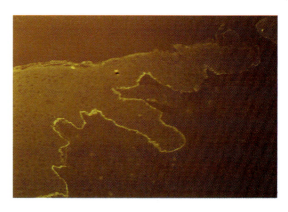

Figure 8.17　Mucous membrane pemphigoid. Deposition of C3 at the epitheliomesenchymal junction is shown by immunofluorescence

Management

The diagnosis can usually be confirmed by biopsy and immunofluorescence microscopy, but it is essential to obtain an intact vesicle or bulla. Nikolsky's sign may be positive, as in pemphigus vulgaris, and a striking clinical finding is that the epithelium may slide away beneath the edge of the knife, however sharp, when biopsy is attempted.

When the diagnosis has been made, the patient should be referred for ophthalmological examination. Scarring leading to impairment or loss of sight is the most serious complication. Rarely,

fibrosis can cause stenosis of the larynx or oesophagus.

When localized to the mouth, mucous membrane pemphigoid can often be controlled with topical corticosteroids for very long periods, if not entirely. This treatment is usually without significant side effects and delays the need for giving systemic steroids with their attendant complications. However, if there is any sign of spread of the disease, particularly to the eyes, systemic corticosteroids should be given and are effective.

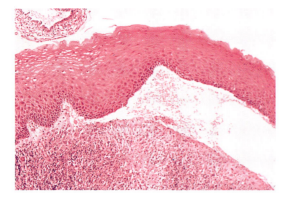

Figure 8.16　Mucous membrane pemphigoid. A subepithelial blister has been formed by separation of the full thickness of the epithelium from the connective tissue, which has become inflamed

Linear IgA disease

Linear IgA disease affects the skin more frequently than the mouth but can closely resemble mucous membrane pemphigoid for which it has frequently been mistaken. Both are characterized by subepithelial bulla formation, but linear IgA disease (as its name implies) shows linear deposition of IgA along the basement membrane zone by immunofluorescence microscopy, and low titres of circulating IgA antibodies to basement membrane zone antigen may be detectable (Chan *et al.*, 1990; Porter *et al.*, 1992).

Linear IgA disease tends to be unresponsive to topical corticosteroids but may be controlled with dapsone or a sulphonamide, although a systemic corticosteroid may also need to be given.

Dermatitis herpetiformis

Dermatitis herpetiformis is of unknown aetiology, but about 70% of patients have histological evidence of coeliac disease, although clinically evident malabsorption is uncommon.

Clinically, males are affected twice as frequently as females and an intensely itchy vesiculopapular rash mainly on the face, scalp, extremities and shoulders is typical. Oral involvement is rare but ranges from mild erythematous patches to painful erosions due to ruptured bullae.

Microscopically, IgA is deposited in the basement membrane zone of the tips of the papillary corium and associated with papillary tip micro-abscesses.

Management

The microscopic and immunofluorescence findings should enable a distinction to be made from linear IgA disease. If the lesions are troublesome, there is a typically dramatic response to dapsone or some-times to a gluten-free diet. The latter is safer but difficult to maintain.

'Desquamative gingivitis'

This is not a diagnosis but a clinical description of diseases which cause the gingivae to appear red or raw. Usually the attached gingiva of varying numbers of teeth is affected. Atrophic lichen planus is the most common cause: less frequent is mucous membrane pemphigoid where the gingivae are typical sites of bulla formation and erosions. Linear IgA disease is a rare cause.

Unlike simple marginal gingivitis, the gingival margins are frequently spared, but the diagnosis should be confirmed by biopsy.

Bullous erythema multiforme (Stevens–Johnson syndrome)

In this mucocutaneous disease the mouth is probably invariably affected, and is often the only site, particularly among patients coming to dental practice, as in 95 patients reported by Lozada-Nur *et al.* (1989).

Aetiology

The cause is not clear, though the disease may be a reaction to a variety of triggering agents. The latter include some infections, notably herpes simplex or mycoplasmal pneumonia and drugs, particularly sulphonamides. Barbiturates and penicillamine have also been blamed, but it is very rare to obtain a positive drug history. Even when drugs are being taken, they are not necessarily the cause.

The disease is regarded by some as being immunologically mediated, but no convincing mechanism has been proposed and in many, if not the majority, of patients no precipitating cause can be found.

Clinical features

Teenagers or young adults, particularly males, are predominantly affected. The most conspicuous feature is often the grossly swollen, crusted and bleeding lips. Within the mouth there are usually widespread irregular erosions with ill-defined margins and widespread erythema.

The eyes are the next most frequently affected site and conjunctivitis of variable severity may be seen. Dermal lesions may consist of widespread erythema alone or characteristic target lesions. These are red macules, a centimetre or more in diameter with a bluish cyanotic centre. In severe cases, large bullae form. The attack usually lasts for three or four weeks, with new crops of lesions developing over a period of about 10 days. Recurrences, usually at intervals of several months, for a year or two are characteristic but occasionally the disease is chronic and persistent.

In the most severe cases the patient is acutely ill after prodromal fever and constitutional distur-bance and the term *Stevens–Johnson syndrome* is applied to this type of disease. Ocular damage can impair sight and rarely cause blindness. Even more rarely, renal damage can be fatal.

Microscopy

The histological appearances are variable. Wide-spread necrosis with eosinophilic colloid change in the superficial epithelium may be an obvious feature. Though not specific, this may progress to intra-epithelial vesiculation (Figure 8.18). Vesicles or bullae can also be sub-epithelial (Figure 8.19) and there is dense infiltration of the corium by inflammatory cells. These may have a perivascular distribution but true vasculitis is absent.

There is no specific treatment. Corticosteroids may give symptomatic relief. Antibiotics are frequently also given in severe cases, with the idea of preventing secondary infection. Lozada-Nur *et al.* (1992) have reported a complete response to levamisole in 31 out of 39 patients.

Reiter's disease

Reiter's disease comprises urethritis, arthritis and conjunctivitis, though the last is present in only about 50% of patients, and many other organ systems can be affected.

The aetiology is unknown and, though often regarded as a sexually transmitted disease, very many cases (as in Reiter's original patient) have followed outbreaks of infective enteritis by a variety of Gram-negative bacilli. Reiter's disease, therefore, appears to be a post-infective reaction with a strong association with HLA B27.

Clinically, men are predominantly affected in the ratio of up to 50 to 1 and are usually aged between 20 and 40 years. Arthritis of the extremities, sometimes intensely painful and often polyarticular, is usually the chief complaint. Skin or mucosal lesions are common, the temporomandibular joint

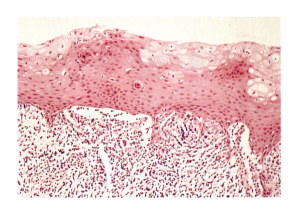

Figure 8.19 Erythema multiforme. There is sub-epithelial vesiculation and an intense neutrophil infiltrate forming micro-abscesses in this specimen

is occasionally involved and facial palsy may be another complication. Fever and loss of weight are associated.

Oral lesions may develop in 20% or more, but are usually so transient and painless as to pass unnoticed. They most typically form rounded red areas with a peripheral, white raised line and can closely resemble stomatitis areata migrans (see below).

Most cases resolve after a few months, but recurrences may follow. The mucosal lesions should not require treatment, but joint pain responds to anti-inflammatory agents.

Acanthosis nigricans

Acanthosis nigricans is so called because of the pigmentation of the skin lesions. It is a well-recognized marker of internal malignancy, but there are several variants either developmental or associated with other types of systemic disease such as insulin-resistant diabetes mellitus or other endocrinopathies. The condition has been extensively reviewed by Sedano and Gorlin (1987).

Clinically, most patients are over the age of 40 years. Approximately 40% of patients with the malignant type of acanthosis nigricans have oral lesions consisting of shaggy thickening or confluent papillomatous overgrowths, particularly of the labial or lingual mucosa. The buccal mucosa may be thickened and velvety in texture, and gingival

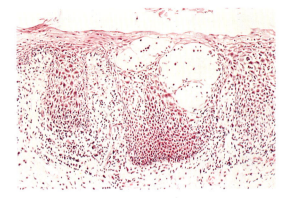

Figure 8.18 Erythema multiforme. There is intra-epithelial vesiculation and acute inflammation

enlargement may be gross. The oral lesions are not pigmented.

The cutaneous lesions consist of multiple pigmented papillomatous or verrucous overgrowths of many sites, particularly flexural surfaces such as the axillae, neck, groin or inner thighs, or umbilical or perianal areas. Palmar and plantar hyperkeratosis is present in approximately 25% of patients.

The neoplasms are mostly of the gastrointestinal tract or its appendages and are highly malignant. Carcinoma of the stomach is most common and found in 60% of patients. Other types of tumours such as lymphomas are occasionally associated.

In a minority, mucocutaneous lesions sometimes precede detection of internal cancers by many years, but more frequently follow it. They may wax or wane as the neoplasm spreads or regresses in response to treatment, only to flourish again as the tumour recurs. This suggests that the mucocutaneous lesions are the response to chemical mediators released by the tumours.

Microscopically, the buccal mucosa is greatly thickened with many vacuolated epithelial cells, giving it a basket-weave appearance resembling white sponge naevus but with a more shaggy surface (Mostofi *et al.*, 1983).

Oral lesions appear to affect only a small minority of the non-neoplastic types of acanthosis nigricans and do not appear to have been fully categorized.

Management

When oral lesions of malignant acanthosis nigricans are the first manifestation, screening of the gastrointestinal tract in particular must be carried out and, if necessary, repeated at intervals to allow early treatment of tumours. The oral lesions respond only to treatment of the underlying malignant disease, but once the latter has developed the average period of survival is no more than 2 years.

Pyostomatitis vegetans

Pyostomatitis vegetans is a rare oral manifestation of inflammatory bowel disease, particularly ulcerative colitis. Thornhill *et al.* (1992) could find only 32 reports since it was originally described in 1949,

but added three more. However, Chan *et al.* (1991) had described two other cases. In approximately 50%, cutaneous lesions (pyoderma vegetans) are associated.

Clinically, the age of those affected ranges from the third to sixth decades, but occasionally the disease has not been recognized until even later. Males predominate in a ratio of 3 to 1. Diarrhoea is usually the first complaint, but ulcerative colitis sometimes continues for several years before oral lesions appear. Occasionally, however, oral lesions are the first sign or diarrhoea may be insignificant.

In the mouth, there are multiple, yellowish miliary pustules typically in a thickened, erythematous mucosa which is sometimes folded or fissured. The pustules readily rupture to release purulent material and leave shallow ulcers. Large irregular, fibrin-covered ulcers may be associated and may extend on to the vermilion borders of the lips. Pustules appear in almost any site within the mouth, particularly the gingival, buccal and labial mucosa, but rarely on the dorsum of the tongue. Other mucous membranes such as those of the genitalia may be affected and pyoderma vegetans, with pustules particularly in flexural areas, may be associated.

Microscopically, the pustules show suprabasal clefting and intra-epithelial vesiculation or abscess formation, but typically lack true acantholysis. They contain many eosinophils and there is a mixed inflammatory infiltrate in the corium. Immunofluorescence sometimes shows intercellular immunoglobulin, usually IgG, in the epithelium. A significant peripheral eosinophilia is usually associated and may amount to 20% of the total leucocyte count.

Management

Pyostomatitis vegetans must be distinguished from pemphigus vulgaris by (a) the pustular oral lesions and, when present, the skin lesions; (b) the association with diarrhoea or frank ulcerative colitis; (c) peripheral eosinophilia; and (d) the benign course. Microscopically, the lack of true acantholysis and the eosinophil content of the intra-epithelial abscesses help to distinguish the oral lesions from pemphigus vulgaris, but may resemble those of pemphigus vegetans.

The main requirement is treatment of troublesome bowel disease. Sulphasalazine or sulphamethoxypyridoxazine may be effective and may cause resolution of the oral lesions. They are probably the treatment of choice. Chronic ulcerative colitis may have to be treated by colectomy and this may allow the oral lesions to heal. However, the latter do not always respond to drug treatment of associated bowel disease. They occasionally respond to topical corticosteroids, but more frequently to systemic prednisolone. Dapsone is frequently also effective but may have to be stopped if haemolysis develops.

'Allergic stomatitis'

Many otherwise harmless substances coming into contact with the skin cause hypersensitization in susceptible subjects. Further contact then causes an inflammatory reaction. A common example is the reaction to a wide variety of household detergents and industrial materials.

Some mucous membranes such as the eyes can also become sensitized in this way, but other parts of the body differ widely in their response. Sulphonamide ointments, for example, are potent skin sensitizers, but are widely used without trouble in the eyes.

The oral mucous membrane appears to show yet other differences and appears to be unable to mount reactions comparable with contact dermatitis and there is no oral counterpart to allergic eczema. Indeed, atopic disease has no oral mucosal manifestations in the 10% of the population who suffer from it. Even patients who are sensitized to a material such as nickel can tolerate it in the mouth; it may then cause a characteristic rash but no oral lesions. Amalgam restorations cause no trouble in patients sensitized to mercury, provided that the unset material does not touch the skin. Similar considerations apply to methylmethacrylate. Those few people who are sensitized to the monomer can wear acrylic dentures with impunity. Inflammation under acrylic dentures, often in the past described as 'acrylic allergy', is usually candidal infection and most so-called allergic reactions of the mouth are probably due to direct irritation.

The number of authenticated cases of contact hypersensitization of the oral mucous membrane is, therefore, so few as to make it questionable whether the oral mucosa can mount this type of reaction. If it does so, it must be phenomenally rare, but examples of what are frequently regarded as oral hypersensitivity reactions are cinnamon-related lesions and plasma cell gingivitis.

Cinnamon-related lesions

Cinnamon or cinnamonaldehyde is a common flavouring agent in foods and toothpastes. It has been incriminated in a variety of intra-oral lesions such as soft tissue swellings due to a granulomatous reaction (Patton *et al.*, 1985), as well as gingivitis, glossitis, cheilitis, swelling or ulceration with non-specific inflammatory changes microscopically (Lamey *et al.*, 1990). By contrast, Miller *et al.* (1992) have reported white keratotic patches on the buccal mucosa in 13 out of 14 cases, and sometimes also in other sites but on the gingivae in only 2. Microscopically, there was ortho- or parakeratosis, acanthosis and a mainly lymphocytic inflammatory infiltrate. Plasma cells were not prominent, but there were dense perivascular infiltrates. Ten of the patients reported by Lamey *et al.* (1990) gave positive delayed reactions on patch testing with cinnamon and the majority experienced recurrences on rechallenge after withdrawal of cinnamon-containing products. Eleven of the 14 patients reported by Miller *et al.* (1992) achieved major or complete resolution of their oral lesions on withdrawal of cinnamon.

Despite the strong suggestion of the involvement of hypersensitivity in the production of these lesions, the disparate nature of the clinical and histological responses to the same substance is difficult to understand.

Plasma cell gingivitis and mucositis

This is another reaction where hypersensitivity mechanisms have been implicated. Sollecito and Greenberg (1992) found that approximately 50 cases of plasma cell gingivitis were reported between 1966 and 1977, mainly in the USA. The disease suddenly then seemed to disappear. Silverman and Lozada (1977) postulated that it had been a reaction to an unidentified allergen in chewing gum, dentifrice or other product.

Clinically, plasma cell gingivitis appears as intense erythema and oedema of the attached gingiva.

Microscopically, there is irregular acanthosis, often with spongiform pustules, and a sub-epithelial infiltrate predominantly of plasma cells extending deeply into the connective tissue. The density of this infiltrate is comparable to that seen in myeloma, but is clearly reactive rather than neoplastic.

Of the two patients reported by Sollecito and Greenberg (1992), one was subjected to skin testing for many common allergens and an exclusion diet. Neither showed objective resolution, but topical corticosteroids were palliative.

In sharp contrast to the lesions of plasma cell gingivitis, White *et al.* (1986) reported a case of *plasma cell orificial mucositis* in an edentulous woman with psoriasis. Despite the microscopic similarities to plasma cell gingivitis, this reaction consisted of a thickened, fissured and erythematous plaque encircling the entire oral orifice, fissuring of the tongue and diffuse irregular thickening of the free edge of the epiglottis. Patch tests to 25 common dental allergens were negative and treatment with corticosteroids was ineffective.

Oral mucosal reactions to drugs

Of the numerous possible mechanisms for oral drug reactions, few have been convincingly clarified. These reactions are not common overall, but may be important as early signs of a dangerous systemic reaction. Nevertheless, a drug being taken is not necessarily the cause of any oral symptoms and coincidence is often difficult to exclude, particularly with common diseases such as lichen planus. The problem is made difficult by multiple drug treatment, but a precise drug history is always essential, as it may be relevant to other aspects of dental treatment. An obvious example is a patient taking systemic corticosteroids who may, as a result, have oral candidosis but is also at risk when subjected to surgery under general anaesthesia.

Local reactions to drugs

Chemical burns An aspirin tablet held against the mucosa close to an aching tooth is a well-known cause of superficial necrosis and a white patch. When the irritant is removed, the dead epithelium is shed and the mucosa heals. Other irritant chemicals are chromic acid, trichloracetic acid, or phenol.

Disturbance of the oral flora and superinfection Prolonged topical use of antibiotics, particularly tetracycline, in the mouth allows resistant organisms, particularly *Candida albicans*, to proliferate, causing thrush. Inhaled corticosteroids can have a similar effect by affecting local immunity.

Systemically mediated reactions to drugs

Depression of marrow function

Anaemia Few drugs significantly depress red cell production alone. The main example is prolonged use of phenytoin which can occasionally cause folate deficiency and macrocytic anaemia. This in turn can produce severe aphthous stomatitis, which responds promptly when folate is given.

Leucopenia Drugs capable of having this effect include antibacterials (particularly co-trimoxazole and chloramphenicol), analgesics (particularly phenylbutazone), phenothiazines and antithyroid agents. Agranulocytosis is characterized by necrotizing gingival and pharyngeal ulceration and can go on to a severe sometimes lethal prostrating illness.

When the main effect is neutropenia, low-grade oral pathogens are able to overcome local resistance and produce necrotizing ulceration, particularly of the gingival margins.

Purpura Drugs may affect haemostasis by depressing platelet production. Drug-induced purpura is often also an early sign of aplastic anaemia caused by drugs which cause general marrow depression, as indicated above. Purpura can produce severe spontaneous gingival bleeding or blood blisters and widespread submucosal ecchymoses.

Clotting function is impaired by other drugs, notably anticoagulants such as the coumarins. In overdose these can cause severe bleeding after oral surgery, but do not otherwise cause abnormal oral signs.

Depression of cell mediated immunity

Immunosuppressive drugs such as corticosteroids and cytotoxic agents greatly enhance susceptibility to infections. Viral and fungal infections of the mouth are common in patients having organ transplants and cytotoxic chemotherapy. Confluent vesiculation due to herpes may clinically be difficult to distinguish from the plaques of thrush, as may bacterial plaques. Recurrent infections such as measles, chickenpox or herpes zoster are also seen.

Many cytotoxic drugs, particularly methotrexate, are liable also to cause mucositis. The latter can range from soreness and erythema to ulceration severe enough to prevent eating.

Lichenoid reactions

As discussed earlier, many drugs, notably gold and antimalarials (both used in the treatment of rheumatoid arthritis or other collagen diseases), and the antihypertensive agents methyldopa and, occasionally, captopril, can produce a disease indistinguishable from lichen planus with characteristic oral signs or sometimes widespread erosions alone.

Bullous erythema multiforme (Stevens–Johnson syndrome)

As mentioned earlier, drugs can occasionally trigger this disease. Those most commonly implicated are long-acting sulphonamides and, rarely, barbiturates, but many cases have no recognizable triggering agent.

Fixed drug eruptions

These sharply circumscribed skin lesions recur in the same site or sites each time the drug is given. Among many drugs capable of causing this reaction, phenolphthalein, a component of purgative mixtures, is well recognized. Involvement of the oral mucous membrane is exceedingly rare.

Exfoliative stomatitis and dermatitis

Exfoliative dermatitis is one of the most dangerous and severe types of reaction to drugs. Comparable changes to those on the skin may develop in the mouth and are seen as widespread erosions due to destruction of the epithelium. Occasionally, oral changes precede or may initially be more severe than the dermal changes and may cause the patient to seek help for the soreness of the mouth. Early diagnosis and treatment is essential as the reaction can be lethal.

Metals are important causes, but gold is the only one at all widely used currently. Several other drugs, particularly phenylbutazone (now restricted), and barbiturates have also been incriminated.

Healing of oral lesions may leave a lichenoid pattern of striae.

Other drug effects

Gingival hyperplasia   Phenytoin and less frequently cyclosporin, nifedipine or its analogues can cause progressive fibrous hyperplasia of the interdental papillae.

Oral pigmentation   (see Chapter 9).

Dry mouth   This is a relatively common side effect of drugs, especially those with an atropine-like action, particularly tricyclic antidepressants (Chapter 11).

Tongue complaints

The tongue can be involved in a generalized stomatitis and develop lesions similar to those in other parts of the mouth, but it is also the site of lesions or a source of symptoms peculiar to itself and, for unknown reasons, can produce the earliest symptoms of latent defects of haemopoiesis. For white lesions of the tongue, see Chapter 9.

Glossitis is used to describe the red, smooth and sore tongue particularly characteristic of anaemia. However, this combination of signs (redness and smoothness) and a symptom (soreness) are by no means consistently associated. Tongues can be sore in the absence of visible changes or smooth but asymptomatic. Sore tongue is an only too common complaint and four clinical variants are recognizable.

Ulceration of the tongue

The tongue may be involved in, or even the main site of, various kinds of stomatitis such as herpes simplex or, more often, lichen planus. The tongue may also be the site of solitary ulcers, particularly carcinoma, which when far back may be difficult to see.

In general, definable lesions such as these, make the diagnosis straightforward by their clinical features and often biopsy.

Glossitis

The tongue is more or less uniformly red (inflamed), smooth (atrophy of the papillae) and sore. The main causes are:

● *Anaemia.* Iron deficiency and pernicious anaemia are the main causes, and women are more frequently affected. The red cell indices are important, as a fall in haemoglobin level may lag behind morphological changes in the red cells. There may, therefore, be glossitis, haematological signs of a deficiency state, but a haemoglobin level within normal limits. Early vitamin B_{12} deficiency can cause peculiar streaky red changes on the dorsum of the tongue (Moeller's glossitis).
● *Candidosis.* The tongue can be red, sore and oedematous due to candidal infection. This is particularly characteristic of acute antibiotic stomatitis and is often then associated with angular stomatitis and other features of candidosis. This condition is rarely seen now that antibiotics are used somewhat less irresponsibly.
● *Other vitamin B group deficiencies.* These are exceedingly rarely seen, but glossitis with angular stomatitis is characteristic of riboflavin and to some extent of nicotinic acid deficiency. The diagnosis of vitamin deficiency should not be made on oral signs alone in an otherwise healthy patient. The giving of B group vitamins is a

common gesture in an attempt to deal with the complaint, but is almost invariably ineffective. However, the lack of response makes it clear that deficiency of these vitamins is not a cause.
● *Lichen planus.* A smooth tongue due to atrophy of the papillae, particularly in long-standing disease, may be seen, but there is then no soreness. There is often a bluish-white sheen to the surface of the tongue, and other signs of lichen planus are likely to be present in other parts of the mouth. Soreness of the tongue in lichen planus is due to atrophic lesions or erosions.

The sore, physically normal tongue

This, the most common and troublesome type, predominantly affects post-menopausal females. In the absence of visible signs, it is often tempting to assume the complaint to be psychogenic, but this is not always the case.

Deficiency states   It is essential to appreciate that pre-anaemic deficiency states can cause soreness of the tongue without any visible abnormality in colour or texture. Women in the age group where sore tongue is most common are also the main group susceptible to pernicious anaemia. The haemoglobin is usually within normal limits, but red cell abnormalities are apparent from routine indices, particularly the mean corpuscular volume (MCV) and may indicate the need for further investigation. Specific treatment for the deficiency will relieve the symptoms.

Psychogenic disorders   Sore tongue unassociated with organic disease is a psychogenic symptom and comparable to atypical facial pain. The great majority of patients are also women of middle age or over, but diagnosis can be difficult. Depression is sometimes the underlying trouble, but is often effectively disguised and replaced by complaint of this physical symptom. In such cases, adequate treatment with antidepressant drugs such as amitriptyline or dothiepin can sometimes abolish the tongue complaint and restore the patient's general sense of well-being.

In a few patients the underlying problem seems to be an anxiety state. This can occasionally be dealt with by reassurance, especially if there is an unfounded fear, particularly of cancer of the mouth. In other cases, the basis for the anxiety seems to be less specific. A short course of an anxiolytic such as diazepam may occasionally be helpful.

As with atypical facial pain, there seem also to be many patients who complain bitterly and persistently of sore tongue, in whom no organic disease can be found and who show no response to psychoactive drugs or any other form of treatment.

Geographical tongue (benign migratory glossitis)

This common condition is characterized by the recurrent appearance and disappearance of red areas, frequently with a white margin, on the tongue.

The cause is unknown, but in some the condition is familial and has been described in several succeeding generations. The abnormality can be seen even in infancy, though probably is often unnoticed, but many cases are seen in middle-aged patients.

Clinically, geographical tongue may appear as irregular, smooth, red areas, usually with sharply defined edges; they extend for a few days, then heal, only to appear again in another area. Alternatively, the areas can be annular with slightly raised whitish margins and can coalesce to form scalloped patterns. *Stomatitis areata migrans* is the term given to similar lesions which occasionally appear in other parts of the mouth. Microscopically, these lesions show a close resemblance to those of psoriasis (Chapter 9) with spongiform intra-epithelial micro-abscesses (Figure 8.20). Morris *et al.* (1992) have confirmed that migratory glossitis is four times, and stomatitis areata migrans five times, more frequent in patients with psoriasis than controls. These lesions may therefore be an oral form of psoriasis.

Most patients with migratory glossitis have no symptoms, but some complain of soreness. Sometimes, perhaps, the patient has suddenly noticed the appearance and become anxious that cancer is the cause. Reassurance is then necessary and may be effective. In others, soreness may be due to a coincidental haematological deficiency and haematological investigation is therefore necessary.

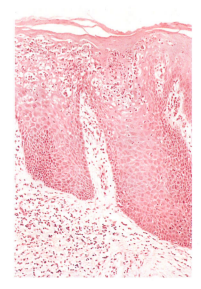

Figure 8.20   Geographical tongue. Intra-epithelial, polymorph micro-abscesses (spongiform pustules) and elongated, square-tipped rete ridges have produced a psoriasis-like picture

However, it would not be surprising if the thinning of the epithelium, together with the inflammatory changes seen histologically, caused symptoms.

Soreness in association with geographical tongue may also be psychogenic and may then respond to appropriate treatment. Some evidence has been produced to show an apparently significant association between geographical tongue and emotional disturbance. However, there remain many where no cause for the soreness can be found and no treatment seems to be effective.

Hairy tongue

This appearance is due to overgrowth of the filiform papillae which become elongated and hair like, forming a thick fur on the dorsum of the tongue. The filaments may be up to half a centimetre long and may be pale brown to black in colour. Adults are affected and heavy smoking, overuse of antiseptic mouthwashes or antibiotics, or a defective diet may be responsible, but the cause is often unclear. The discoloration is caused by pigment-producing bacteria.

Treatment is unsatisfactory unless a cause can be found and eliminated. The measure most likely to succeed is probably that of persuading the patient to scrape off the hyperplastic papillae and vigorously cleanse the dorsum of the tongue using a firm toothbrush. This dislodges many microbes mechanically and, by removing the overgrown papillae, makes conditions less favourable for their proliferation.

Sometimes the dorsum of the tongue may become black without overgrowth of the papillae. This may merely be staining by drugs such as iron compounds used for the treatment of anaemia, but is then transient. Alternatively, it may have similar causes to black hairy tongue (see Chapter 9).

Furred tongue is a coating with desquamating cells and debris. It is a typical sign in systemic infections, when the mouth becomes dry and little food is taken. It is often seen in the childhood fevers, especially scarlet fever.

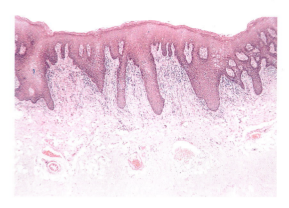

Figure 8.21   Median rhomboid glossitis. Elongation, branching and fusion of the rete ridges are shown

Median rhomboid glossitis

Median rhomboid glossitis is a lesion of the midline of the dorsum on the tongue at the junction of the anterior two-thirds with the posterior third, and for long it was believed to be the result of persistence of the tuberculum impar. However, this view is no longer widely accepted: the anomaly appears to be very rare in children, but is seen in adults.

Clinically, the appearance is variable. There is sometimes a red or pink rhomboid (lozenge-shaped) area of depapillation, the area may be white or pink and it may be lobulated. It is typically symptomless.

Microscopically, the appearances are also variable and include irregular (pseudo-epitheliomatous) hyperplasia (Figure 8.21), with an inflammatory infiltrate. There is sometimes candidal infection (the white variant) (Figure 8.22), and occasionally the lesion proves to be a granular cell tumour.

The chief importance of median rhomboid glossitis is that it has been mistaken for a carcinoma both clinically and histologically and treated accordingly (Ogus and Bennett, 1978). Carcinoma hardly ever develops in this site, but competent histological assessment is necessary. The candidal variant can be treated with antifungal drugs; otherwise, reassurance is frequently all that is required.

Foliate papillitis

The foliate papillae are small lymphoid follicles separated by shallow crypts on the posterior lateral margins of the tongue. They may become mildly enlarged and red. They may then be noticed by and alarm patients who inspect their tongues. Reassurance that this is not a tumour can readily be provided by showing the patient the similar foliate papilla on the opposite side of the tongue.

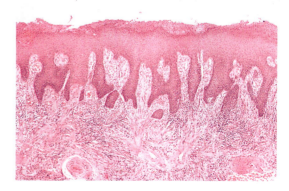

Figure 8.22   Median rhomboid glossitis with candidosis. The hyperkeratotic plaque shows psoriasiform changes with epithelial hyperplasia and a heavy chronic inflammatory infiltrate in the corium

Acute glossitis

Acute glossitis is rare, but there have been several reports between 1965 and 1984, as reviewed by Stoddard and Deshpande (1991). Most cases have been in infants or children. *Haemophilus influenzae* has been the most frequently identified cause, but with current immunization schedules, many such cases may be prevented. Typically, the tongue is red, swollen, oedematous and may protrude from the mouth. In severe cases the airway may be endangered. Some examples have been categorized as cellulitis of the tongue, while others have progressed to abscess formation.

Management

Prompt treatment is necessary because of the threat to the airway, and early intubation may be advisable. Exudate should if possible be obtained for culture and sensitivities, and empirical anti-microbial treatment given until sensitivity findings dictate a change. Intravenous cefotaxime may be a suitable choice in view of the possibility that *H. influenzae* may be responsible.

Ischaemic necrosis of the tongue

Despite its excellent blood supply, ischaemic necrosis of the tongue is a rare but recognized entity and Sofferman (1980) reported 3 cases. It is virtually diagnostic of giant cell arteritis, and Missen (1961), in autopsy examinations of 10 patients with giant cell arteritis, found bilateral involvement of the lingual arteries in 9 cases. Rarely also this disease can cause ischaemic necrosis of the lip, other parts of the face or the scalp.

Giant cell arteritis has been described in Chapter 7. In some cases, treatment of the head-ache of this disease with ergotamine may have worsened the ischaemia. Ischaemia of the tongue is heralded by severe pain and swelling and may be accompanied by other signs of temporal arteritis or polymyalgia. The tongue becomes blanched, cold and painful to move. It then may become cyanotic and undergo necrosis. The whole of the anterior half of the tongue may slough away or has to be excised once a line of demarcation has become clear.

Treatment with corticosteroids, if started before ischaemia is too far advanced, may possibly prevent further deterioration. They should in any case be given as soon as the diagnosis is suggested by the symptoms, a greatly raised erythrocyte sedimentation rate and inflamed scalp vessels. Dare *et al.* (1981) report a case where the tongue had become blanched, swollen and painful but there was no early response to corticosteroids (prednisolone 120 mg/day). Resolution followed anticoagulation with intravenous heparin and Rheomacrodex but, because of previous reports where lingual ischaemia had not progressed to gangrene, Dare and colleagues were uncertain whether their treatment had achieved the desired effect or whether the ischaemia was self-limiting.

References

Centers for Disease Control (1987) Revision of the CDC surveillance case definition for the acquired immuno-deficiency syndrome. *MMWR*, **36** (Suppl. 1), 1S–15S

Chan, L.S., Regezi, J.A. and Cooper, K.D. (1990) Oral manifestations of linear IgA disease. *Journal of the American Academy of Dermatology*, **22**, 362–365

Chan, S.W.Y., Scully, C., Prime, S.S. *et al.* (1991) Pyostomatitis vegetans. Oral manifestation of ulcerative colitis. *Oral Surgery, Oral Medicine and Oral Pathology*, **72**, 689–692

Dare, B., Byrne, E. and Robertson, A. (1981) Acute lingual ischaemia complicating temporal arteritis. *Medical Journal of Australia*, **1**, 534

Eisen, D. and Ellis, C.N. (1990) Topical cyclosporine for oral mucosal disorders. *Journal of the American Academy of Dermatology*, **23**, 1259–1264

Eisen, D., Ellis, C.N., Duell, E.A. *et al.* (1990) Effect of topical cyclosporine rinse on oral lichen planus. A double-blind analysis. *New England Journal of Medicine*, **323**, 290–294

French, P.D., Birchall, M.A. and Harris, J.R.W. (1991) Cytomegalovirus ulceration of the oropharynx. *Journal of Laryngology and Otolaryngology*, **105**, 739–742

Goon, W.W.Y. and Jacobsen, P.L. (1988) Prodromal odontalgia and multiple devitalised teeth caused by a herpes zoster infection of the trigeminal nerve: report of case. *Journal of the American Dental Association*, **116**, 500–504

Holmstrup, P. (1992) The controversy of a premalignant potential of oral lichen planus is over. *Oral Surgery, Oral Medicine and Oral Pathology*, **73**, 704–706

Holmstrup, P., Thorn, J.J., Rindum, J. *et al.* (1988) Malignant development of lichen planus-affected oral mucosa. *Journal of Oral Pathology and Medicine,* **17,** 219–225

Jonsson, R., Mountz, J. and Koopman, W. (1990) Elucidating the pathogenesis of autoimmune disease: recent advances at the molecular level and relevance to oral mucosal disease. *Journal of Oral Pathology and Medicine,* **19,** 341–350

Karjalainen, T.K. and Tomich, C.E. (1989) A histopathologic study of oral mucosal lupus erythematosus. *Oral Surgery, Oral Medicine and Oral Pathology,* **67,** 547–554

Lamey, P.-J., Lewis, M.A.O., Rees, T.D. *et al.* (1990) Sensitivity reaction to the cinnamonaldehyde component of toothpaste. *British Dental Journal,* **168,** 115–118

Lamey, P.-J., Rees, T.D., Binnie, W.H. *et al.* (1992) Oral presentation of pemphigus vulgaris and its response to systemic steroid therapy. *Oral Surgery, Oral Medicine and Oral Pathology,* **74,** 54–57

Lozada-Nur, F., Cram, D. and Gorsky, M. (1992) Clinical response to levamisole in thirty-nine patients with erythema multiforme. An open prospective study. *Oral Surgery, Oral Medicine and Oral Pathology,* **74,** 294–298

Lozada-Nur, F., Gorsky, M. and Silverman, S. (1989) Oral erythema multiforme: clinical observations and treatment of 95 patients. *Oral Surgery, Oral Medicine and Oral Pathology,* **67,** 36–40

Macleod, R.I. and Munro, C.S. (1991) The incidence and distribution of oral lesions in patients with Darier's disease. *British Dental Journal,* **171,** 133–136

MacPhail, L.A., Greenspan, D., Feigal, D.W. *et al.* (1991) Recurrent aphthous ulcers in association with HIV infection. Description of ulcer types and analysis of T-lymphocyte subsets. *Oral Surgery, Oral Medicine and Oral Pathology,* **71,** 678–683

Miller, R.L., Gould, A.R. and Bernstein, M.L. (1992) Cinnamon-induced stomatitis venenata. Clinical and characteristic histopathologic features. *Oral Surgery, Oral Medicine and Oral Pathology,* **73,** 708–716

Mintz, S.M. and Anavi, Y. (1992) Maxillary osteomyelitis and spontaneous tooth exfoliation after herpes zoster. *Oral Surgery, Oral Medicine and Oral Pathology,* **73,** 664–666

Missen, G.A.K. (1961) Acute massive gangrene of the tongue. *British Medical Journal,* **1,** 1393–1394

Morris, L.F., Phillips, C.M., Binnie, W.H. *et al.* (1992) Oral lesions in patients with psoriasis. *Cutis,* **49,** 339–344

Mostofi, R.S., Hayden, N.P. and Soltani, K. (1983) Oral malignant acanthosis nigricans. *Oral Surgery, Oral Medicine and Oral Pathology,* **56,** 372–374

Ogus, M.D. and Bennett, M.H. (1978) Carcinoma of the dorsum of the tongue: a rarity or misdiagnosis. *British Journal of Oral Surgery,* **16,** 115–124

Patton, D.W., Ferguson, M.M., Forsyth, A. *et al.* (1985) Oro-facial granulomatosis: a possible allergic basis. *British Journal of Oral and Maxillofacial Surgery,* **23,** 235–242

Porter, S.R., Bain, S.E. and Scully, C.M. (1992) Linear IgA disease manifesting as recalcitrant desquamative gingivitis. *Oral Surgery, Oral Medicine and Oral Pathology,* **74,** 179–182

Porter, S.R., Scully, C. and Flint, S. (1988) Hematologic status in recurrent aphthous stomatitis compared with other oral disease. *Oral Surgery, Oral Medicine and Oral Pathology,* **66,** 41-44

Sedano, H.O. and Gorlin, R.J. (1987) Acanthosis nigricans. *Oral Surgery, Oral Medicine and Oral Pathology,* **63,** 462–467

Scully, C. and Porter, S.R. (1989) Recurrent aphthous stomatitis: current concepts of etiology, pathogenesis and management. *Journal of Oral Pathology and Medicine,* **18,** 21–27

Silverman, S. and Lozada, F. (1977) An epilogue to plasma-cell gingivostomatitis (allergic gingivostomatitis). *Oral Surgery, Oral Medicine and Oral Pathology,* **43,** 211–217

Sircus, W., Church, R. and Kelleher, J. (1957) Recurrent aphthous ulceration of the mouth. A study of the natural history, aetiology and treatment. *Quarterly Journal of Medicine,* **XXVI,** 235–249

Sofferman, R.A. (1980) Lingual infarction in cranial arteritis. *Journal of the American Medical Association,* **243,** 2422–2423

Sollecito, T.P. and Greenberg, M.S. (1992) Plasma cell gingivitis. Report of two cases. *Oral Surgery, Oral Medicine and Oral Pathology,* **73,** 690–693

Stoddard, J.J. and Deshpande, J.K. (1991) Acute glossitis and bacteremia caused by *Streptococcus pneumoniae*: case report and review. *American Journal of Diseases of Children,* **145,** 598–599

Thornhill, M.H., Zakrzewska, J.M. and Gilkes, J.J.H. (1992) Pyostomatitis vegetans: report of three cases and review of the literature. *Journal of Oral Pathology and Medicine,* **21,** 128–133

Voute, A.B.E., de Jong, W.F.B., Schulten, E.A.J.M. *et al.* (1992) Possible premalignant character of oral lichen planus. The Amsterdam experience. *Journal of Oral Pathology and Medicine,* **21,** 326–329

Wechsler, B. and Piette, J.C. (1992) Behçet's disease. Retains most of its mysteries (Editorial). *British Medical Journal,* **304,** 1199–1200

White, J.W., Olsen, K.D. and Banks, P.M. (1986) Plasma cell orificial mucositis. Report of a case and review of the literature. *Archives of Dermatology,* **122,** 1321–1324

Wright, J.T. (1990) Comprehensive dental care and general anesthetic management of hereditary epidermolysis bullosa. *Oral Surgery, Oral Medicine and Oral Pathology,* **70,** 573–578

Wright, J.T., Fine, J.-D. and Johnson, L.B. (1991) Oral soft tissues in hereditary epidermolysis bullosa. *Oral Surgery, Oral Medicine and Oral Pathology,* **71,** 440–446

9

White, red and pigmented lesions of the oral mucosa

Oral white lesions

The appearance of most oral white lesions is due to hyperkeratosis. Apart from the lingual filiform papillae, visible keratinization of any significant degree is abnormal in the mouth. Any excess keratin, becoming sodden with saliva, appears white. *Leucoplakia* literally means no more than a white plaque, but in the past was widely but incorrectly regarded as virtually synonymous with premalignancy. The term 'leucoplakia' should therefore be used only as defined by a World Health Organisation committee as 'a white patch or plaque which cannot be characterized clinically or pathologically as any other condition'.

A minority of white lesions can undergo malignant change, but hyperkeratosis *per se* is of no significance, except in so far as it may be associated with epithelial dysplasia. By no means all leucoplakias are premalignant, nor are all premalignant lesions white. As discussed later, erythroplastic (red) lesions are more frequently dysplastic than white lesions.

White sponge naevus

White sponge naevus is a developmental anomaly inherited as an autosomal dominant trait.

Clinically, the appearance is distinctive. The affected mucosa is white, soft and irregularly thickened. Unlike other white lesions, this anomaly can spread so widely as to involve the whole oral mucosa. It lacks well-defined borders and its edges fade imperceptibly into normal tissue. The anus and vagina can also be affected.

Microscopy

The epithelium is hyperplastic, with uniform acanthosis and the rete ridges having a smooth lower border. Shaggy hyperparakeratosis and intracellular oedema with abnormally prominent cell membranes produce a so-called basket-weave appearance (Figures 9.1 and 9.2). There is no dysplasia and inflammatory infiltration in the corium is typically absent.

Management

The appearance is readily recognized, particularly when there is widespread mucosal involvement. A positive family history is virtually confirmatory. If there is any doubt, a biopsy will confirm the diagnosis. Occasionally, patients relate that antibiotic treatment has caused the whiteness to

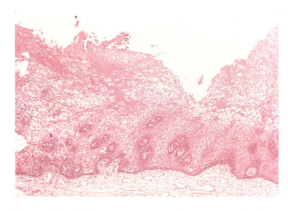

Figure 9.1 White sponge naevus. Low power showing acanthosis, ballooning degeneration of the spinous layer and thick, irregular parakeratosis

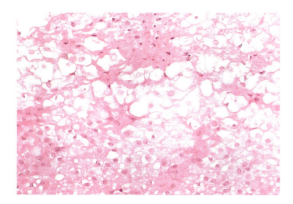

Figure 9.2 White sponge naevus. Higher power showing vacuolated superficial cells

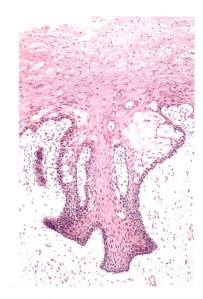

Figure 9.3 Pachyonychia congenita showing vacuolated cells and irregular parakeratosis

disappear, but any such response is unreliable. The main requirement is to reassure the patient of the benign nature of the anomaly.

Pachyonychia congenita

Pachyonychia congenita is an uncommon congenital disorder, characterized by hypertrophy of the nail beds, skin lesions (particularly hyperkeratosis of the palms and soles) and oral white lesions. Premature eruption, including natal teeth, may be associated.

The oral lesions typically comprise areas of soft whitish mucosal thickenings (leucokeratosis). Typically, the leucokeratosis appears as widespread, translucent thickening of the mucosal surface, sometimes with localized white plaques. Leucokeratosis may be present in infancy but becomes prominent, especially in areas subject to trauma, over years. White sponge naevus, by contrast, produces considerably more diffuse and widespread white mucosal thickening and lacks ungual or cutaneous abnormalities.

Microscopically, the oral plaques show acanthosis and widespread hyperparakeratosis. The epithelial cells show intracellular vacuolation, somewhat like those of white sponge naevus (Figure 9.3), but in a more limited zone in the spinal cell layer and surrounded by normal cells (Figure 9.4). No treatment other than reassurance is required.

Fordyce's spots

Sebaceous glands may appear in the oral mucosa as creamy white spots a few millimetres in diameter.

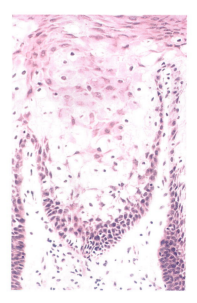

Figure 9.4 Pachyonychia congenita showing ballooning, vacuolated cells in the stratum spinosum

They are soft, symmetrically distributed and, increasing in number and size with age, may become conspicuous. The buccal mucosa is the main site, but sometimes the lips and rarely even the tongue are involved.

If these glands are mistaken for disease, patients can be reassured.

Dyskeratosis congenita

Dyskeratosis congenita is heritable as a rare recessive or dominant trait. Dysplastic lesions of the oral mucosa, dermal pigmentation, dystrophies of the nails and, occasionally, aplastic anaemia are the main features.

Clinically, oral white patches are seen in over 80% of patients or there may be inconspicuous erythematous areas. The cutaneous pigmentation is greyish brown, reticulate and predominantly affects the neck, arms and upper chest. The nails become dystrophic early and, by adolescence, may be completely destroyed. Alopecia is present in over 30% and haematological abnormalities in 51% of patients. Many patients also appear to be immunodeficient or have other abnormalities: the findings in 104 cases of the disease have been reviewed by Davidson and Connor (1988).

Microscopy
However slight the symptoms and however innocent oral lesions appear clinically, they frequently show epithelial atypia microscopically and the risk of carcinomatous change is high. Multiple oral carcinomas can result and the expectation of life is poor. Close observation and repeated biopsies should be prompted by the slightest symptoms to enable each tumour to be treated as early as possible.

The management is the same as for other dysplastic lesions, as discussed later, but overall the prognosis is poor. The mean expectation of life is less than 25 years. Causes of death include cancers of the mouth or other sites, and bleeding (gastrointestinal or cerebral), but in 50% of cases from infections, which are frequently opportunistic.

Frictional keratosis and cheek biting

This is caused by prolonged mild abrasion of the mucous membrane by such irritants as a sharp tooth, cheek biting or dentures.

Clinically, in the early stages the patches are pale and translucent, but later become dense and white, sometimes with a rough surface. Habitual cheek-biting causes an area of buccal mucosa to appear patchily red and white with a rough surface.

Microscopy
The epithelium is moderately hyperplastic with a prominent granular cell layer and thick hyperkeratosis but no significant dysplasia (Figure 9.5). There are often scattered chronic inflammatory cells in the corium.

Management
Removal of the irritant causes the patch quickly to disappear and should make biopsy unnecessary. Frictional keratosis is completely benign, and there is no evidence that continued minor trauma alone has any carcinogenic potential.

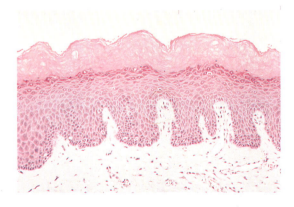

Figure 9.5 Hyperkeratosis. The epithelium has a thick keratinized layer and prominent granular cell layer. There is no significant dysplasia

Smoker's keratosis ('nicotinic stomatitis')

Smoker's keratosis is seen among heavy, long-term pipe smokers and some cigar smokers. The appearances are distinctive in that the palate is affected, but any part covered by a denture is spared. Changes are then seen only on the soft palate.

The lesion has two components, namely hyperkeratosis and inflammatory swelling of minor mucous glands; either may predominate, but typically, white thickening of the palatal mucosa is associated with small umbilicated swellings with red centres. The white plaque is sometimes distinctly tessellated.

Microscopy

The white areas show hyperorthokeratosis and acanthosis with a variable inflammatory infiltrate beneath. The diagnostic feature is the swollen, inflamed mucous glands with hyperkeratosis extending up to the duct orifice.

Management

The clinical appearances and history are so distinctive that biopsy should not be necessary. Though epidemiological evidence suggests that pipe smoking increases the risk of cancer, when oral cancer develops in association with pipe smoking it typically appears not in the keratotic area on the palate (one of the least common sites for cancer), but low down in the mouth, often in the lingual retromolar region. This may be the result of carcinogens pooling and having their maximal effect in drainage areas of the mouth. It also suggests that there are different causes for the hyperkeratosis and any carcinomatous change.

By contrast, there is no characteristic type of hyperkeratotic lesion associated with cigarette smoking. The role of tobacco in the aetiology of oral cancer is discussed in Chapter 10.

The main requirement is to persuade the patient to stop smoking. The lesion then resolves remarkably quickly. Persuasion is reinforced by warning of the risk of malignant change and pointing out the damage already done.

Snuff dipper's keratosis and other smokeless tobacco lesions

Tobacco chewing or snuff dipping (holding flavoured tobacco powder in an oral sulcus) causes a white hyperkeratotic lesion. Oral snuff appears to cause more severe changes than tobacco chewing (Daniels *et al.*, 1992) and is probably the main way in which smokeless tobacco is currently used in Western countries.

Clinically, the habit of snuff dipping may be maintained for decades and gives rise to keratoses in the area against which the tobacco is held – in the buccal or labial sulcus. Early changes are erythema and mild, whitish thickening. Long-term use gives rise to extensive leucoplakia-like thickening and wrinkling of the buccal mucosa.

Microscopy

The main changes are thickening of the epithelium with plump or squared-off rete ridges. There are varying degrees of hyperorthokeratosis or parakeratosis. Chevron keratosis is sometimes regarded as characteristic, but was seen in only 17% of 132 biopsies examined by Daniels *et al.* (1992). Dysplasia may eventually be seen and, occasionally, malignant change can follow several decades of use. A high proportion of these carcinomas are verrucous.

The heaviest users of oral snuff in the Western world are in Sweden, but Larsson *et al.* (1991), in an extensive study, found no carcinomas among them and stated that they have never been seen in the great number of biopsies from all parts of Sweden over many years.

Management

Diagnosis is based on the history of snuff use and the leucoplakia-like lesion in the area where the tobacco is held. Biopsy is required to exclude dysplasia or early malignant change.

Larsson *et al.* (1991) have shown that snuff dipper's lesions will resolve on stopping the habit, even after 25 years of use. This therefore is the main measure. If this fails, regular follow-up and biopsies are required.

Syphilitic leucoplakia

Leucoplakia of the dorsum of the tongue is a characteristic complication of tertiary syphilis but is of little more than historical interest now.

Clinically, syphilitic leucoplakia has no distinctive features, but typically affects the dorsum of the tongue and spares the margins. The lesion has an irregular outline and surface. It is usually regarded as having a high risk of malignant change, and cracks, small erosions or nodules may be foci of invasive carcinoma. Carcinoma developing near the centre of the dorsum of the tongue is typically a sequel to syphilitic leucoplakia and, as a consequence of the great decline in late-stage syphilis, is exceedingly rare in this site now.

Microscopy

In addition to hyperkeratosis and acanthosis, often with dysplasia, the characteristic late syphilitic chronic inflammatory changes, with plasma cells predominating, may be seen. Giant cells and, rarely, more or less well-formed tuberculoid granulomas may be present. Endarteritis of small arteries is particularly characteristic. However, any distinctive features of a syphilitic tissue reaction may be totally lacking.

Management

The diagnosis is confirmed mainly by the serological findings. However, even if positive, biopsy is still essential, as minute areas of malignant change may be found, and the management is affected accordingly. In particular, the presence of syphilitic endarteritis may be a contraindication to radiotherapy.

Antibiotic treatment of syphilis does not cure the leucoplakia, which persists and can undergo malignant change even after serology has become negative.

Candidosis

Candidosis can cause acute and chronic whitish lesions (thrush and chronic hyperplastic candidosis) and also red lesions such as denture stomatitis, as discussed later.

Thrush

Thrush, a disease recognized in infants by Hippocrates, can also affect adults and is then, as it was termed in the nineteenth century, a 'disease of the diseased'. This has been dramatically confirmed by its frequency in HIV infection.

Factors predisposing to thrush or chronic candidosis include immunodeficiency, anaemia and suppression of the normal flora of the mouth by antibacterial drugs. However, any adult male who develops thrush without apparent cause should be suspected of having HIV infection.

Clinically, the distinctive feature of thrush is that the patches can be wiped off to expose an erythematous mucosa. The patches are soft, friable, and creamy in colour. Their extent varies from isolated small flecks to widespread confluent plaque.

Microscopy

A Gram-stained smear shows large masses of tangled hyphae, detached epithelial cells and leucocytes. Biopsy shows hyperplastic epithelium infiltrated by inflammatory oedema and cells, predominantly neutrophils. Staining with PAS shows many candidal hyphae growing down through the epithelial cells to the junction of the plaque with the spinous cell layer (Figure 9.6). At this level there is a concentration of inflammatory exudate and inflammatory cells forming, in places, micro-abscesses. More deeply, the epithelium is hyperplastic but attenuated, with long slender processes extending down into the corium, surrounded by a light, predominantly lymphoplasmacytic infiltrate.

The microscopic appearances explain both the friable nature of the plaques of thrush and their ready detachment.

Management

If any local cause such as topical antibiotic treatment can be controlled, this alone may allow thrush to resolve. If not, a course of nystatin, amphotericin lozenges or miconazole gel should

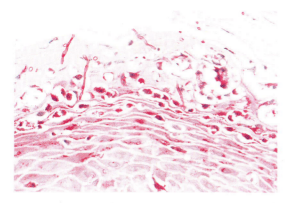

Figure 9.6 Thrush. The superficial epithelial layers are infiltrated by polymorphs to form micro-abscesses (spongiform pustules) and candidal hyphae are extending down through the superficial parakeratinized epithelial cells. PAS stain

allow the oral microflora to return to normal. If the patient has HIV infection, the infection may respond to fluconazole or itraconazole, but candidosis is indicative of a poor prognosis.

Chronic hyperplastic candidosis (candidal leucoplakia)

Clinically, chronic oral candidosis produces a plaque, distinguishable only by biopsy from other leucoplakia-like conditions and may have malignant potential.

Adults, typically males of middle age or over, are affected. The usual sites are the dorsum of the tongue and the post-commissural buccal mucosa. The plaque is variable in thickness and often rough or irregular in texture, or nodular with an erythematous background, giving it a speckled appearance. Angular stomatitis may be associated, is sometimes continuous with intraoral plaques and suggests the candidal nature of the lesion.

Microscopy
The plaque cannot be wiped off, but fragments can be detached by firm scraping and, when Gram stained, shows clumps of epithelial cells with embedded hyphae.

Like thrush, the plaque of chronic candidosis is parakeratotic, but more coherent, containing only

beads of inflammatory exudate which give it a psoriasiform appearance. In haematoxylin and eosin stained sections, hyphae appear as no more than clear or faintly basophilic tracks through the upper epithelium. Periodic acid–Schiff stain clearly shows the hyphae growing (as in thrush) through the full thickness of the plaque to the glycogen-rich zone where the inflammatory exudate tends to be more concentrated and can form micro-abscesses (Figures 9.7a and 9.7b).

Electron microscopy shows *Candida albicans* to be an intracellular parasite growing within the epithelial cytoplasm (Cawson, 1972): the hyphae, therefore, grow in relatively straight lines and do not follow a tortuous path along the intercellular spaces (Figure 9.8).

Acanthosis of the epithelium can sometimes be extensive with rounded down-growths, and there may be dysplasia. Induction of epithelial proliferation by *C. albicans* infection has been demonstrated experimentally (Cawson, 1973).

The chronic inflammatory infiltrate in the corium is variable in density, but may not break into the deeper epithelium. The basement membrane then remains intact and may appear to be thickened.

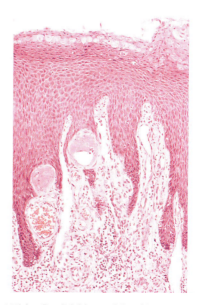

Figure 9.7(a)   Candidal leucoplakia (chronic candidosis) showing superficial parakeratotic infected plaque, psoriasiform acanthosis and striking fibrin deposition round superficial vessels

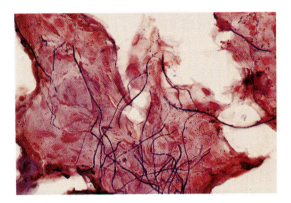

Figure 9.7(b) Candidal leucoplakia. Scraping showing candidal hyphae embedded in detached epithelial cells (Gram stain)

This unusual feature in an oral keratotic lesion is typical of chronic candidosis.

Management

After confirmation of the diagnosis by biopsy, treatment should be with a systemically acting antifungal agent such as fluconazole, but this may have to be continued for several months. Other factors likely to perpetuate candidal infection should be controlled. Stopping the patient from smoking and elimination of candidal infection from under an upper denture are important. Any iron deficiency should also be treated.

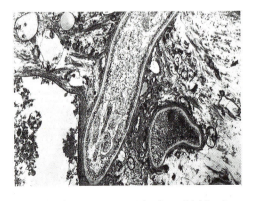

Figure 9.8 Electron micrograph of candidal hypha illustrating its intracellular growth as it extends through the cytoplasm of an epithelial cell

Excision of candidal plaque alone is of little value, as the infection can recur in the same site even after skin grafting. Vigorous antifungal therapy is therefore essential, but sometimes some residual (uninfected) plaque may persist after treatment and probably, once the process has been initiated, it may become (as in syphilitic leucoplakia) autonomous.

Chronic mucocutaneous candidosis (CMCC) syndromes

These syndromes are all rare, but difficult to manage. The following classification is mainly based on that of Higgs and Wells (1974):

● familial (limited) type
● diffuse type (candida 'granuloma')
● endocrine candidosis syndrome
● late onset (thymoma syndrome).

Clinically, these syndromes differ from each other mainly in their extraoral features. Only the diffuse type shows significantly more severe candidal infection and may, therefore, be distinguishable from the others clinically. The microscopic features are essentially as described above.

The main features of these variants are as follows:

Familial (limited) mucocutaneous candidosis Inheritance is by an autosomal recessive trait, though rarely the trait may be dominant. The onset is in infancy, with thrush-like plaques in childhood. Later the oral lesions become indistinguishable from those of sporadic cases of chronic hyperplastic candidosis, but there may be mild cutaneous involvement and sideropenia is characteristically associated.

Diffuse-type mucocutaneous candidosis Most cases are sporadic, but there appear to be rare familial cases. This is the most severe type and was earlier termed 'monilial granuloma' by Hauser and Rothman (1950) because of the extensive, warty and often disfiguring overgrowths on the skin. However, there is no granuloma formation microscopically. Rather, the lesions are produced by epithelial proliferation and an extreme expression of the same process that produces oral epithelial plaques in response to candidal invasion.

These patients are usually also abnormally susceptible to bacterial diseases, particularly pulmonary and superficial suppurative infections.

Endocrine candidosis syndrome In this variant, chronic mucocutaneous candidosis is associated with multiple glandular deficiencies and organ-specific autoantibody production. Nevertheless, there is no direct cause-and-effect relationship between the candidosis and the endocrine deficiency. The candidal infection can precede the onset of endocrine deficiency by as long as 15 years, but occasionally this sequence is reversed. Treatment of the candidosis does not affect the endocrine deficiency and vice versa.

The most common associated endocrine deficiency is hypoparathyroidism. For quite different reasons, hypoparathyroidism and chronic candidosis may also be associated in Di George's syndrome. A myth has therefore arisen that hypoparathyroidism confers susceptibility to candidosis.

Endocrine candidosis syndrome is a manifestation of type I chronic polyendocrinopathy. In the latter, Addison's disease and hypoparathyroidism are present in the great majority, and other glandular deficiencies can develop, but candidosis is often so mild as to pass unnoticed.

Late onset mucocutaneous candidosis This syndrome has a clear immunological basis, in that there is a persistent defect of cell-mediated immunity produced by a thymoma. In the full syndrome, myasthenia gravis and pure red cell aplasia are associated.

Management of mucocutaneous candidosis syndromes

Microscopic diagnosis of the candidal infection has been described earlier, but precise categorization may have to await development of other features of one of these syndromes, such as endocrine deficiency or elucidation of a relevant family history.

Immunological investigation, apart from detection of autoantibodies to glandular tissues in the endocrine candidosis syndrome, is not generally helpful, though detection of impaired or absent cell-mediated immunity to *C. albicans* strongly

suggests that the patient has one of the muco-cutaneous candidosis syndromes rather than limited oral chronic hyperplastic candidosis.

The principles of management are, therefore, to treat the candidal infection with antifungal drugs such as itraconazole and to deal with associated disorders as appropriate. Thus, antibacterial chemotherapy is necessary in diffuse-type CMCC, and endocrine replacement is essential in endocrine candidosis.

Lichen planus

Lichen planus occasionally causes plaque-like lesions, particularly on the dorsum of the tongue and in long-standing cases. The plaques may be thick, are characteristically snowy white and may have ill-defined margins giving them a fluffy or cottonwool-like outline. The microscopic features, management and possible risk of malignant change have been discussed in Chapter 8.

Lupus erythematosus

Both discoid and systemic lupus erythematosus can produce white lesions. These are rarely plaque-like, but are often associated with erosions. However, occasional cases of carcinoma developing in long-standing lesions of lupus erythematosus have been reported (Chapter 8).

Sublingual keratosis

A white soft plaque with a wrinkled surface, with an irregular but well-defined outline and sometimes with a butterfly shape, may appear in the sublingual region. The plaque typically extends from the anterior floor of the mouth to the undersurface of the tongue. There is usually no associated inflammation (Figure 9.9).

Microscopically, sublingual keratosis is not distinctive, but malignant change was associated in 24% of 29 cases reported by Kramer *et al.* (1978).

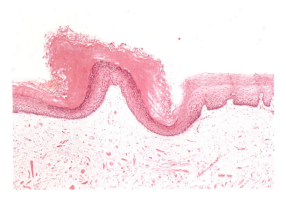

Figure 9.9   Sublingual keratosis. There is sharply demarcated epithelial atrophy and severe hyperkeratosis

Such a high risk of malignant change has not been widely confirmed and it is puzzling that more than 20 years should elapse between the reporting of this potential and the description of sublingual keratosis as a harmless naevus by Cooke (1956).

Psoriasis

Psoriasis is a common skin disease estimated to affect 2% of the population. Oral psoriatic plaques are rare, but there is a significant association between both benign migratory glossitis (geographical tongue) and stomatitis areata migrans (the counterpart in other parts of the oral mucosa), and cutaneous psoriasis, which these lesions closely resemble histologically.

Clinically, oral psoriatic plaques are typically associated with severe pustular psoriasis but occasionally with psoriasis vulgaris. The appearance of the oral lesions is variable. Whitish translucent plaques are most characteristic or there may be the circinate white lesions of migratory glossitis or stomatitis areata migrans. Macules, diffuse erythema and pustules may occasionally be seen. Oral lesions are frequently asymptomatic and probably often unnoticed.

Microscopy
Oral lesions have essentially the same appearance as dermal lesions. There is parakeratosis, superficial spongiosis and an inflammatory infiltrate which can form spongiform pustules (Monro microabscesses) superficially in the epithelium (Figure 9.10). There may also be the characteristic pattern of acanthosis with long, slender, square-tipped or club-shaped epithelial downgrowths. The inflammatory infiltrate in the corium is usually sparse.

Like migratory glossitis, chronic candidosis and Reiter's disease can have a psoriasiform microscopic appearance. The diagnosis of oral psoriasis should only, therefore, be made when it has the characteristic microscopic features and is associated with cutaneous psoriasis.

Management
Since oral psoriatic plaques are so rare, biopsy should be carried out for any oral white plaque in a patient with psoriasis to exclude a coincidental disease. If, however, microscopy confirms the oral lesion to be psoriasis, no more than reassurance is required.

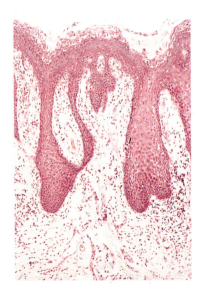

Figure 9.10   Oral psoriasis showing elongated rete ridges with club-shaped tips, spongiform pustules in the superficial epithelium and vascular, oedematous papillary corium

HIV-associated hairy leucoplakia

Patients with HIV infection may develop a clinically and histologically distinctive type of leucoplakia. The lateral margins of the tongue are usually affected, and the plaque is soft, white and usually asymptomatic. The surface is vertically corrugated but only occasionally has hair-like filamentous projections of keratin.

Microscopically, hairy leucoplakia is characterized by hyperkeratosis with a ridged surface or, sometimes, hair-like extensions of keratin (Figure 9.11). Secondary invasion of the surface by candidal hyphae is relatively common, but microscopic features of candidosis are lacking (Figure 9.12). More important is the presence of *koilocytes*, which are vacuolated and ballooned prickle cells with pyknotic nuclei surrounded by a clear halo. There is little or no inflammatory infiltrate in the corium.

Epstein–Barr virus (EBV) capsid antigen can be identified in the epithelial cell nuclei and viral particles resembling EBV can be seen by electron microscopy. This finding appears to be unique to hairy leucoplakia, and the likelihood that the EBV is the aetiological agent is suggested by reports by Resnick *et al.* (1988), among others, that hairy leucoplakia responds to treatment with acyclovir or its analogues. Langerhans cells may be few or absent, so that a defect of local immunity may contribute to the development of this lesion.

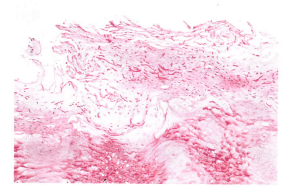

Figure 9.12   Hairy leucoplakia. Specimen stained to show numerous candidal hyphae in the superficial epithelium. PAS stain

Management

The differential diagnosis is from other types of leucoplakia and from candidosis in particular. Other features of HIV infection or serum positivity are strongly suggestive, but biopsy is necessary if confirmation is required or serology is not permissible. Hairy leucoplakia can rarely be seen in immunodeficient patients such as those receiving renal transplants and is not completely unique to HIV infection. However, patients with hairy leucoplakia are, with rare exceptions, HIV positive and 60–70% of them develop the full syndrome of AIDS within very few years. HIV-associated hairy leucoplakia is, therefore, an indication of a poor prognosis. Hairy leucoplakia does not appear to be precancerous, but the short expectation of life may preclude the realization of any such potential. Hairy leucoplakia has a remittant course and can regress spontaneously. If troublesome, acyclovir may be beneficial but Lozada-Nur and Costa (1992) recommend topical application of podophyllum resin sol as safe and avoiding the risk of development of tolerance to acyclovir.

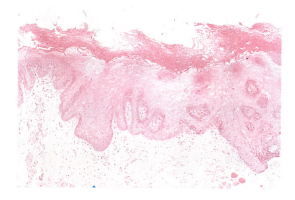

Figure 9.11   Hairy leucoplakia. Irregular parakeratotic plaque overlies acanthotic vacuolated stratified squamous epithelium. There is no inflammation of the underlying corium

Oral keratosis of renal failure

Leucoplakia-like oral lesions are an occasional and unexplained complication of long-standing renal failure.

The plaques are soft, have a crenated surface and are typically symmetrically distributed.

Microscopy

The features do not appear to be sufficiently distinctive to enable a diagnosis to be made without knowledge of the underlying disease; there is irregular acanthosis with mild atypia of the epithelial cells and moderate parakeratosis. The appearances are somewhat similar to those of hairy leucoplakia (see Figures 9.11 and 9.12). Biopsy may be useful also to distinguish these lesions from adherent bacterial plaques, which may also develop in patients with renal failure.

Management

Since these plaques are secondary to renal failure, correction of the latter by effective dialysis or renal transplantation resolves the lesion spontaneously. No local treatment is necessary or likely to be effective.

Verruciform xanthoma

Verruciform xanthoma is a rare proliferative lesion which can have a white, hyperkeratotic surface.

Clinically, verruciform xanthoma is most common in the fifth to seventh decades. It is usually found on the gingiva but can form in almost any site in the mouth. It can be white or red in colour, be sessile or pedunculated, have a warty surface, and range in size from one to several centimetres across. It may be mistaken for a papilloma, leucoplakia or carcinoma clinically, but is readily recognizable histologically.

Microscopically, the warty surface is due to the much infolded epithelium which, in white variants, is hyperkeratinized, but may be merely parakeratinized (Figure 9.13). In haematoxylin and eosin stained sections, the parakeratin layer stains a distinctive orange colour. The rete ridges are uniformly elongated and extend to a straight, well-defined lower border.

The diagnostic feature is the large, foamy, xanthoma cells which fill the connective tissue papillae but extend only to the lower border of the

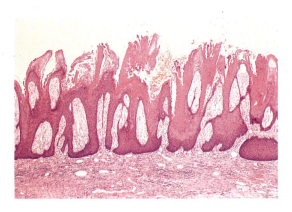

Figure 9.13   Verruciform xanthoma showing a verrucous, parakeratinized plaque with pale cells in the papillary corium

lesion (Figure 9.14). These cells contain lipid and PAS-positive granules.

Management

Verruciform xanthoma is benign and has no known associations with diseases such as hyperlipidaemia or diabetes mellitus associated with cutaneous

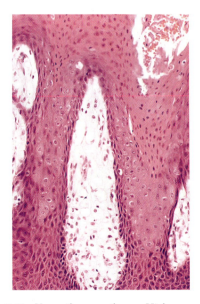

Figure 9.14   Verruciform xanthoma. Higher power view shows foamy cells in the papillary corium and the parakeratinized superficial plaques extending into the spinous layer

xanthoma formation. Simple surgical excision is curative.

Oral submucous fibrosis

In oral submucous fibrosis (Chapter 8), affected areas of the oral mucosa such as the palate or buccal mucosa appear almost white. This is not a leucoplakia-like lesion, but the mucosa is typically smooth, thin and atrophic, and the pallor due to the underlying fibrosis and ischaemia, is symmetrically distributed. However, the epithelium may show dysplasia and leucoplakia may be associated. Murti *et al.* (1985) reported the development of oral carcinoma in 7.6% of 66 patients with submucous fibrosis followed up for a median period of 10 years (Chapter 10).

Idiopathic (including dysplastic) leucoplakia

No aetiological factor can be identified for the majority of persistent white plaques. The histopathology is also highly variable, ranging from hyperkeratosis and hyperplasia to severe dysplasia.

The most extensive follow-up studies on leucoplakia suggest that this idiopathic group now has the highest risk of developing cancer. In most lesions of definable cause, the risk of malignant change is low, especially now that late-stage syphilis forms a negligibly small group.

Though there is no doubt about the malignant potential of leucoplakias, the level of risk cannot be accurately assessed from the histopathology. The largest study was carried out by Einhorn and Wersall (1967) and based on no fewer than 782 cases of histologically unspecified oral white lesions followed for an average of 12 years; of these, only 2.4% underwent malignant change in 10 years and less than 5% after 20 years. However, even this low rate represents a risk of malignant change 50–100 times that in the normal mouth. It was also conspicuous that in this large study the rate of malignant change in oral leucoplakias was 10 times higher in non-smokers than in smokers. By contrast, in a study of 257 patients with leucoplakia

who had been followed for an average of 8 years, Silverman *et al.* (1984) found malignant transformation in 17.5%. However, malignant change was also more frequent among non-smokers. Earlier, Silverman *et al.* (1976) had reported transformation rates of 0.12% in India and 6% in the USA. Other, smaller, series have suggested rates of 30% or more, though in many cases no time scale has been indicated, and the wide variation in the rate of malignant change in these different series suggests that the findings have been significantly affected by selection of cases.

It must be emphasized that these large-scale studies have been on histologically unspecified oral keratoses. Because of the rarity of dysplastic oral lesions there are very few studies, and none on a large scale, that have followed their progress for adequate periods. In the study by Mincer *et al.* (1972), 45 patients with oral dysplastic lesions were followed for up to 8 years. Only 11% underwent malignant change in this period and up to 30% of them regressed or even ultimately disappeared spontaneously. Eveson (1983), in a review of published surveys, found that dysplastic lesions appeared to regress more frequently than to undergo malignant change. As a consequence, it is not possible to prognosticate solely on the basis of the histopathological changes. An additional problem is that, apart from the subjective nature of the assessment, if part is taken for biopsy purposes, there is no certainty that it is representative of the whole. The aetiology of cancer and of precancerous lesions overlaps on many points and they are therefore discussed in the next chapter.

Clinical features
Idiopathic leucoplakias and dysplastic lesions do not have any specific clinical appearance. Small and innocent-looking white patches are as likely to show epithelial dysplasia as large and irregular ones. However, red (erythroplastic) lesions or erythroplasia in leucoplakias (speckled leucoplakia) are usually dysplastic or frank carcinomas.

Microscopy
The epithelium may or may not be hyperplastic and is often thinner than normal (Figures 9.15a–c). The plaque may show hyperortho- and parakeratosis in different parts, and the two may alternate along

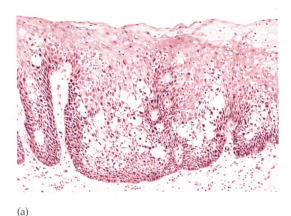

(a)

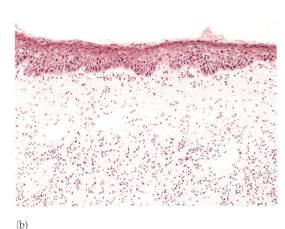

(b)

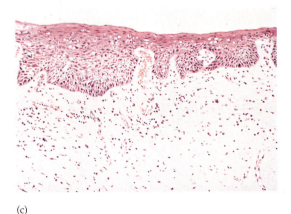

(c)

Figure 9.15(a–c)   Epithelial dysplasia. A series of photomicrographs to show some of the varied appearances

the length of the specimen. The epithelium is characterized by any of the cytological changes of dysplasia, namely:

- *Nuclear hyperchromatism.* The nuclei stain more densely due to increased nucleic acid content.
- *Nuclear pleomorphism and altered nuclear/cytoplasmic ratio.* The nuclei are variable in size, out of proportion to that of the cell; there may then be little cytoplasm surrounding the nucleus.
- *Mitoses.* They may be frequent or abnormal and at superficial levels.
- *Loss of polarity.* The basal cells in particular may lie higgledy-piggledy at angles to one another.
- *Deep cell keratinization.* Individual cells may start to degenerate long before the surface is reached and show eosinophilic change deeply within the epithelium. The term *dyskeratosis* applies only to this particular cellular change.
- *Differentiation.* The organization of the individual cell layers becomes lost and no clearly differentiated basal and spinous cell layers can be identified. Drop-shaped rete ridges are regarded as a particularly adverse feature.
- *Loss of intercellular adherence.* The boundaries of the cells may become separated.

A lymphoplasmacytic infiltrate of highly variable intensity is usually present in the corium.

Carcinoma-in-situ

Carcinoma-in-situ is a controversial term used for severe dysplasia where the abnormalities extend throughout the thickness of the epithelium – a state sometimes graphically called 'top-to-bottom change'. All the cellular abnormalities characteristic of malignancy may be present; only invasion of the underlying connective tissue is absent.

Top-to-bottom epithelial dysplasia, like other dysplastic lesions, has no characteristic clinical appearance. Erythroplasia, however, as discussed below, often proves to be carcinoma-in-situ or early invasive carcinoma.

Management of dysplastic lesions
The management of dysplastic oral lesions remains controversial, as their relative rarity has made it

impossible as yet to accumulate enough data to make reliable predictions. It is frequently also assumed that dysplasia is no more than an early stage in the development of carcinoma which will subsequently behave like any other carcinoma. This leads to the assumption that treatment of dysplastic lesion provides an opportunity to treat carcinoma at an exceptionally early, and potentially curative, pre-invasive stage.

In contrast to an optimistic viewpoint of this sort, are the findings (discussed earlier) in the large survey where Einhorn and Wersall (1967) discovered, after prolonged follow-up, that lesions which had been treated by surgery more frequently became frankly malignant than those which had not. Though selection of patients may have biased these results, they certainly do not endorse the value of surgery.

From the histological viewpoint it is also noticeable that the degree of atypia in many dysplastic lesions is considerably more severe than that seen in many frank carcinomas of the mouth. This may possibly be an indicator (on the assumption that the degree of differentiation of carcinomas is a guide to prognosis) of particularly aggressive behaviour.

Further, small dysplastic lesions, despite excision, can be followed by multiple carcinomas and a fatal outcome, as confirmed by the report of Shibuya *et al.* (1986) of 522 cases of carcinoma or carcinoma-in-situ (severe dysplasias) of the tongue. They found that the risk of multiple carcinomas was 5 times greater in patients with carcinoma preceded by leucoplakia than those carcinomas which had no such precursor. This large study, therefore, appears to confirm the possibility that some dysplastic leucoplakias may have a worse prognosis than isolated carcinomas without leucoplakia. Though such phenomena may be described as 'field change', this hardly helps either the patient or the surgeon.

By contrast, there is the evidence, discussed earlier, that many dysplastic lesions can regress spontaneously. It is clear, therefore, that the behaviour of dysplastic lesions is unpredictable and that there is no reliable protocol of management. If they are of manageable size, it is tempting to excise them – this can presumably do no harm, but it is essentially a treatment of hope rather than certainty. Prolonged, close follow-up is therefore essential. Even then, the prognosis may be poor. An alternative policy is to avoid surgical inter-ference unless there are signs of progression and deterioration.

Another approach is cryotherapy ablation. In the short term the area usually heals rapidly to leave an apparently normal mucosa. However, there is some uncertainty about the risk of invasive carcinomas subsequently arising in sites previously treated by cryotherapy. Carbon dioxide laser ablation has also been advocated, but the same objections may apply.

Treatment with systemic or topical retinoids has also been tried. Topical retinoids are largely ineffective and though a proportion of white lesions resolve with systemic treatment, the toxic effects are usually unacceptable. Further, lesions which resolve with treatment, recur on withdrawal of the drugs. More recently Lippman *et al.* (1993) have reported that high-dose induction followed by low-dose systemic isotretinoin did not cause an unacceptable degree of toxicity, stabilized the majority of lesions and was more effective than beta-carotene in preventing malignant change in oral leucoplakia. This seems an approach worth pursuing for lesions which are so readily accessible for clinical and pathological assessment of progress.

With regard to possible predictors of malignant change in leucoplakias, there is good evidence that such change is more common in women. This also appears to apply to malignant change in lichen planus, as discussed earlier.

In summary, frequent clinical observation, preferably with photographic records, and immediate biopsy of any suspicious or changing areas is the best that can be offered.

Speckled leucoplakia

This term applies to lesions consisting of white flecks or fine nodules on an atrophic erythematous base. They can be regarded as a combination of or transition between leucoplakia and erythroplasia; speckled leucoplakia also more frequently shows dysplasia than lesions with a homogeneous surface. The histological characteristics are usually, therefore, intermediate between leucoplakia and erythroplasia.

Many cases of chronic candidosis have this appearance.

Erythroplasia ('erythroplakia')

In contrast to the foregoing lesions, erythroplasias are red. The surface is frequently velvety in texture and the margin may be sharply defined. Lesions of this type typically do not form plaques (hence the term 'erythroplakia' is inappropriate) but, instead, their surface is often depressed below the level of the surrounding mucosa. Erythroplasia is uncommon in the mouth.

Microscopy

Erythroplastic lesions usually show epithelial dysplasia which may be severe. In other cases, there may be micro- or frankly invasive carcinoma. The risk of development of cancer is, therefore, highest in these lesions if they are not already carcinomas.

Early squamous cell carcinoma

Occasionally, early carcinomas produce sufficient surface keratin to appear as white plaques. They should not be confused with carcinomatous change in pre-existing leucoplakia. These carcinomas are always small (5–7 mm across), since further progress produces a more typical mass or ulcer.

Red, purple and pigmented mucosal lesions

One of the most important considerations is to exclude erythroplasia as the cause of a localized red area by biopsy. Other possible causes include the following:

Vitamin B$_{12}$ deficiency Exceptionally rarely, pernicious anaemia can cause red areas simulating erythroplasia. However, they are transient, only to reappear in another site. These are associated with a raised mean corpuscular volume in the blood picture or, later, the typical haematological features of pernicious anaemia.

More characteristic of pernicious anaemia is a pattern of red streaks on the dorsum of the tongue (Chapter 8). Generalized redness of the dorsum of the tongue can be seen in any type of anaemia.

Candidosis Candidal infection can cause patchy or widespread erythema according to the following circumstances. Angular stomatitis may be associated with any of them and is a sign of candidosis.

- *Denture-induced stomatitis*. Occlusion of the mucosa under a well-fitting upper denture cuts it off from the protective effects of saliva and creates a localized area of xerostomia. In susceptible patients this can promote candidosis. This is seen as an area of erythema sharply limited to the area of mucosa covered by the upper denture. Microscopically, direct Gram-stained smears show candidal hyphae and some yeast forms which have proliferated in the interface between denture base and mucosa. Histologically, there is mild acanthosis with prominent blood vessels superficially and a mild chronic inflammatory infiltrate. There is no plaque formation unless anaemia or any immune defect promotes the formation of patches of thrush in the erythematous area or elsewhere.
- *Generalized candidal erythema*. Xerostomia promotes candidal infection and in conditions such as Sjögren's syndrome, the whole of the oral mucosa becomes red and sore. Resolution follows use of nystatin suspension or miconazole gel held in the mouth.

  A clinically similar condition, *antibiotic stomatitis*, can follow overuse or topical oral use of antibiotics, especially tetracycline, as a result of suppression of normal, competing oral flora, but is infrequently seen now. Resolution may follow withdrawal of the antibiotic, but is accelerated by topical antifungal treatment.
- *Erythematous candidosis*. Though this term can be, and sometimes is, applied to any of the foregoing forms of candidosis, it is frequently now restricted to patchy, red mucosal macules due to this infection in HIV-positive patients. It is a sign of depletion of T-helper lymphocytes

and may precede any of the other types of candidosis. If resistant to topical nystatin, resolution may be obtained with fluconazole or itraconazole, but development of full-blown AIDS must be anticipated within a few years.

Amelanotic melanoma As discussed below, approximately 15% of oral melanomas are amelanotic and appear red but are equally malignant.

Haemangiomas These may form localized purple malformations, but mucocutaneous angiomatosis (Chapter 13) typically forms large red areas of mucosa sharply delimited by the midline.

Isolated haemangiomas form flat or nodular lesions which are typically sharply defined and blanch on pressure. If small, this can readily be demonstrated by compressing them with a glass microscope slide.

Kaposi's sarcoma This tumour must be excluded in any patient with a red or purple area or nodule on the palate or any other mucosal site. Kaposi's sarcoma in a male below the age of about 50 who is not having immunosuppressive treatment is pathognomonic of HIV infection (Chapters 13 and 14).

Telangiectases Telangiectases are small, localized abnormalities of superficial blood vessels. They are usually either a manifestation of hereditary haemorrhagic telangiectasia (HHT) or may be the result of previous irradiation. HHT is readily recognizable by the multiple small (pinhead) purplish lesions scattered about the oral mucosa and also on the lips and skin. Significant oral bleeding from this cause is rare. Irradiation telangiectasia is recognizable not merely from the history but also by the pallor of the surrounding mucosa due to ischaemia secondary to obliterative endarteritis and fibrosis.

Lingual varices Varices form on the underside of the tongue in the elderly and if they are noticed and alarm the patient, reassurance should be given.

Purpura and blood blisters Purpura can cause blood blisters or more extensive macular ecchymoses in the oral mucosa, particularly where there is pressure, as under the post-dam line of an upper denture. Haematological investigation and assessment of haemostatic function are necessary to find the underlying cause before there is a more severe bleeding episode, and to start treatment if necessary. The main conditions to be considered are idiopathic (autoimmune) thrombocytopenic purpura, acute leukaemia or drug-associated purpura. Autoimmune thrombocytopenic purpura is typically more common in women, but when AIDS-associated, is more frequent in men.

Localized oral purpura In this harmless condition, blood blisters form in the oral mucosa as a result of minor or unnoticed trauma without any abnormality of haemostasis. It is probably due to abnormal fragility of oral mucosal blood vessels.

Rupture of these blisters leaves a sore area, but healing is otherwise uneventful. Occasionally such blisters can form in the palate or throat and cause a choking sensation ('angina bullosa haemorrhagica'). A long history of recurrent oral blood blisters without either skin purpura or any other haemorrhagic episodes is usually enough to exclude systemic purpura. However, the latter should be excluded by haematological examination and the patient can then be reassured.

Bullous diseases In bullous diseases, particularly mucous membrane pemphigoid, the blisters can become filled with blood. Biopsy should make the diagnosis clear (Chapter 8) and it is rarely necessary to have a blood picture to exclude purpura.

Melanomas and pigmented naevi

Malignant melanoma of the oral cavity has a poor prognosis and must be distinguished from other pigmented lesions such as naevi and the common amalgam tattoos.

Terminology Melanocytes are of neuroectodermal origin, but migrate to the basal cell layer of the skin and oral mucosa where they form variable amounts of melanin and transfer it via dendritic processes to adjacent keratinocytes (Figure 9.16).

Heavier pigmentation may be due to more rapid synthesis and formation of coarser granules of melanin (as in coloured races) or to proliferation of melanocytes, or both.

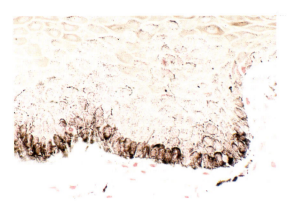

Figure 9.16 Melanin in melanocytes and keratinocytes. Fontana stain

Junctional activity is the term given to proliferation of melanocytes at the epitheliomesenchymal junction and protrusion of such foci into the corium (Figure 9.17). In adults, junctional activity suggests the possibility of malignant change.

Compound naevi show junctional activity together with clusters of naevus cells in the corium. In such cases, melanocytes appear to be dropping off the basal layer. Compound naevi are benign, but intraoral malignant melanomas are invariably compound in character.

Oral melanotic naevi

Pigmented naevi far more frequently affect the skin than the mouth. They are well circumscribed and most commonly macular or slightly raised and only very rarely polypoid. They can be brown, bluish, grey or almost black and only about 15% are non-pigmented and reddish. The palate is the most common site and women seem to be affected in the ratio of 2 to 1.

Microscopically, most melanotic naevi are intra-mucosal and show the naevus cells lying freely or in circumscribed groups (theques) in the corium.

Compound mucosal naevi (Figure 9.18) are rare and may be difficult to distinguish from malignant melanoma if trauma has induced proliferative cellular activity. Junctional naevi of the oral mucosa are even more uncommon.

Blue naevus

Blue naevi form about 35% of all oral naevi and are characterized by normal epithelium, but spindle-shaped pigmented melanocytes and melanin-containing macrophages (melanophages) are loosely grouped together in the corium and are typically well separated from the epithelium (Figures 9.19 and 9.20).

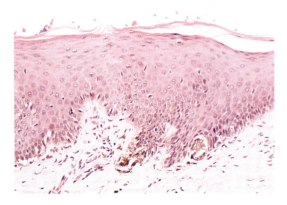

Figure 9.17 Junctional activity in a mucosal naevus. There are focal collections of heavily pigmented melanocytes at the epitheliomesenchymal junction

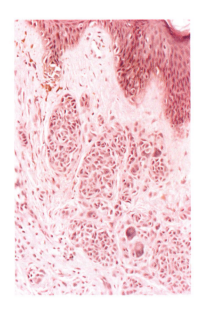

Figure 9.18 Compound naevus showing foci of junctional activity and underlying nests of naevus cells

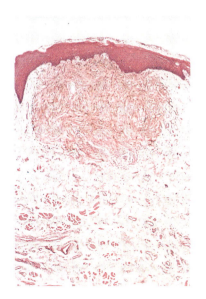

Figure 9.19   Blue naevus showing a discrete island of pigmented, spindle-shaped cells in the corium

Oral melanotic macule

These freckle-like pigmented macules are most commonly of the lip or buccal mucosa.

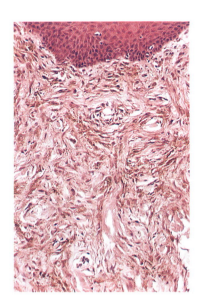

Figure 9.20   Blue naevus at higher power showing densely pigmented spindle-shaped cells close to the overlying epithelium

Microscopically, pigmentation is confined to the basal cell layer or immediately adjacent keratinocytes, but the epithelium and corium are otherwise normal (Figure 9.21).

Oral and labial melanotic macules may be associated with HIV infection and have been found in 2–6% of these patients.

Melanoacanthoma

Melanoacanthoma is an exceptionally rare pigmented lesion which may also show papillomatous proliferation. It may be a sequel to trauma, and may regress after incomplete excision. Melanoacanthoma may, therefore, be reactive rather than neoplastic.

Microscopically, the epithelium is acanthotic and contains clear cells and melanin-producing melanocytes with dendritic processes (Figures 9.22 and 9.23).

Management of benign pigmented lesions
All pigmented lesions need to be treated by excision biopsy to exclude the possibility of malignant melanoma. Since most benign lesions are small, excision is curative. As a general guide, naevi are more common in younger people (aged up to 40 years), are usually small, and appear to be static.

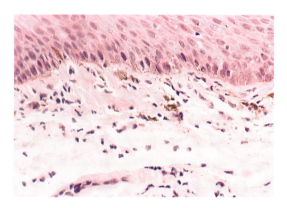

Figure 9.21   Melanotic macule showing increased melanotic pigmentation of basal melanocytes and melanophages in the superficial corium

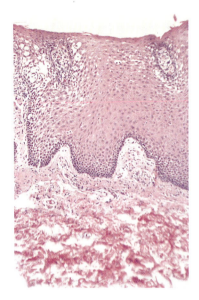

Figure 9.22 Melanoacanthoma showing acanthosis and spongiosis

Malignant melanoma

Oral melanomas are rare. The peak age incidence is between 40 and 60 years; nearly 50% are on the hard palate and about 25% are on the upper gingivae. About 30% of melanomas are preceded by an area of hyperpigmentation, often by many years. Pigmentation varies from black to brown, while rare non-pigmented melanomas (15% of oral melanomas) are red. Oral melanomas may be flat but are usually raised or nodular, and asymptomatic initially, but may later become ulcerated, painful or bleed. Because of their rapid growth, most oral melanomas are at least a centimetre across, and approximately 50% of patients have metastases at presentation.

Microscopically, malignant melanocytes invade both epithelium and connective tissue. Malignant cells may be round, spindle-shaped or both and there may be associated pseudoepitheliomatous hyperplasia (Figure 9.24).

Superficially spreading melanomas, which are considerably more rare in the mouth than on the skin, have a pre-invasive phase when atypical melanocytes with clear areas of cytoplasm (pagetoid cells) are clustered along the epitheliomesenchymal junction. Growth is radial rather than invasive, and there may be a few scattered melanocytes in the superficial corium associated with sparse inflammatory cellular infiltrate. Active invasion follows after a variable period.

Lentigo maligna, although not uncommon in the facial skin, is an exceptionally rare oral variant of melanoma, and is distinguished only by its microscopic features. A better prognosis for this variant when in the mouth has not been confirmed.

Prognosis and management

Clinically, size and rapid growth, particularly if associated with destruction of underlying bone or

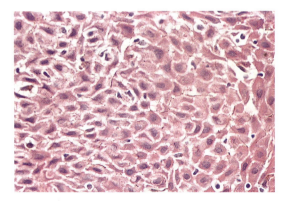

Figure 9.23 Melanoacanthoma. A higher power shows spongiosis and the dendritic processes of melanocytes in the stratum spinosum

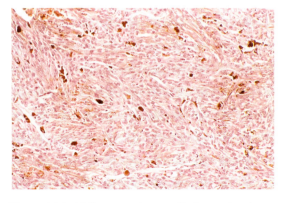

Figure 9.24 Malignant melanoma. Both round and spindle-shaped malignant melanocytes are present; some of them contain conspicuous amounts of melanin

presence of metastases, are obvious indicators of a poor outcome (Figure 9.25).

Microscopically, tumour thickness, measured in millimetres from the granular cell layer to the deepest identifiable melanocyte (the Breslow thickness), is the main guide to prognosis. With cutaneous melanomas the 5-year survival rate is inversely proportional to the Breslow thickness. The poor prognosis of oral melanomas is probably due to their later detection than more conspicuous skin tumours.

Other indicators of poor prognosis are malignant melanocytes in blood vessels and multiple, or atypical, mitoses. The morphology of the melanocytes or the amount of melanin does not appear to affect the outcome.

Once the diagnosis has been confirmed, the only hope of cure is provided by the widest possible excision followed by radical radiotherapy. There is no evidence that chemotherapy is of significant value except for palliation. The overall 5-year survival rate appears to be about 5%.

Secondary melanomas

Secondary melanomas have very occasionally been reported in the oral cavity and in the parotid gland. If unpigmented and anaplastic, they may pass unrecognized if the possibility is not suspected. S-100 protein is a marker for melanocytes, but not specific to these cells. More specific antibodies such as HMB 45 are now available.

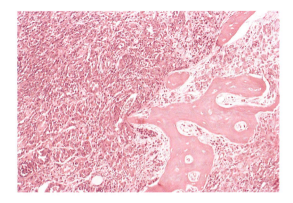

Figure 9.25   Melanoma of mandible invading bone

Melanotic neuroectodermal tumour of infancy (progonoma)

This rare tumour appears almost exclusively in the first year of life. It is intraosseous but the pigmentation may show through the mucosa and appear as a purplish area. It has been discussed more fully in Chapter 5.

Miscellaneous oral pigmentations

Amalgam tattoo

Amalgam tattoos are the most common cause of localized oral pigmentation. They form painless, bluish black macules usually less than a centimetre in diameter, with well-defined, or diffuse and irregular, margins. The mucosa close to the teeth or floor of the mouth are the common sites. They usually arise from mucosal abrasions during cavity preparation contaminated with amalgam fragments, from fractured restored teeth at the time of extraction, or from apicectomies sealed with retrograde amalgam restorations.

Microscopy typically shows dark, refractile particles of amalgam in the corium. The granules are black or brownish and tend to be deposited along collagen bundles and around small blood vessels (Figure 9.26). They are also found in nerve sheaths, around elastic fibres and in muscle, and may be present in the cytoplasm of macrophages, multinucleated giant cells or fibroblasts (Figure 9.27). Frequently there is no tissue reaction, but in about 30% of cases there may be a foreign body reaction or macrophage accumulations.

Intraoral radiographs with low penetration may sometimes show a small fragment of amalgam within the lesion and, when present, confirms the diagnosis. The only importance of these pigmentations is to distinguish them from naevi or melanomas and for this reason they should be excised for microscopy whenever there is doubt.

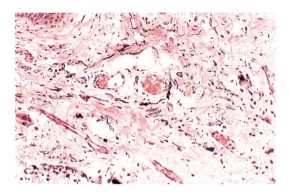

Figure 9.26   Amalgam tattoo showing dark granules of amalgam deposited along collagen bundles and around vessels

Peutz–Jeghers syndrome

This syndrome comprises intestinal polyposis and melanotic macules of the face, mouth and less commonly of hands and feet. It is inherited as an autosomal dominant characteristic, but only about half the patients have a family history of the syndrome.

There are multiple freckles on the lips and oral mucosa, particularly the mucosal aspect of the lower lip and the buccal mucosa and around the nares. Facial pigmentation is mainly around the mouth, eyes and nose; it usually fades after puberty, but the mucosal pigmentation persists. Microscopy shows increased melanin in the basal keratinocytes.

Polyps may be present throughout the gastro-intestinal tract, and in the small bowel can cause

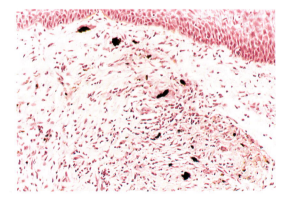

Figure 9.27   Amalgam tattoo showing black, refractile amalgam and an associated giant cell reaction

recurrent abdominal pain and minor intestinal obstruction. The polyps, which are hamartomas, have a low malignant potential and malignant transformation is rare.

Addison's disease (hypoadrenocorticism)

Addison's disease is rare. Bilateral destruction of the adrenal cortices was usually due to tuberculosis in the past, but the majority of cases are now due to organ-specific autoimmune disease or to histoplasmosis in immunodeficient patients. Addison's disease, therefore, occasionally now appears in AIDS patients as a result of opportunistic infections of the adrenal glands.

Clinically, pigmentation of the skin and oral mucosa is an early sign. The skin becomes bronzed, particularly in exposed parts, areas subjected to friction or trauma, skin folds and scars. Occasionally vitiligo is the predominant feature.

Oral pigmentation varies from light brown to almost black and can affect the gingivae, tongue (particularly the lateral margins), buccal mucosa and lips. Microscopy shows increased melanotic pigmentation, mainly of basal keratinocytes.

Weakness, lassitude, gastrointestinal disturbances, weight loss and hypotension may develop. Occasionally, oral white lesions of chronic muco-cutaneous candidosis are present and indicative of polyendocrinopathy syndrome type I, as discussed earlier.

Investigation typically shows low serum levels of sodium and chloride but raised potassium and urea. The diagnosis can be confirmed by a tetracosactrin (a synthetic ACTH-like polypeptide) test to measure the plasma cortisol response half an hour after an injection. Low plasma cortisol ($<5~\mu g/dl$) is diagnostic. However, Addison's disease is probably the least common cause of intraoral pigmentation, and such investigations should not be initiated in the absence of other suggestive clinical features.

Mucosal pigmentation in AIDS

Diffuse oral pigmentation can be seen in some patients with HIV infection. Pigmentation may be drug-associated or due to Addison's disease. In others, no cause other than HIV infection can be found. As mentioned earlier, oral melanotic macules may also be seen.

Racial pigmentation

This is the most common cause of widespread oral mucosal pigmentation and is seen particularly in Blacks, Asians and people of Mediterranean origin. Brown to almost black pigmentation is symmetrically distributed on the gingivae, palate, buccal mucosa and elsewhere, but its intensity is not directly related to the darkness of the skin. About 5% of adult Caucasians show similar pigmentation. Microscopy shows increased melanin pigmentation of the basal, and to a much lesser extent, suprabasal, keratinocytes (Figure 9.28).

Lichen planus

Degenerative changes in the basal keratinocytes may lead to pigmentary incontinence, particularly in coloured races, and this can result in an area of brownish pigmentation which persists long after the lichen planus has resolved (Figure 9.29).

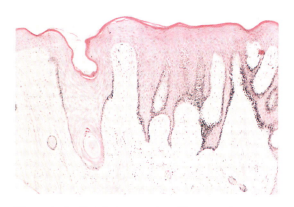

Figure 9.28 Racial pigmentation. There is a dense, linear increase in melanotic pigmentation of basal and, to a lesser extent, suprabasal keratinocytes

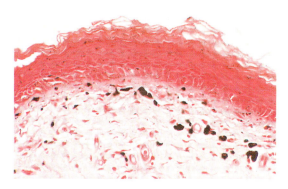

Figure 9.29 Pigmentary incontinence. Melanin in sub-epithelial macrophages is seen in a case of long-standing lichen planus. Fontana stain

Oral pigmentation and lung disease

Pigmentation of the soft palate may develop in patients with malignant or suppurative lung disease and is seen in nearly 25% of patients with bronchogenic carcinoma. Although most such patients are long-term smokers, the incidence of oral pigmentation appears to be much higher than in smokers without lung cancer.

Drug-associated pigmentation

Gingival pigmentation by heavy metals (mercury, lead, antimony, bismuth) was, in the past, a feature of industrial or therapeutic exposure to these agents. These metals caused blue, brown or black lines typically just short of the gingival margins and due to formation of sulphides as a result of reaction with plaque products. The cytotoxic drug cisplatin can cause a bluish gingival platinum line. Drugs which may cause diffuse mucosal pigmentation include the antimalarials, amodiaquine, chloroquine and mepacrine, busulphan, some contraceptive pills and phenothiazines. In patients with HIV infection, zidovudine, clofazimine, ketoconazole and pyrimethamine have been implicated in mucosal pigmentation.

Antibiotics and antiseptics used topically may cause pigmentation, particularly of the dorsum of the tongue due to overgrowth of pigment-forming bacteria.

Smoker's melanosis, with increased melanin formation, particularly in the attached gingivae, has been described but is less common or conspicuous than might be expected from the number of habitual smokers (Figure 9.30).

Black hairy tongue

This condition (see Chapter 3) is due to elongation of the filiform papillae which form hair-like overgrowths and become stained brown or black due to proliferation of chromogenic microbes. The causes are unknown, but heavy smoking and the use of antiseptic mouthwashes may contribute. The dorsum of the tongue may also become blackened without overgrowth of the filiform papillae in patients using antibiotic mouthwashes, particularly tetracycline.

Black hairy tongue only rarely resolves on stopping the underlying habit or antibiotic. Treatment is largely ineffective but the patient should be instructed to scrub the dorsum of the tongue daily with a toothbrush.

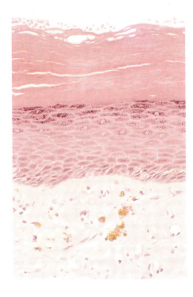

Figure 9.30   Smoker's keratosis and melanosis

References

Cawson, R.A. (1973) Induction of epithelial hyperplasia by *Candida albicans. British Journal of Dermatology,* **89,** 497–503

Cawson, R.A. and Rajasingham, K.C. (1972) Ultrastructural features of the invasive phase of *Candida albicans. British Journal of Dermatology,* **87,** 435–443

Cooke, B.E.D. (1956) Leukoplakia buccalis and oral epithelial naevi. *British Journal of Dermatology,* **68,** 151–174

Daniels, T.E., Hansen, L.S., Greenspan, J.S. *et al.* (1992) Histopathology of smokeless tobacco lesions in professional baseball players. Associations with different types of tobacco. *Oral Surgery, Oral Medicine and Oral Pathology,* **73,** 720–725

Davidson, H.R. and Connor, J.M. (1988) Dyskeratosis congenita. *Journal of Medical Genetics,* **25,** 843–846

Einhorn, J. and Wersall, J. (1967) Incidence of oral carcinoma in patients with leukoplakia of the oral mucosa. *Cancer,* **20,** 2189–2193

Eveson, J.W. (1983) Oral premalignancy. *Cancer Surveys,* **2,** 403–424

Hauser, F.V. and Rothman, S. (1950) Monilial granuloma. Report of a case and review of the literature. *Archives of Dermatology and Syphilology,* **61,** 297–310

Higgs, J.M. and Wells, R.S. (1974) Classification of chronic muco-cutaneous candidosis. Clinical data and therapy. *Hautartz,* **25,** 159–165

Kramer, I.R.H., El-Labban, N. and Lee, K.W. (1978) The clinical features and risk of malignant transformation in sublingual keratosis. *British Dental Journal,* **144,** 171–180

Larsson, A., Axéll, T. and Andersson, G. (1991) Reversibility of snuff dippers' keratosis in Swedish moist snuff users: a clinical and histologic follow-up study. *Journal of Oral and Pathological Medicine,* **20,** 258–264

Lippman, S.M., Batsakis, J.G., Toth, B.B. *et al.* (1993) Comparison of low-dose isotretinoin with beta carotene to prevent oral carcinogenesis. *New England Journal of Medicine,* **328,** 15–20

Lozada-Nur, F. and Costa, C. (1992) Retrospective findings of the clinical benefits of podophyllum resin 25% sol on hairy leukoplakia. Clinical results in nine patients. *Oral Surgery, Oral Medicine and Oral Pathology,* **73,** 555–558

Mincer, H.H., Coleman, S.A. and Hopkins, K.P. (1972) Observations on the clinical characteristics of oral lesions showing histologic epithelial dysplasia. *Oral Surgery, Oral Medicine and Oral Pathology,* **33,** 389–399

Murti, P.R., Bhonsle, R.B., Pindborg, J.J. *et al.* (1985) Malignant transformation rate in oral submucous fibrosis over a 17-year period. *Community Dentistry and Oral Epidemiology,* **13,** 340–341

Resnick, L., Herbst, J.S., Ablashi, D.V. *et al.* (1988) Regression of oral hairy leukoplakia after orally administered acyclovir therapy. *Journal of the American Medical Association,* **259,** 384–388

Shibuya, H., Amagasa, T., Seto, K.-I. *et al.* (1986) Leukoplakia-associated multiple carcinomas in patients with tongue carcinoma. *Cancer,* **54,** 843–846

Silverman, S., Bhargava, R., Mani, N.J. *et al.* (1976) Malignant transformation and natural history of oral leukoplakia in 57,518 industrial workers in Gujarat, India. *Cancer,* **38,** 1790–1795

Silverman, S., Gorsky, M. and Lozada-Nur, F. (1984) Oral leukoplakia and malignant transformation: a follow-up study of 257 patients. *Cancer,* **53,** 563–568

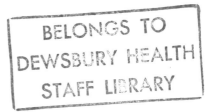

10

Epithelial tumours and cancer of the mouth

Papilloma

Squamous cell papillomas are relatively common oral mucosal tumours and usually clinically recognizable by their warty surfaces or long, papillary finger-like processes. They are white when keratinized or pink if not. Adults between the ages of 20 and 50 years are predominantly affected, but their age and site distribution and other characteristics have been analysed in detail by Abbey *et al.* (1980).

Human papilloma virus (particularly HPV 6 or 11) can be isolated from papillomas by DNA hybridization. However, unlike infective warts discussed below, evidence of viral proliferation is not seen by light microscopy. Moreover, simple papillomas appear not to be infective and have no tendency to spread by auto-inoculation to other sites.

Florid oral papillomatosis

This is a rare condition of widespread oral papilloma formation, which may involve the whole of the buccal mucosa, lip or other sites which become pebbly in character. It has been reported in Down's syndrome (Eversole and Sorenson, 1974), and massive oropharyngeal papillomatosis causing obstructive sleep apnoea in a child has been reported by Brodsky *et al.* (1987). Surgical excision may be justified, particularly for effects such as the latter, or for cosmetic reasons when the lips are affected, but the condition is otherwise benign.

It should be differentiated particularly from naevus unius lateris.

Microscopy
Papillomas have a branching structure consisting of a vascular connective tissue core, supporting a thick hyperplastic epithelium, which is often heavily keratinized (Figure 10.1). Occasionally, the epithelium shows mitotic activity but malignant change in oral papillomas is virtually unknown.

Management
Excision is curative. For patients reluctant to accept surgery, cryotherapy is equally effective but often followed by severe postoperative oedema.

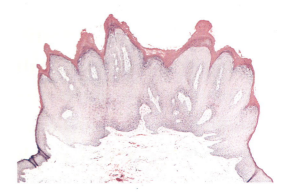

Figure 10.1 Squamous papilloma with sessile base, acanthosis and irregular warty hyperkeratosis

Papillary hyperplasia of the palate

Palatal papillary hyperplasia consists of multiple soft tissue nodules giving a coarsely granular or cobblestone texture to the vault of the palate. It is frequently regarded as response to trauma from or infection under a denture. However, it may occasionally be seen in the absence of a denture, but the latter aggravates the condition, particularly when harbouring *Candida albicans*. The papillae are then red and oedematous.

Microscopically, papillary hyperplasia consists of multiple, closely set, rounded nodules of connective tissue covered by hyperplastic epithelium and infiltrated by varying numbers of chronic inflammatory cells.

Management

If a denture is worn, the main requirement is to correct any defects and to treat candidal infection, if present, with topical nystatin or miconazole. There is little or no justification for surgical intervention.

Cowden's (multiple hamartoma) syndrome

Cowden's syndrome is a rare autosomal dominant, genetic disorder characterized by hamartomas in almost any site and, later, of malignant neoplasms. The mouth, skin, thyroid, breast, gastrointestinal tract and reproductive system are most frequently involved and papular facial lesions may bring the patient to seek attention.

Clinically, the disease often remains unrecognized until middle age, though the patient may have had treatment for what seemed to be disparate conditions for several years. Skin lesions are concentrated round the centre of the face and consist of fine, hyperkeratotic papular lesions which can give a toad-skin appearance. Oral lesions are present in most patients and consist of multiple, often almost confluent, small papules on the lips, buccal mucosa, gingivae, tongue or uvula, resembling florid oral papillomatosis. The tongue

may also be scrotal. The papules are initially painless, but may be so many as to interfere with mastication and if abraded become sore. Due to incomplete penetrance, relatives may have minor manifestations such as telangiectasia. The oral and systemic manifestations have been reviewed by Swart *et al.* (1985).

Microscopically, the oral papules consist of a fibrous core which may be highly vascular, covered by acanthotic epithelium.

Management

Diagnosis depends on the clinical orofacial features and usually also a history of removal of multiple, initially benign tumours, particularly in the sites mentioned earlier. Oral lesions require no treatment unless they trouble the patient. If so they can be excised, but Devlin *et al.* (1992) reported persistent bleeding as a complication. Continued observation is required to enable internal cancers to be recognized and treated as early as possible.

Verruca vulgaris

Infective warts occasionally affect the oral mucosa, particularly in children with warts of the fingers.

Clinically, oral warts are white and similar in appearance to papillomas. HPV 2a–e can be found in common warts and HPV 6a–f can be found in oral warts.

Microscopy

Warts are similar to papillomas, but distinguishable by the presence of intranuclear inclusion bodies.

Excision is treatment of choice, but further lesions may develop as a result of repeated auto-inoculation.

Condyloma acuminatum

Condyloma acuminatum is a sexually transmitted lesion seen mainly in the anogenital region. It is rare in the mouth but increasingly frequently seen in the mouth in patients with AIDS as an opportunistic infection, probably transmitted by orogenital contact. DNA of HPV 6 and 11 has been identified in 85% of condylomata acuminata by DNA hybridization, though HPV 11 may be found in all types of papilliferous lesions.

Clinically, condyloma acuminatum appears as a white or pink nodule with prominent papillary processes, larger and broader than those of papillomas. It is usually sessile and may be single or multiple.

Microscopy

The epithelium is thrown up into folds or broad papilla, giving a clefted appearance, and supported by a vascular stroma with a scanty, chronic inflammatory infiltrate. There is parakeratosis with a clear zone in the upper levels of the epithelium due to vacuolated koilocytic cells with pyknotic nuclei. Acanthosis is characterized by broad, long rete ridges. However, there are no reliable histological criteria for distinguishing condyloma acuminatum from infective warts.

Molluscum contagiosum

The molluscum contagiosum virus is a member of the poxvirus family and spreads by contact. It causes pearly umbilicated nodules on the skin, particularly of the neck, limbs and trunk. The nodules can reach 1 cm in diameter. They are exceedingly rare in the mouth (Barsh, 1966), but may be seen in the perioral region in those with HIV infection.

Microscopically, molluscum contagiosum consists of a goblet-shaped mass. The proliferating epithelium forms compressed papillae pushing down into the corium and surrounding a central cavity open to the surface. The superficial epithelial cells are distended by molluscum bodies which are large, hyaline, eosinophilic inclusion bodies containing enormous numbers of the virus. The contents of the central cavity are mainly desquamating keratin with molluscum bodies.

Verruciform xanthoma

This rare lesion can appear as a papilloma-like warty swelling with a whitish surface, but is readily recognizable histologically by the large sub-epithelial xanthoma cells (Chapter 9).

Focal epithelial hyperplasia (Heck's disease)

Focal epithelial hyperplasia is an HPV-associated disease, but possibly dependent on a genetic predisposition. It was first noted among American Indians and an Eskimo boy. The reported incidence in various racial groups was reviewed by Praetorius-Clausen (1973), who showed that it may be seen in up to 20% of Greenlandic Eskimos and nearly 34% of Venezuelan Indians. It is rare in Britain, but isolated cases have been reported from many parts of the world including Africa. HPV 13 and HPV 32 appear to be virtually specific to this disease.

Clinically, focal epithelial hyperplasia appears as creamy, slightly elevated, nodular, soft masses usually about 6–7 mm across. They are asymptomatic and frequently noticed by chance. The labial and buccal mucosa are typical sites, but the palate appears to be spared. Almost any age and either sex may be affected.

Microscopy

The epithelium is hyperplastic, mildly parakeratotic and with vacuolated, koilocyte-like cells with pyknotic nuclei just below the surface. The rete ridges are broad and often confluent. Virus-like particles can be identified by electron microscopy and viral protein identified by DNA hybridization.

Management

The diagnosis is confirmed by biopsy. Treatment is not normally required and may be impractical if lesions are widespread. Spontaneous resolution has also been seen.

Adenomas and adenocarcinomas

These tumours arise from minor intra-oral salivary glands and can, therefore, appear in the oral mucosa as submucosal nodules or swellings, most commonly on the palate, in the lip or buccal mucosa. They are discussed in Chapter 12.

Cancer and precancerous lesions

Definitions

Cancer refers here to squamous cell carcinoma which is by far the most common oral mucosal malignant tumour. However, the definition of premalignant lesions is more difficult. In practice, lesions can only be termed precancerous after malignant change has developed, since there is, as yet, no means of identifying with certainty the risk of cancerous transformation before the event. Cancerous change is well recognized, but by no means inevitable, in chronic white or red lesions. Even severely dysplastic lesions can undergo spontaneous regression as discussed earlier (Chapter 9). The histological findings, therefore, indicate no more than that a lesion has a malignant potential, but cannot be used as a firm prediction that malignant change will develop.

Clinically, the main lesions with malignant potential are idiopathic keratoses, speckled leucoplakias and erythroplasias. Microscopically, the main predictive feature is epithelial dysplasia.

Epidemiological aspects

Oral cancer is a disease of the elderly, having a peak incidence in the sixth or seventh decades. Overall, mouth cancer is uncommon in the UK, when compared with other sites. Although there are regional variations, oral cancer is also uncommon in most parts of the world where reliable data is available. The main exception is the Indian sub-continent, where the figure reaches 40% in some areas, and the mouth is one of the most common sites of cancer in any part of the body.

Incidence In England and Wales, in 1984 (latest available figures), the number of registrations for intra-oral cancer was 1329 and for cancer of the lip was 250. Together these accounted for 2.4% of all malignant neoplasms.

For comparative purposes, it is more useful to express incidence rates as annual age-adjusted rates per 100 000 population. Where reliable national cancer registries exist, these figures may be used for international comparisons. However, in India, where oral cancer has been reported to account for 40% of all cancers, this does not apply to all areas and figures for the country as a whole may not be reliable. Within Europe, the incidence varies from 2.5 in southern Britain to 16.5 per 100 000 in Malta where there is an unusually high incidence of lip cancer, probably due to the strong sunlight. The different incidence rates for rural and metropolitan Poland and Spain are probably similarly explained by the exposure of rural workers to sunlight. Binnie *et al.* (1972) remarked on the exceptionally high mortality from oral cancer in France, where there appeared to be an association between oral cancer, cirrhosis and the consumption of immature pot-still spirits containing toxic by-products of distillation.

In Northern America and Canada there appear to be even greater variations in incidence than in Europe. Newfoundland has the highest rate for oral cancer in the Western world. Again, this high incidence may be explained by the high rate of lip cancer among fishermen in Canada. The chances of a fisherman in Newfoundland of developing lip cancer is 4.4 times higher than that of a comparable male in other occupations. In the USA the incidence of oral cancer varies considerably between States and between Whites and Blacks. This might be explained by the low incidence of lip cancer among Blacks. National figures are not, however, available for the USA.

As previously mentioned, figures for Asia are also less reliable due to the absence of national cancer registries. Waterhouse *et al.* (1976) quote an incidence of only 19.6 per 100 000 for Bombay. This figure is considerably lower than that quoted by other studies undertaken in different areas of India such as 33 in Ernakulam, 25.2 in Gujarat, 22 in Srikakulam and 21.4 in Uttar Pradesh. There are conspicuous differences in incidence rates between the various races in Singapore, with the highest rate among Indians. Though this may be due to tobacco and betel chewing, submucous fibrosis (Chapter 7) or genetic factors cannot be excluded.

Age

Oral cancer is largely a disease of the elderly. Seventy-seven per cent of all oral cancers develop between the ages of 55 years and 77 years. In Britain, the mean age for oral cancer is 64 years for males and 61 for females.

Sex incidence and trends

Cancer of the mouth is traditionally regarded as a disease predominantly of males. The Registrar General's figures for 1921, for example, showed that the male to female ratio for deaths from mouth cancer was 13 to 1 in England and Wales. The magnitude of this difference is all the more remarkable if account is taken of the heavier female predominance in the population as a whole at that time, as a result of the losses in the 1914–1918 war.

Recent figures for England and Wales, however, show, for cancer of the tongue, a male to female ratio of no more than 1.5 to 1. Moreover, in most sites within the mouth, this ratio is even smaller, but for cancer of the floor of the mouth, the male to female ratio is 2.7 to 1. This change is due to a fall in the incidence in males, while the incidence in females has remained virtually constant.

Site
The floor of the mouth, bounded by the lateral and ventral aspects of the tongue and the mandibular alveolus, forms a horseshoe-shaped sump into which any soluble carcinogens could pool. Although this area is only 30% of the surface area of the oral cavity, it accounts for 70% of carcinomas and this fact suggests that an exogenous carcinogen may operate.

By contrast, cancer is so rare in the centre of the vault of the palate as to be a clinical curiosity. Cancer of the centre of the dorsum of the tongue is also rare that an isolated case is sufficiently remarkable to be reported in the international literature, and a retrospective survey of the microscopy of six such cases (Ogus and Bennett, 1978–79) showed that the histological diagnosis had been incorrect in all of them.

Though squamous cell carcinoma of the mouth does not show any significant variation in its histological features in different areas of the mouth, there are differences in behaviour and in prognosis according to site. The following sites are usually, therefore, identified.

- lip (vermilion border) (ICD 140)
- tongue (ICD 141)
- alveolar ridge or gingival margin (ICD 143)
- floor of the mouth (ICD 144)
- buccal mucosa
- palate.

For cancer registration and data on a national or international scale, the International Classification of Diseases is used, and in Britain at least, only the first four of these sites are considered in terms of incidence and survival. The remaining two sites are categorized as 'Other and unspecified' (ICD 145).

Frequency in different sites
The tongue is the single most frequently affected site. In women, the lip is one of the least frequently affected sites. The reason for the considerable and persistent difference in the incidence of cancer of the floor of the mouth between men and women is unknown.

In the South Thames Cancer Registry area (covering a population of approximately 6.5 million), of 589 mouth cancers registered in one year, 83% of the tongue tumours were histologically confirmed squamous cell carcinomas, while for the gum and floor of the mouth and other unspecified sites the figures were 78%, 83% and 60%, respectively. These figures are slightly low because not all diagnoses were histologically verified, and in some cases the type of carcinoma was not specifically categorized as epidermoid.

Aetiology

Much has been written about, but relatively little is known for certain, of the aetiology of cancer of the mouth or of precancerous conditions. Though the two are discussed together here, it must be emphasized that oral carcinoma developing in an identifiable precancerous lesion is found in only a minority of cases. In a careful study of 77 patients over the period 1935 to 1984, of the association between leucoplakia and cancer, Bouquot *et al.* (1988) found leucoplakia juxtaposed to intra-oral carcinoma in 1–9% of cases according to the site, though they found juxtaposition to be more frequent (66%) on the vermilion border of the lip. More puzzling is that in a study of 212 patients with oral cancer, Hogewind *et al.* (1989) found that 48% of them had *separate* white lesions. Moreover, as discussed earlier (Chapter 9), precancerous (dysplastic) lesions are usually of unknown cause.

The matter has been greatly confused by use of the term 'head and neck' cancer. To lump together such diverse types of neoplasia as mouth, salivary gland, nasopharyngeal, laryngeal or thyroid neoplasms – to name but a few – in terms of aetiology is, to say the least, to confuse the issue. Nevertheless, it is common to refer to 'head and neck' cancer without specifying which precise sites are being examined, both in epidemiological as well as clinical studies. Cancers, even in sites so close as the lip and intra-oral tissues, have different aetiologies and epidemiological studies on 'head and neck' cancer as a consequence often have little, if any, meaning.

Conditions or factors related to or thought to be involved in the aetiology of cancer of the mouth include the following:

- Possible carcinogens, direct or indirect:
  Tobacco
  Alcohol
  Areca ('betel') nut
  Experimental carcinogens
  Industrial hazards:
    woollen textile work
    some chemical industries.
- Infections (possibly with co-carcinogens):
  Syphilis
  Candidosis
  Viruses.
- Genetic (specific syndromes):
  Dyskeratosis congenita
  Fanconi's anaemia.
- Mucosal or mucocutaneous diseases:
  Iron deficiency (Paterson Kelly syndrome)
  Lichen planus
  Lupus erythematosus
  Oral submucous fibrosis (Chapter 7)

Dysplastic leucoplakias and erythroplaksias.
- Physical agents: sunlight (lip cancer only).

Race and actinic radiation

Dark-skinned ethnic groups have very low lip cancer rates in comparison with fair-skinned people living in the same areas. Anderson (1971) has shown that melanin acts as a protector, either as a physical barrier which blocks the passage of ultraviolet rays or by the chemical absorption of carcinogens released by ultraviolet radiation. This protective influence of melanin is not confined to Blacks. Belamarie (1969) reported that among the Chinese in Hong Kong the incidence of lip cancer formed only 4% of mouth cancers in contrast to 25–30% reported in the Western world.

Dorn and Cutler (1959) also showed that the incidence of lip cancer in the USA increased from the north-eastern States to the south-western States in line with the sunnier weather. This finding has been generally confirmed in countries such as America and Australia where immigrant populations with fair complexions are exposed to stronger sunlight than in their country of origin. The protective function of skin pigmentation is suggested by the lower incidence of lip and skin cancer in such countries among the indigenous populations.

In Britain, lip cancer has a higher incidence in Scotland than in England and Wales, and this too may possibly be explained by the higher proportion of fair- and red-haired Scots than English or Welsh. The amount of exposure to sunshine or the degree of protection from it among outdoor workers is nevertheless difficult to assess. Thus, there are many fewer hours of strong sunshine during the year in Britain than in Texas, but in Texas the wearing of an unusually broad-brimmed ('ten gallon') hat is traditional. By contrast, Lindquist and Teppo (1978) have reported an inverse relationship between the mean annual amount of solar radiation and lip cancer incidence in Finland, but this is exceptional and unexplained. In general, therefore, the incidence of lip cancer is greater in rural than in urban populations living in the same area, and outdoor occupational workers carry a higher risk of developing lip cancer. Sunlight is usually implicated as the causative factor and microscopically cancer of the lip is typically associated with a wider area of actinic damage (solar elastosis, cholastic change).

Though genetically determined racial skin pigmentation has a protective effect against lip and skin cancer in tropical climates, a genetic factor in some races may confer susceptibility to intra-oral cancer. This is suggested by the exceptionally high incidence of oral cancer in the Indian subcontinent. Oral submucous fibrosis contributes to some extent to this high incidence and a genetic influence is suggested by the high frequency of HLA10, DR3 and DR7 (Caniff *et al.*, 1986). Murti *et al.* (1985) report a malignant transformation rate of 7.6% in 66 patients with oral submucous fibrosis, observed over a median period of 10 years.

Tobacco use

Pipe smoking

Historically, it has been claimed that there is a link between clay pipe smoking and lip cancer. For example, the decline in pipe smoking in Britain has been associated with a steady decline in mouth cancer in males. However, as this habit is now rare in most countries, evidence is lacking to prove or refute this claim. A high incidence of lip cancer in one region of Czechoslovakia has been attributed to a combination of actinic radiation, spicy food and the use of the tschibuk, a short-stemmed clay pipe.

In Gujarat, India, the hookli, a short-stemmed clay pipe, is widely used. Mehta *et al.* (1969) noted that 7% of hookli smokers developed labial leucoplakia as a result of this habit.

Conventional pipe smoking can also cause a characteristic leucoplakia of the palate, but as discussed earlier (see Chapter 9), any associated carcinoma develops in another part of the mouth.

Cigarette smoking

Unfortunately, few workers have attempted to distinguish between the effects of cigarette smoking and other tobacco habits in the aetiology of mouth cancer. Wynder *et al.* (1957) and Keller (1967) both demonstrated a relationship between tongue and floor of mouth cancer and total tobacco smoked. Martinez (1969) estimated that in Puerto Rico the risk of developing oral cancer

was 2.5–5 times higher for heavy smokers than for non-smokers, but no distinction was made between different smoking habits. Graham *et al.* (1977), in the USA, have shown that heavy smokers (more than 20 cigarettes or 5 cigars daily) are six times more likely to develop oral cancer than those who do not smoke.

Although cigarette smoking is widely believed to play a major role in the onset of oral cancer, its influence must be limited. In several countries, the incidence of oral cancer has been declining during the same period when cigarette smoking has increased. In Britain, in particular, where detailed and accurate national data are available, the steady increase in cigarette smoking since the beginning of the century has been associated with a steady decline in the incidence of mouth cancer in males and no increase in this disease in females.

Moreover, unlike pipe smoking, there is no recognized or consistently found lesion caused by long-term cigarette smoking. Detailed follow-up studies have also shown that malignant change in leucoplakias is more common in non-smokers than in smokers.

More recently, data from several countries has suggested that there has been a significant but unexplained rise in the incidence of tongue cancer, particularly in persons under 45 years old.

Other smoking habits

Wynder *et al.* (1957) have also presented some evidence to link pipe and cigar smoking and oral cancer. Cheroot smoking is a common habit among Danish females, and Pindborg *et al.* (1972) have shown that floor of the mouth leucoplakia is associated with cheroot smoking.

In the Indian sub-continent, cancer of the hard palate is common and this has been linked with the reverse smoking of chuttas, with the burning end in the oral cavity. However, in the Caribbean, where a similar habit is practised, there is no link with oral cancer.

Bidi smoking, as practised in India, is related to oropharyngeal cancer. A bidi consists of a small amount of Nipani tobacco rolled up in a dried temburni leaf. Hoffman *et al.* (1974) have shown that bidi smoke has a higher content of carbon monoxide, ammonia, hydrogen cyanide, phenol and carcinogenic hydrocarbons than cigarette smoke. Pindborg *et al.* (1967) have shown a high incidence of commissural leucoplakia with bidi smoking and that 16% of bidi smokers had leucoplakia.

Tobacco chewing

There is a high prevalence of oral cancer in India, where chewing a betel quid containing tobacco is widespread. Attempts have therefore been made to assess the role of this habit. There is a greater prevalence of oral cancer:

- among individuals who chew betel quid compared with those who do not
- in the site where betel quid is habitually held
- among individuals who used betel for prolonged periods or particularly frequently.

Hirayama (1966) has confirmed that oral cancers form at the sites where the quid is habitually held.

The composition of the betel quid also varies from district to district, but usually contains tobacco, slaked lime, catachu and areca nut wrapped in a betel leaf. Recent epidemiological surveys have shown that it is only in those areas where tobacco is present in the quid that oral cancer is associated with the habit, though potential carcinogens such as arecoline have been identified in areca nuts.

Jaftarey and Zaidi (1976) have shown that in Pakistan the combination of betel chewing (with tobacco) and smoking enhances the risk of developing oral cancer by 23 times in men and 35 times in women. Others have shown a relationship between smokeless tobacco and oral cancer in the USA, as discussed below.

Snuff dipping and use of smokeless tobacco

In the south-eastern States of the USA, lower gingival and alveolar ridge carcinoma is common and women account for 45% of such cases (Winn and Blott, 1985). This has been linked with the widespread habit of so-called snuff dipping among women, over many years. Relatively recently, Skoal Bandits (small permeable paper bags, resembling teabags but containing tobacco) have been introduced.

Link *et al.* (1992) compared oral carcinomas in a small group of smokeless tobacco users with those in non-users. Among 874 patients with squamous cell carcinomas, 1.4% were smokeless tobacco users, while of 129 patients with verrucous carcinomas, 7.7% were smokeless tobacco users. The numbers at risk from smokeless tobacco use are unknown, but it is noticeable that, as Link and colleagues confirmed, both squamous cell and verrucous carcinomas far more frequently affected the buccal mucosa where the tobacco was held. More remarkably, they found that cancers developed later in users than in non-users. The mean age of smokeless tobacco users developing either type of carcinoma was 70.5 years and of non-users was 64.2 years. Moreover, the squamous cell carcinomas in users were, overall, better differentiated than those in non-users. Any carcinogenic potential for smokeless tobacco, therefore, appears to be low. Indeed, in Sweden where the use of smokeless tobacco is reputedly heaviest, Larsson *et al.* (1991), in reporting the findings from no fewer than 252 biopsies from regular snuff dippers, emphasized that over a period of many years they have never seen a carcinoma developing in a pre-existing snuff dipper's lesion. In short, despite the fact that tobacco-specific carcinogens can be identified, a relatively low proportion of long-term snuff users develop carcinomas. If malignant change develops, it is only likely to follow several decades of use.

Alcohol

Wynder *et al.* (1957) calculated that heavy drinkers (more than 6 ounces daily of spirits or equivalent) had a 10 times higher risk of developing oral cancer than occasional drinkers. However, it should be realized that many heavy drinkers are also heavy smokers. It is difficult to separate these risks and Lemon *et al.* (1964) found a low mortality from oral cancer among Seventh Day Adventists, a group who abstain from both alcohol and tobacco. By contrast, Binnie *et al.* (1972) noted that there was no association in Britain between alcohol consumption and oral cancer. Both alcohol and tobacco consumption had grown considerably during the previous 40 years, but during this time the incidence of oral cancer had been progressively falling in Britain. Binnie (1976) also noted that any association between alcohol consumption and oral cancer in the USA and France could be related to consumption of unmatured pot-stilled spirits containing toxic by-products.

Other authors have found an association between cirrhosis and oral cancer. They have suggested that alcohol-induced liver damage helps to initiate or accelerate malignant changes in the oral mucosa. Protzel *et al.* (1964) have shown, in animal experiments, that alcohol may be an aetiological factor in oral cancer through a systemic effect and that other substances which damage the liver can potentiate the action of carcinogens on the oral mucosa.

Infections and immunological factors

Syphilitic leucoplakia holds pride of place as a precancerous disease, in that reports suggest a rate of malignant change between 30% and 100%. However, the condition has become so rare that investigation of possible mechanisms has now become impossible.

The role of chronic candidosis is also obscure. The evidence rests on the facts that, first, *Candida albicans* is an intracellular parasite (Cawson and Rajasingham, 1972) and also candidal infection induces epithelial hyperplasia experimentally (Cawson, 1973). Secondly, chronic candidosis (candidal leucoplakia) is frequently speckled in character clinically and dysplasia is frequently associated. Thirdly, Cawson (1966) found that in randomly selected leucoplakias, in which the microscopic features of chronic candidosis were later found, the incidence of malignant change had been exceptionally high. Finally, cancer developing in cases of chronic candidosis have been reported. The possible role of candidosis in the aetiology of oral cancer has been summarised by Cawson and Binnie (1980), but even if chronic candidosis does promote malignant change, it accounts for relatively few cases.

Currently, there is active consideration of the oncogenic potential of viruses and some evidence has been produced to suggest the herpes virus genome or more recently human papilloma virus (particularly HPV 16) genomes can be found, incorporated into mouth cancer cells. The importance of this finding is as yet unclear, especially as HPV is equally frequently found in normal mucosa.

There is no evidence of any increased susceptibility to intra-oral cancer among patients who are deeply immunosuppressed or who have AIDS. However, the former have high rates of lip cancer if exposed to strong sunshine.

Various immunological abnormalities have been described among 'head and neck cancer' patients, but again their significance is as yet uncertain.

Genetic syndromes and oncogenes

The susceptibility to mouth cancer is significantly increased in dyskeratosis congenita (Chapter 9) and Fanconi's anaemia, as mentioned earlier, and is occasionally seen in Bloom's syndrome (telangiectatic erythema with growth retardation). A strain of rat with a high genetic susceptibility to cancer has also been described. However, the low incidence of mouth cancer in the population at large suggests that any genetic component in the aetiology is insignificant, though the possibility cannot be discounted that it may contribute to the high incidence of the disease in the Indian subcontinent.

Fanconi's anaemia
Fanconi's anaemia is a rare genetic chromosomal defect typically characterized by progressive bone marrow failure leading to pancytopenia and various congenital anomalies. Oral squamous cell carcinomas developed in 57% of 14 cases reviewed by Kennedy and Hart (1982). Carcinomas affected the oesophagus or other sites in the remainder.

Bone marrow failure usually starts to become apparent before the age of 10 and most die of anaemia or leukaemia within the next 10 years. In those where the marrow failure is mild or less rapidly progressive, carcinomas appear in the teens and usually before the age of 30.

Treatment of the oral carcinomas is according to accepted protocols but the long-term prognosis is probably limited by marrow failure which if mild at first may be accelerated by stress such as infection.

Oncogenes and anti-oncogenes
Currently, there is great interest in the p53 tumoursuppressor gene which may undergo mutation to contribute to the development of cancer. Mutant p53 proteins are stable and their concentration in cancer cells is considerably higher than that of normal p53 protein in non-neoplastic cells. Ogden *et al.* (1992) found that 55% of 20 oral cancers

expressed the stable p53 protein, but failed to identify it in what they termed normal, benign or premalignant mucosa.

Dental factors

Poor oral hygiene, rough restorations, sharp edges of teeth and ill-fitting dentures have often been implicated in the aetiology of oral cancer, particularly in the past. Indeed, it is uncommon to find a patient with oral cancer with a well-preserved dentition. However, the incidence of these dental irritants is so high that it is hard to prove a causal relationship with oral cancer.

Renstrup *et al.* (1962) have demonstrated that chronic irritation enhances oral carcinogenesis in experimental animals. Graham *et al.* (1977) attempted to assess dental status using a 'Dentition Index', and they found a greater risk of oral cancer to be associated with a low dental status. They found that men who smoked heavily, drank large quantities of alcohol and had a poor dentition had a risk eight times higher than matched controls.

The well-established improvement in dental health over the years in Britain has also been associated with an overall decline in oral cancer, though strangely not in women. Also, the lowest socioeconomic groups who have the lowest standards of dental health also are at highest risk for oral cancer. However, like so much of the data already discussed, any evidence for the role of oral sepsis in the aetiology of mouth cancer is circumstantial.

Mucosal diseases

The precancerous potential of various mucosal diseases has been discussed earlier (Chapter 8). Of these, the only common condition with a small but significant risk of malignant change is lichen planus. In the less frequently seen diseases lupus erythematosus and epidermolysis bullosa, there is also a risk of malignant change, but the overall contribution of such diseases to oral cancer must be small. Of other diseases listed, Paterson–Kelly syndrome appears to have strong precancerous potential, both for the mouth and oesophagus, but the importance of iron or other haematinic deficiency in this process is unclear. Moreover, the condition has become rare both in Britain and Sweden, and both this and other mucosal diseases, in so far as they may be premalignant, contribute little to the incidence of mouth cancer overall.

Clinical presentation of oral cancer

The clinical diagnosis of oral cancer is usually straightforward. Compared with most other sites within the body, the oral cavity is relatively easily examined without special equipment. Oral tumours, unlike many other sites, also cause early symptoms, and patients can become aware of, and often complain about, minute lesions within the mouth. Nevertheless, between 27% and 50% of patients present for treatment with late lesions. Many of these patients are elderly and frail, and therefore delay the effort of visiting their doctor or dentist. Many such patients wear dentures and may accept discomfort or ulceration and see no urgency in seeking treatment. Furthermore, the practitioner himself may not be suspicious that a lesion is malignant, and initial empirical treatment with antifungal therapy, antibiotics, steroids or mouthwashes may delay confirmation of the diagnosis and treatment. One survey suggested that medical practitioners are more likely to do this than dental practitioners.

It is essential that any clinician should use a thorough and methodical technique for examining the oral cavity. All areas of the oral mucosa should be inspected meticulously, and any suspicious lesion palpated for texture, tethering to adjacent structures and induration of underlying tissues.

Finally, the neck from the submandibular region to the clavicles should be carefully palpated in order to detect any lymphadenopathy.

Clinical presentation by site
Tongue   The majority of tongue cancers affect the middle third of the lateral margin and extend early in the course of the disease into the ventral aspect and floor of the mouth. Approximately 25% affect the posterior third of the tongue, 20% the anterior third and only 4% the dorsum. Rare cancers of the dorsum of the tongue are usually secondary to syphilitic glossitis.

Early tongue cancer may manifest itself in a variety of ways, but is typically painless at first. Often the growth is exophytic with areas of ulceration. It may appear as an ulcer in the depths of a fissure, or as an erosion, sometimes with infiltration into underlying muscle. White patches may or may not be associated with the primary lesion. A minority of tongue cancers may be asymptomatic but arise in an atrophic depapillated area with an erythroplastic patch or peripheral streaks or areas of leucoplakia.

Later, a more typical malignant ulcer usually develops and may reach several centimetres in diameter. The ulcer is hard, with heaped-up and often everted edges. The floor is granular, indurated and bleeds readily. Often there are areas of necrosis. The growth infiltrates the tongue progressively with increasing pain and stiffening, causing difficulty with speech and swallowing. By this stage pain is often severe and constant, radiating to the neck and ears. Lymph node metastases at this stage are common and 50% may have palpable nodes at presentation. The lymphatics from the tip of the tongue drain first to the submental nodes and from there directly to the jugulodigastric nodes deep in the neck. From the dorsum and lateral margins drainage is via the submandibular glands to the jugulodigastric group of nodes. The posterior third of the tongue drains via the jugulodigastric nodes to the upper deep cervical glands. Carcinoma on the tip, dorsum and posterior third may metastasize quite readily to the contralateral side. Due to the tendency to early lymphatic spread of tongue cancer, 12% of patients may present with no symptoms other than a lump in the neck.

Floor of the mouth   The floor of the mouth is the second most common site for intra-oral cancer, and accounts for 17% of cases in England and Wales. Most tumours in this site affect the anterior segment of the floor of the mouth to one side of the midline. Although arising in an anatomically distinct area, namely the U-shaped area between the lower alveolar ridge and the ventral surface of the tongue, carcinomas in this site quickly involve the tongue and lingual aspect of the mandible. This early involvement of the tongue often leads to a characteristic slurring of speech. The lesion usually starts as an indurated mass which ulcerates early. The clinical extent of infiltration is deceptive but may reach the gums, tongue and genioglossus

muscle. Subperiosteal spread is rapid once the mandible is reached. Lymphatic metastasis, although early, is less common than with tongue cancers. Spread is usually to the submandibular and jugulo-digastric nodes and may be bilateral.

More commonly than at other sites, oral carcinoma at this site is associated with pre-existing leucoplakia. Kramer *et al.* (1978) have reported that leucoplakia in the floor of the mouth has a much greater frequency of malignant transformation than those at other sites, though this has not been widely confirmed.

Gingiva and alveolar ridge   Few authors distinguish between carcinomas arising from the alveolar mucosa and those arising from the gingival margins. However, they have quite different clinical presentations. In England and Wales, carcinoma of the 'gum' (ICD 143) accounts for about 20% of oral cancers, is rather more frequent in males, and is three times more frequent in the mandible than the maxilla. The disease is more common in the USA and particularly in the south-eastern States where women account for 45% of cases, particularly those with the habit of snuff dipping.

In the dentate patient, gingival carcinoma is likely to be misdiagnosed by the dentist as the signs may closely mimic dental sepsis and periodontal disease, even when radiographs show bone destruction. The usual features are soft tissue proliferation at the gingival margin or superficial gingival ulceration. Loosening of the related teeth due to early spread of the tumour along the periodontal ligament can follow.

On the edentulous ridge, a carcinoma often appears as an indolent superficial ulcer adjacent to or within an area of leucoplakia. Occasionally, the lesion may be proliferative and again mimic fibrous denture hyperplasia. Because of these presentations, gingival and alveolar carcinomas are frequently unrecognized and often there is a history of extraction in an attempt to resolve so-called dental sepsis. Even in the absence of radiographic changes, the underlying bone is invaded in 50% of cases and this has important consequences for management.

Regional metastases are common at presentation and found in 30–84% of cases.

Buccal mucosa   The buccal mucosa extends from the upper down to the lower alveolar ridge, and from the commissure anteriorly to the ramus and retromolar region posteriorly. In general, the prognosis for this site is probably better than elsewhere in the oral cavity. This may be due to several factors. Bone is involved late in the disease, and unlike other sites, fewer tumours are typical squamous cell carcinomas. Verrucous carcinoma, although accounting for only about 5% of oral cancers overall, most frequently affects this site.

The majority of carcinomas of the buccal mucosa are posteriorly situated. The onset of the disease may then be insidious, with trismus due to deep infiltration of the buccinator muscle. The tumours are also subject to occlusal trauma, with consequent early ulceration and secondary infection. Extension posteriorly involves the anterior pillar of the fauces and soft palate with consequent worsening of the prognosis.

Infiltrative lesions can later involve the overlying skin of the cheek, resulting in multiple sinuses, and metastasize to the submental submandibular, parotid and lateral pharyngeal nodes.

Microscopy

Approximately 90% of cancers of the mouth are squamous cell carcinomas, and are usually well differentiated. The characteristic microscopic features are the retention of an obvious epidermoid character (sheets of polygonal cells with intercellular bridges) by all but the most peripheral cells of the tumour processes, loss of definition or disappearance of the basal lamina, nuclear pleomorphism and hyperchromatism, deep cell keratinization and invasion of normal structures in the tumour's path. There is almost invariably an inflammatory reaction (predominantly lymphoplasmacytic) around the tumour margins, and many believe that this represents an immunological defence against the disease.

Abnormal keratinization frequently leads to formation of whorls of keratin (cell nests) within the tumour processes. In addition to deep keratinization, these tumours, in their earlier stages at least, occasionally produce significant amounts of surface keratin and this can cause them to be mistaken clinically for leucoplakia.

As tissue destruction progresses, the surface usually ulcerates, and the ulcer typically has thickened margins infiltrated by the tumour.

In less well-differentiated neoplasms, cell nests are absent, prickle cells become less obvious and there is increasing atypia. The most obvious features of the latter are the increased nuclear cytoplasmic ratio, so that the tumour may consist largely of closely packed, hyperchromatic nuclei of variable shape and size. However, there is frequently variation in the degree of differentiation from one area of the tumour to another, and this inevitably makes grading – a subjective assessment at best – even more difficult, as discussed later.

Anaplastic carcinomas are rare in the mouth and, by definition, lack features indicative of their epidermoid origin, and prickle cells cannot be identified. They can, therefore, be difficult to distinguish by light microscopy, from metastases, or even from lymphomas. However, with the use of immunocytochemistry and epithelial markers, particularly cytokeratins, it is possible to identify epithelial tumours with more certainty.

Examples of these variations in microscopic differentiation are more satisfactorily illustrated (Figures 10.2–10.7) than described.

Classification, staging and prognosis

The practice of dividing cancer cases into stages arose from the finding that survival was better when the tumour was localized than for those which had extended beyond the immediate site of

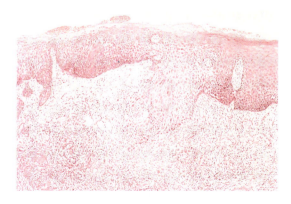

Figure 10.2 Very early squamous cell carcinoma showing micro-invasion in an area of severely dysplastic epithelium.

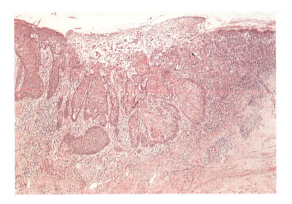

Figure 10.3   Early invasive well-differentiated squamous cell carcinoma

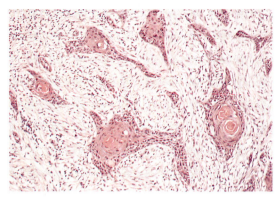

Figure 10.5   Well-differentiated squamous cell carcinoma also with conspicuous keratin pearl formation

origin. Subsequent observation suggested that even for a tumour confined to its site of origin, its dimensions also influenced the prognosis. Small, localized tumours are referred to as 'early' cases, though this implies that all cancers grow at the same rate.

There are many possible bases for classification, such as the anatomical site and size of the tumour, the duration of symptoms or signs, the sex and age of the patient, or the histological grade. All of these variables influence the outcome of the disease.

The TNM classification is based on clinical assessment of the anatomical extent of disease, and as a consequence, subjective and dependent upon the personal experience and skills of the clinician. The TNM classification had as its primary aim the clinical staging of tumours without addi-

tional diagnostic aids. This was achieved by recording the size and degree of infiltration of the primary tumour (T), the presence and condition of the associated regional lymph nodes (N) and the presence or absence of distant metastases (M). When precisely evaluated, these variables should give an indication of the prognosis and help the clinician in his choice of treatment.

After more than 10 years of research, the TNM classification, although extensively modified, faces essentially the same problems that were inherent in the original method, namely:

1. Is it possible to evaluate with sufficient accuracy the dimensions of the primary tumour, involvement of the regional lymph nodes and any metastases?

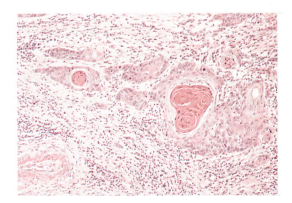

Figure 10.4   Well-differentiated squamous cell carcinoma with fibroblastic, inflamed stroma

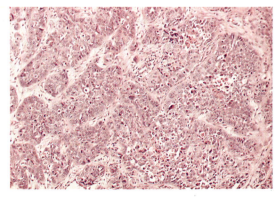

Figure 10.6   Moderately well-differentiated squamous cell carcinoma showing dyskeratosis but no keratin pearls

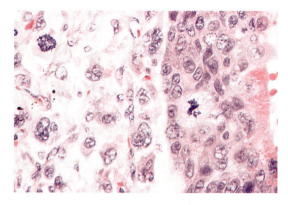

Figure 10.7　Poorly-differentiated squamous cell carcinoma showing extreme pleomorphism and bizarre mitotic figures

2. Are these criteria sufficient to formulate a prognosis, and if so, how accurately?
3. As most clinical cancer research is based upon retrospective rather than prospective studies, are the recorded data sufficiently detailed and reliable?
4. How consistent is the quality of the data from different centres, even when the same criteria are apparently used?

The need for staging

Before starting treatment for a patient with oral cancer, that patient's disease must be fully evaluated. Assessment includes an exhaustive history, physical examination, and laboratory and imaging studies, to determine the extent of the tumour and the presence or absence of lymph node or distant metastases. Every tumour should be biopsied and the histopathological diagnosis must be confirmed before the start of treatment. Because carcinomas arising from different sites in the oral cavity have distinctive clinical features, courses and prognoses, the therapeutic approach must be tailored to each patient. The many approaches to oral cancer suggest that a universally applicable form of treatment does not exist. The selection of the most effective treatment for a specific tumour at a particular stage, in any individual patient, is entirely dependent upon a meaningful comparison of the end results of adequate numbers of similar cases reported from different centres. For these reasons a classification

system is essential, but it has to be admitted that, though the TNM system is widely used, an ideal system does not as yet exist, as discussed earlier.

Modality of treatment must be presumed to affect the outcome, and data have been available on a national scale for the survival rates for surgery as opposed to radiotherapy. However, such information is biased by selection, since cases too advanced or too unfit for surgery are likely to receive radiotherapy. Moreover, there are so many other unmeasurable variables, such as the skill of the operator and the thoroughness of the excision, that it may not be possible to draw any conclusions from different published series except to note that from some centres better results are reported than from others. However, personal series, though usually too small to overcome the inherent variables affecting prognosis, may be of value, because more details about both the tumours and patients are available.

The size of the sample　As discussed below, so many variables affect survival rates that when this aspect is under consideration, data on anything less than several thousand cases are rarely of value.

The country of origin　It is common to extrapolate data from the USA to Britain, but though this may be justified, the wide variations in site, sex and other aspects of cancer in different countries make such extrapolations difficult to validate. Some differences may be related to genetic factors, but environmental influences are likely also to play a part.

Accuracy of site identification　This is one of the most common sources of confusion, since, as mentioned earlier, 'head and neck cancer' encompasses a wide variety of tumours, most of which are likely to have different aetiologies, and certainly have different survival rates. Frequently, because overall numbers are small, cancer registries find it convenient to include pharyngeal cancer with mouth cancers (oropharyngeal cancer) and may even include lip and salivary gland tumours. Aetiologies and survival times certainly vary widely even for this relatively restricted group of sites. Often these facts are not made clear, and it may be assumed that the data applies to mouth cancer only. In addition, it has been shown that even for oral cancer there are significant variations in survival times according to the site within the mouth. Broadly speaking, the further posteriorly the tumour, the poorer the prognosis.

Tumour size   Few surgeons make more than an approximate visual assessment of the maximum diameter of a tumour. In addition to any inaccuracies in such assessments, they can only take account of the visible surface of the tumour and cannot take into account the extent to which it may be undermining the surrounding tissues and extending deeply. Moore *et al.* (1986), for example, found that with tumours between 2 and 4 cm in surface diameter, there was little correlation with behaviour as depth of invasion was not taken into account. It seems inescapable that invasion has a significant impact on survival, but such information is not available until the specimen is examined histologically.

Reliability of histological grading methods
It is considered virtually axiomatic that well-differentiated tumours do better than poorly differentiated ones. Any staging procedure should logically, therefore, take the histological grade into account. The difficulty is that assessments of grade are also largely subjective and different systems take into account different microscopic features. Further, a biopsy may provide an unrepresentative area since the cell populations of tumours are frequently heterogeneous. For this last reason, the long-established Broders' 1927 classification has been reported to be unreliable, but the number of grading systems published since then testifies to the difficulties involved. In addition to attempting to assess degrees of differentiation, other microscopic variables such as intravascular invasion may be taken into account. The latter has been correlated with the incidence of lymph node metastases (Close *et al.*, 1987) and more recently has been found to have a considerable impact on survival as well as on the incidence of recurrence or metastases.

Anneroth *et al.* (1987) have carried out a detailed comparison of histological grading systems since Broders' contribution, and proposed yet another. The latter provides a point system for assessing degrees of (a) keratinization, (b) nuclear pleomorphism, and (c) numbers of mitosis. In addition, assessment is also made of tumour–host relationship in terms of (a) pattern of invasion, (b) depth of invasion, and (c) lymphoplasmacytic response. Anneroth *et al.* (1987) also recommended exclusion

of assessment of vascular invasion because of the difficulties in defining and recognizing it.

More recently still, Bryne *et al.* (1989) proposed a grading system modified from that proposed by Anneroth *et al.* (1987) and applied only to the most invasive areas of the tumour. Using this method for 68 oral carcinomas, these workers found a strong correlation between the histological score and survival. By contrast, they found no correlation between Broders' grade and survival. The site and size of the tumour were also found to affect the outcome.

As more refined techniques develop, so further methods of grading tumours must be anticipated. In a study of 176 oral carcinomas by Tytor and Olofsson (1992), the findings from DNA cytometry were compared with more conventional staging procedures and correlated with outcome. In brief, their findings were that a high microscopic malignancy grading correlated with DNA non-diploidy and with a higher frequency of lymph node metastasis and bone invasion. Non-diploid tumours also had a shorter history. Aneuploid tumours responded better to preoperative radiotherapy than diploid or polyploid tumours. Bryne (1991) reviewed the various molecular and cellular factors used to assess the prognosis of oral carcinomas. He suggested that histopathological grading, tumour thickness and tumour DNA content formed independent markers for prognosis which might be useful clinically and that the features of cells from the invading margins were probably of greater prognostic value than others. He also summarized the research on other cellular and serum markers at that time. However, in contrast to many earlier reports, Stell (1992), on the basis of an unusually large personal series of 842 tumours of the oral cavity, of which 512 were histologically proven squamous cell carcinomas, found that the histological grade appeared to be unimportant and that the only identifiable host factors determining survival were greater age and worsening performance status, although survival was similar for either sex.

Earlier, in an attempt to overcome the deficiencies of TNM classifications and their modifications, Rapidis *et al.* (1977) and Langdon *et al.* (1977) proposed an expanded classification applicable primarily to tumours of the oral cavity. They also developed a staging system which circumvented the problems of having large subgroups of the permutations of T, N and M and aimed to provide a more accurate indication of the prognosis.

Rapidis *et al.* (1976) proposed a revised classification, for intra-oral carcinoma, consisting of S (site), T (tumour dimensions), N (lymph node involvement), M (distant metastases) and P (histopathology), and therefore termed the STNMP system. In this, the anatomical site of the primary tumour (S) was subdivided into nine different categories, although only five of these (tongue, cheek, palate, floor of mouth and alveolar process) were intra-oral.

The STNMP classification has since been applied to a larger series of patients and compared with the TNM classification. Evans *et al.* (1982) developed a new statistical approach, using life tables and applying actuarial methods to compute survival times and confirmed that the STNMP scoring system was an accurate predictor of survival and was a significant improvement over TNM systems. However, Rich and Radden (1984) were unable to confirm that the STNMP system was of any greater value than TNM in estimating prognosis in a series of 118 patients. They considered that the probable explanation was that the weighting system used in the STNMP system, and indeed in any system where a subjectively measurable variable is given an arbitrary score, is difficult to manipulate statistically to enable valid comparisons to be made.

Evans *et al.* (1982) computed yet another variable – the velocity of growth (V) – by dividing the area of the tumour at presentation by the time elapsed since symptoms were first noted. The area of the tumour was assessed as three-quarters of the length × the breadth of the lesion (a rough estimate of the area of an ellipse). Their analysis showed that this estimate of velocity of growth was even more important than the size of tumour at presentation.

Estimates of the delay between the onset of symptoms and a definitive diagnosis are highly subjective, since they rely on the memory of the patient. Nevertheless, even an estimated velocity of tumour growth appears to have important prognostic significance.

Conclusions

Staging is clearly important in planning treatment, assessing prognosis and advising patients accordingly. Further, if a valid set of measurable features could be devised, accurate staging would be of immense value in assessing different approaches to treatment. However, it is clear that so many variables are involved that it would require immense numbers of patients, each of whose disease would have to have been equally accurately graded, to provide any useful information. The number of grading systems that have been devised and their increasing complexity is an indication of the problems involved and it is likely that most surgeons, unless they have unusually small workloads, will continue to rely on simple, essentially traditional, staging systems when deciding on the treatment of any individual patient.

In summary, it is difficult to say more than that the prognosis is poorer for cancer of the tongue, for men, for the elderly, for poorly differentiated tumours, for late (extensive) disease and for those with nodal involvement.

Management

Overall, cure rates in terms of 5-year survival rates are probably similar for surgery or radiotherapy, and the choice of treatment modality must be made for the individual patient. Combined treatment with radiotherapy before or after surgery is the optimal treatment for most T2/T3 tumours. For some sites – particularly when bone is involved – surgery is normally preferred, whereas for the tongue particularly, where retention of good function is critical, radiotherapy may be preferred. For such reasons, patients with 'head and neck cancer' should be managed in joint clinics with suitable surgical and radiotherapy representation, as well as other specialists such as oral hygienists and speech therapists.

Despite anecdotal reports of cures, there is not as yet any evidence that the use of chemotherapy, either alone or in combination with surgery and/or radiotherapy, confers any benefit. The toxic effects of chemotherapy itself also confer a significant mortality and Stell (1990) has shown that it reduces survival when compared with conventional treatment. It is probably, therefore, at best a treatment of last resort, though clinical trials to evaluate it still continue.

Surgery

With current surgical techniques it is possible to resect most tumours in the head and neck region.

Thus, the vast majority of head and neck cancer patients are potentially treatable by surgery, but many of them should not be because of advanced age, general disability or its mutilating effects. Before the decision to operate is made, four principles must be considered

1. There must be a reasonable prospect of cure.
2. The entire tumour must be removed.
3. Although normal anatomy and function should be retained or restored whenever possible, this consideration should not compromise the excision.
4. To the patient, the most important consideration will often be whether the final result is cosmetically acceptable. What the patient will tolerate is often very different from what the surgeon may require. The patient should, therefore, be carefully advised of the problems involved and possible complications.

The surgical techniques used today for excision of oral cancer were largely perfected before 1950. The last 30 years have yielded very little improvement in cure rate, but there have been considerable improvements in immediate surgical mortality and reconstruction.

Reil *et al.* (1975) analysed the surgical mortality figures for head and neck resections over a 20-year period, and showed a reduction from 16% to 2.5%. The quality of life following excision has greatly improved, largely due to new techniques for reconstruction. Although in historical terms axial flaps, such as the forehead flap and deltopectoral flap, were great advances, the more recent development of myocutaneous flaps (pectoralis major, latissimus dorsi and trapezius flaps) and microvascular, free flaps (particularly the radial forearm flap and compound groin flap) have revolutionized reconstruction and rendered it a one-stage procedure.

Spread of carcinoma of the mouth

The critical feature of carcinomas is their capacity to invade local structures and to spread into the neck through the lymphatics and beyond. Control of the disease in the mouth and neck dominates all aspects of management.

Knowledge of patterns of spread of oral cancer is clearly important if excision is to be complete but

within practical limits. Nevertheless, there are obvious difficulties in the way of adequately defining such patterns. It must, therefore, be appreciated that, despite all the research so far carried out, the following account should be regarded only as a general guide and that cancers can behave unpredictably. It is essential, as described below, to check that resection margins are clear of tumour.

Local spread
Invasion of soft tissues   Mouth cancers often infiltrate widely into adjacent connective tissues. Particularly in the tongue, extensive infiltration beneath intact mucosa is common and very difficult to detect preoperatively. The risk is, therefore, of encroachment of tumour into resection margins which, of necessity, are often very narrow in the oral cavity. Meticulous frozen section control of all soft tissue margins is, therefore, important during resections and, when radiotherapy is used, any such local extension must be taken into consideration in determining the volume of tissue to be excised.

Carcinomas penetrate deeply between and occasionally within the intrinsic muscle bundles of the tongue, but extension through the mylohyoid and hyoglossus muscles in the floor of the mouth is uncommon. In the tongue, infiltration is usually more extensive posteriorly than anteriorly. Tumours arising more posteriorly in the region of the linguotonsillar groove may, however, spread behind the mylohyoid and enter the submandibular space.

These natural soft tissue barriers and pathways become obliterated by previous surgery and/or irradiation, by progressive fibrosis. Under such circumstances, the extent and direction of local spread becomes unpredictable.

Invasion of perineural spaces
Perineural spread in the head and neck region is particularly characteristic of adenoid cystic carcinoma, but may also be seen with squamous cell carcinomas. Once within perineural spaces, tumour cells can track long distances both distally and proximally. Such centripetal infiltration of tumour along branches of the mandibular nerve (inferior dental, long buccal, lingual) may lead to direct intracranial extension. For this reason, whenever the mandible is resected for control of carcinoma,

the inferior dental bundle should be taken as high as possible. Similarly, whenever a rim resection is being considered, the excised portion of the mandible must include the inferior dental canal.

Invasion of vessels Intravascular tumours cells are usually seen as small clumps lying either freely in the vessel lumen or within thrombi. Close *et al.* (1987) demonstrated a significant correlation between vascular invasion and the incidence of nodal metatases, and extended this work (Close *et al.*, 1989) to show a correlation between microvascular invasion and survival from oral and oropharyngeal cancer. The assessment of microvascular invasion in stage determination may, therefore, be important and has been discussed earlier. Paradoxically, no consistent association has been established between penetration of the internal jugular vein and the presence of systemic blood-borne metastases. Invasion of arteries is rare. Infiltrating carcinomas tend to grow around arteries, leaving a distinct peri-adventitial clear zone. Even in patients with carotid rupture, infiltration of the arterial wall is rare. The main predisposing factors are previous irradiation of the neck, necrosis of skin flaps, infection and salivary fistulas.

Thrombi containing tumour cells are rarely seen in lymphatics and evidence of direct permeation along the lumen is uncommon.

Invasion of bone The principal mode of access to the facial bones is by direct extension. Invasion is facilitated by anatomical openings such as the inferior dental canal and incisive and palatine foramina. Access of tumour by periosteal lymphatics is probably not important. Despite its dense cortical plates, mandibular invasion is more common than maxillary invasion. It has been suggested that this is due to the persistence of nutrient vessels running vertically and perforating the crest of the alveolar ridge, even in the edentulous mandible. Reference has already been made to the mylohyoid acting as a barrier to deep invasion. This observation that invasion spreads downwards from the alveolar crest indicates that rim resection of the mandible is a sound procedure in selected cases, provided that the resection includes the inferior dental canal and its contents throughout its length.

The mechanism of bone invasion is mainly by induction of host osteoclasts. Direct erosion of bone

by tumour cells is only a very late feature. The osteoclasts are stimulated by a combination of osteolytic factors – such as prostaglandins E_2 and F_2 – and others such as interleukin 2. These mediators are formed both by the tumour cells and also by host tissues. There is no correlation between the extent of bone destruction or the presence of distant skeletal metastases with hypercalcaemia. There is presumptive evidence that such tumours produce humoral calcium-mobilizing factors.

Preoperative assessment of early bone involvement is difficult. Gilbert *et al.* (1986) have compared the value of clinical assessment, radiography and bone scans, and correlated the frequency of mandibular involvement with spread to lymph nodes. A possible reason for the difficulties in assessing the extent of bone involvement is that it is produced in different ways. Lukinmaa *et al.* (1992) have shown that oral cancers invade bone either by non-uniform infiltration or on a broad front, and that the extent of infiltration of bone can considerably exceed their superficial dimensions. By contrast, some large tumours with clinical fixation to the mandible may not have invaded bone. There was also no clear correlation between the degree of differentiation and bone invasion.

As to visualizing the extent of bone invasion, Millesi *et al.* (1990) correlated the findings of conventional radiography, sonography, CT and MRI and technetium scintigraphy and concluded that ultrasonography provided the most reliable diagnosis in most areas of the mandible. Bahadur (1984) also compared radiography, CT and isotope scans, found none of them to be completely reliable and recommended resection of the superior margin of the mandible for all carcinomas close to, even when not visibly involving, the bone. By contrast, Ator *et al.* (1990) claim that using T_1 and T_2 sequences on a small group of patients, MRI was the most reliable method of determining the full extent of mandibular marrow invasion and superior to CT scanning and conventional imaging methods.

Metastases to regional lymph nodes
Clinical assessment of cervical lymph nodes is unreliable. Crile, as long ago as 1906, observed that 'palpable glands may be inflammatory and impalpable glands may be carcinomatous'. However, the distribution of nodal metastases from

cancers of the mouth and jaws is reasonably predictable. Cancers of the tongue, floor of the mouth and alveolar ridges metastasize principally to the ipsilateral submandibular, jugulodigastric and middle deep cervical nodes. Cancers of the retromolar trigone spread to the submandibular, jugulodigastric and upper and middle deep cervical nodes. The parapharyngeal nodes may also be invaded but are not accessible to conventional radical neck dissection. Cancers of the lip and tip of the tongue spread to submental and submandibular nodes. Lesions of the tongue, lip and floor of mouth close to the midline metastasize to nodes on both sides of the neck.

The number of involved nodes is usually small, but extensive involvement of nodes along the entire length of the jugular chain is more frequent with aggressive tongue cancers which also spread to nodes in the posterior triangle.

Important prognostic factors are multiple involved nodes, metastases in the low cervical nodes and extension of carcinoma beyond the node capsule. The degree of histological differentiation in nodal metastases and in the primary tumour is usually similar and both are equally sensitive, or resistant, to radiotherapy. Extranodal spread results in infiltration of local muscles, the carotid sheath and its contents, bone, salivary glands, skin and prevertebral fascia.

Distant spread

This is discussed below.

Radiotherapy

Radical radiotherapy aimed at cure may be used as the sole treatment or combined with surgery. The object is local control, namely complete destruction of the tumour. This requires the killing of all tumour cells, while at the same time leaving sufficient normal cells in the adjacent tissues to allow repair. In general, radiotherapy is more effective against small tumours, although it is often advocated for the large, so-called inoperable tumour. The larger the tumour, the more likely are tumour cells to survive irradiation and produce a recurrence. Also, as a tumour grows, it tends to outstrip its blood supply; more cells become hypoxic and therefore radioresistant.

Palliative radiotherapy is used to relieve symptoms – such as bleeding, pain and obstruction – without attempting cure. Only a moderate dose is administered (e.g. 20 Gy) given over a short period (e.g. 5 days) to avoid producing other symptoms due to the acute tissue reaction.

The major argument in favour of radical radiotherapy as primary treatment is that many patients can be cured without surgery, and therefore will be spared the possible hazards of deformity and disability. A few of those in whom radiotherapy fails can be treated successfully by surgery (though surgery is made more difficult), but the converse is not true – radiotherapy rarely cures a patient who develops a recurrence after surgery.

Planned operative radiotherapy aims to improve surgical cure. Its basic assumption is that local recurrence or metastases result from dissemination of tumour cells at operation. Preoperative radiotherapy (40–45 Gy) will kill well-oxygenated peripheral tumour cells without causing surgical complications, but though there is some evidence that it improves local control, it is often difficult to arrange and rarely used.

The purpose of postoperative radiotherapy is to destroy small numbers of malignant cells which may be left behind or implanted into the operative field at the time of radical resection. However, after radical surgery, fibrosis progresses rapidly, resulting in local ischaemia. To be effective, postoperative radiotherapy must be instituted within 6 weeks of surgery and should be given whenever tumour extends beyond resection margins, or there is multiple node involvement or extracapsular spread.

Interstitial radiotherapy

Interstitial radiotherapy, in which solid sources of radiation, such as iridium wires, are implanted directly into the tumour, produces a high intensity of radiation in the immediate vicinity of the source, while the dose to the surrounding tissues is low because of rapid fall-off. Side effects such as xerostomia, taste loss and bone necrosis are much less than with external radiation. Radiation sources must, however, encompass the whole lesion with a margin of at least 1 cm all round. This technique is, therefore, applicable only to smaller tumours confined to the soft tissues (tongue, cheek, floor of mouth), but gives very good local control rates.

Fast neutron therapy

After enthusiastic claims for the value of fast neutron therapy based on small numbers of patients with various types of head and neck cancer, it seems that the complications outweigh any suggested benefits. Stafford *et al.* (1992) found that complications were more severe and persisted longer than after conventional radiotherapy. Complications developed, on average, 5.5 years after fast neutron therapy and included airways obstruction, intractable dysphagia and osteoradionecrosis. Remedial surgery to the irradiated area was compromised by greatly impaired wound healing.

Salvage surgery

Where radical radiotherapy fails and there is residual or recurrent tumour, salvage surgery may offer hope. Following radical radiotherapy, the tissues tend to have a much reduced blood supply, be fibrotic and heal poorly. Consequently, salvage surgery carries a higher risk of complications such as delayed wound healing, fistula formation, wound breakdown and carotid artery rupture. These hazards increase with time and surgery is best undertaken within 3 months of completion of radiotherapy.

Management of the neck

Patients staged N0 The regional lymph nodes, although clinically impalpable, sometimes contain occult foci of malignant cells. It seems reasonable to expect, therefore, that removal or treatment of regional lymph nodes, even when clinically clear, would improve cure rates. Alternatively, it can be argued that treatment of the regional nodes in all cases is unnecessary, as only a minority have metastases in the nodes.

The arguments expressed in favour of elective block dissection are:

- the incidence of histologically involved nodes in N0 necks varies from 25% to 65%
- survival rates are considerably lower in patients who develop node metastases

- the recurrence rate following block dissection is higher in advanced disease when there is extracapsular spread or multiple nodes
- by waiting for clinically detectable disease to develop, many patients will have a worse prognosis
- some patients fail to attend regular follow-up and may not appear again until nodal metastases are extensive
- block dissection of the neck carries negligible mortality and an acceptable morbidity
- retrospective reviews confirm that patients undergoing elective neck dissection have higher survival rate
- failure to control nodal metastases is a frequent cause of death.

The arguments against elective neck dissection are that:

- it is rare for treatment to fail in the neck when the primary is controlled – only 4.5% in one large series
- the incidence of histologically positive nodes in elective neck dissections exceeds the incidence of subsequent clinical nodal metastases, suggesting that some microscopic foci are destroyed by the body's defences
- the primary may recur or a second primary develop and metastasize into the dissected neck, making subsequent management very difficult
- elective neck dissection gives no guarantee against recurrence of the tumour in the neck
- block dissection has a considerable morbidity
- removal of regional lymph nodes may remove a barrier to the further spread of disease
- there is no prospectively controlled trial to support the argument that elective neck dissection does improve the prognosis.

On balance, the weight of these arguments is against prophylactic neck dissection. However, advanced tumours in some sites undoubtedly have a very high incidence of nodal disease, and as the submandibular triangle has to be opened as part of the resection of the primary, function-sparing elective neck dissection is recommended for tumours in the floor of the mouth and lower alveolar ridge with bone involvement. This dissection, in which structures such as the accessory nerve, internal jugular vein and sternocleido-mastoid muscle are preserved, can be justified. Further, a survey by Shah (1990) showed that of

501 cancers of the oral cavity, 34% of nodes were found to be positive after elective radical neck dissections. Over 96% of these histologically positive nodes would have been removed by a supra-omohyoid dissection.

The operation should preferably be seen as a staging procedure from which the decision is made to give radical postoperative radiotherapy.

An alternative approach is elective irradiation of the clinically negative neck, and indeed there is some evidence that this is of some benefit in preventing subsequent nodal disease. Certainly, elective irradiation to 40 Gy carries less morbidity than elective neck dissection.

Patients staged N1/N2a/N2b   At present, evidence suggests that the treatment of choice is radical neck dissection, either alone or combined with post-operative radiotherapy if multiple nodal involve-ment or extracapsular extension is found in the resected specimen. In those patients unfit for radical surgery, radical external beam irradiation is indicated.

Patients staged N2c   It is uncommon for patients with oral cancer to present with bilateral nodes. When they do so, there is often a large inoperable primary tumour which is best treated by external radiation. It therefore seems logical to treat the neck also by irradiation. Occasionally, particularly in a young patient, bilateral neck dissection can be justified. A full radical neck dissection is under-taken on the ipsilateral side and the internal jugular vein is spared if possible on the contralateral side. Most often, postoperative radiotherapy will be required for multiple nodal involvement or extra-capsular spread. In such situations, severe post-treatment oedema or congestion of the face and tongue may be anticipated.

Patients staged N3   N3 indicates massive involve-ment, usually with fixation. Large fixed nodes are often associated with advanced primary disease with a poor prognosis. Surgery is not normally advisable: removal of the common or internal carotid artery with replacement, or extensive resection of the base of the skull, although technically feasible, is seldom advisable. Treatment is most often by external radiotherapy. In a few younger patients with resectable primaries, it is worth rendering a fixed mass in the neck operable by preoperative radiotherapy.

Nodal metastases appearing after primary treatment

Provided that follow-up at regular intervals is rigorously maintained, it should be possible to detect a lymph node metastasis while it is still relatively small and therefore operable. Aspiration cytology is particularly useful in this situation to confirm that the palpable node is a carcinoma rather than reactive. Whenever positive, or if there is any doubt, a radical neck dissection is performed, followed by external irradiation if multiple involved nodes or extracapsular spread are found.

Trends in mortality due to metastatic disease

Crile (1906) considered that 'the collar of lympha-tics of the neck forms an extraordinary barrier through which cancer rarely penetrates'. Clinically apparent distant metastases are relatively un-common, but such deposits are found in about 50% of autopsies of patients dying with cancer of the mouth and jaws. The usual sites are the lungs, liver, bones (vertebrae, skull, ribs) and thoracic nodes. Such skeletal deposits are usually osteolytic. Pulmonary metastases diagnosed on chest X-ray should be carefully evaluated as there is a 15% risk of developing separate primary squamous carcino-mas of the lung, pharynx, larynx and oral cavity in these patients.

Since the more widespread introduction of combination therapy, there has been a change in the pattern of failure for oral cancer (Vikram, 1984). The overall survival rate has remained essentially static, but more effective control of the local disease has resulted in greater numbers of deaths from distant metastases and the emergence of second primary tumours. Distant metastases were rarely a problem in the past, as recurrence of locoregional disease was usually responsible for the patient's death. Thus in the past, only 4% died of distant metastases, although autopsy studies showed that up to 50% had metastases present at the time of death (O'Brien *et al.*, 1971). More recently, Luna (1983) has described a rise in deaths due to metastatic disease from 17% to 32%. Distant metastases have therefore become a major cause of death in oral cancer.

Multiple primary carcinomas The tendency to develop multiple primary carcinomas is a significant problem with oral cancers. In resected specimens of oral cancer, it is possible to find separate islands and foci of carcinoma-in-situ and invasive carcinoma in the adjacent epithelium, thus lending support to the theory of field change in oral cancer. Approximately 10% of patients may have two or more carcinomas in the aerodigestive tract. Many of these are within the oral cavity. Among 176 oral cancers described by Tytor *et al.* (1990), 21 (8%) developed second primary tumours of the upper aerodigestive tract and other workers have confirmed this high incidence. Indeed, whenever a patient with oral cancer develops an unusual or unexpected metastasis, the possibility of a second primary tumour should be considered. Adequate treatment for such a second primary may occasionally give a prognosis far better than that for an oral cancer with metastases.

Verrucous carcinoma

This uncommon variant of squamous cell carcinoma characteristically appears as a raised or cauliflower-like, white, warty lesion, and has a more benign course than the more common squamous cell carcinoma. Elderly males are most commonly affected. In the USA, particularly, it is seen as a consequence of prolonged tobacco chewing or snuff dipping.

Microscopy
Verrucous carcinoma typically has a heavily keratinized or parakeratinized, irregular clefted surface (Figure 10.8) with parakeratin extending deeply into the clefts. The prickle cell layers show bulbous hyperplasia, but for a considerable time at least, the tumour has a well-defined lower border and basal lamina (Figure 10.9). Atypia is minimal and there is usually a sub-epithelial inflammatory infiltrate.

Verrucous hyperplasia

A distinction has been made between verrucous hyperplasia and verrucous carcinoma by Shear and

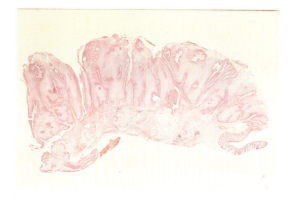

Figure 10.8 Verrucous carcinoma showing heaped-up papillary masses and the characteristic 'pushing' margin

Pindborg (1980). Verrucous hyperplasia is said not to extend more deeply than, or is superficial to, the surrounding normal epithelium. Verrucous carcinoma, by contrast, extends more deeply and pulls down the adjacent normal epithelium at its margins. However, verrucous hyperplasia is said to show dysplasia in the majority of cases, and can develop into verrucous carcinoma or squamous cell carcinoma, and it is widely agreed that the two – if they are separate entities – cannot reliably be

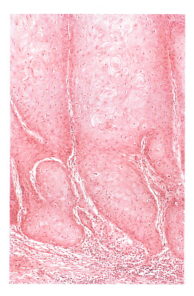

Figure 10.9 Verrucous carcinoma. High-power view shows well-differentiated epithelium and inflammation in the underlying connective tissue

distinguished and may coexist. The distinction does not seem to be of any great significance, even if it can be made, and in practical terms the management is the same.

Behaviour and treatment

Verrucous carcinoma grows slowly, becomes invasive only later and metastasizes later still. The regional lymph nodes may be enlarged, but usually as a result of inflammation. Ultimately, if neglected or mismanaged, deeper tissues are invaded and metastases appear.

Wide surgical excision should be curative. Despite earlier claims, there is no evidence that radiotherapy induces dedifferentiation and invasive behaviour of verrucous carcinomas. However, any individual palpable lymph nodes should be removed, but block dissection is not justified except on the rare occasions when involvement is confirmed histologically.

Keratoacanthoma

Keratoacanthoma ('self-healing carcinoma') is a relatively common lesion of the skin and sometimes of the lips, but rarely affects the oral cavity. Clinically, Habel *et al.* (1991), in a review of intra-oral keratoacanthomas, found the age of those affected to range from 12 to 80 years and out of 10 reported cases, 6 patients were less than 40 years old. There also appeared to be a strong predilection for males. The lesion appears as a painless cratered nodule. Even more rare is the eruptive variant which lacks the keratin-filled crater and more closely resembles a neoplastic ulcer clinically. Spontaneous regression over a period of 4–6 months, leaving a small scar, is characteristic, but unusual confidence is required to leave such a lesion untreated.

Microscopy

At low power, keratocanthoma has a characteristic goblet-shaped form (resembling in some respects an 'invaginated' verrucous carcinoma), with normal mucosa forming the lips of the cup, and showing an abrupt change to the carcinoma-like epithelium (Figures 10.10 and 10.11). There is typically

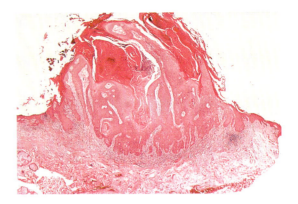

Figure 10.10 Keratoacanthoma. The deep central keratin-filled pit is surrounded by hyperplastic, dysplastic epithelium and a dense inflammatory infiltrate in the stroma

significant epithelial atypia and despite the absence of deep invasion, there is poor demarcation of the peripheral epithelium from the stroma. Habel *et al.* (1991), in reporting what may be the first case of an intra-oral eruptive keratoacanthoma, confirmed the difficulty of reliably distinguishing the central part of these lesions from a squamous cell carcinoma microscopically. They considered the most distinctive microscopic feature to be the elevation of the normal mucosa at the margin of the lesion and the abrupt change to hyperplasia.

In view of possible difficulties in differentiating keratocanthoma from squamous cell carcinoma histologically, account should also be taken of the

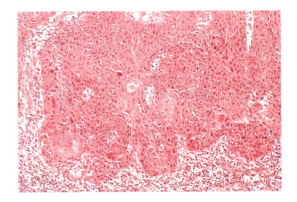

Figure 10.11 Keratoacanthoma. A high-power view shows an appearance identical to that of a well-differentiated squamous cell carcinoma

former's clinical features, particularly its more rapid growth, which usually extends over 6–12 weeks and its more frequent appearance in children or young adults.

Other variants of oral carcinoma

Spindle cell (Figure 10.12) and adenoid squamous carcinomas (Figure 10.13) have been rarely reported in the oral cavity. Too little is known of their behaviour to make any useful practical comments. Basaloid squamous carcinoma is another rare entity showing both basaloid and squamous cells in lobular or trabecular configurations. It appears to behave particularly aggressively.

Epidermoid carcinoma can very occasionally arise from minor oral salivary glands, forming about 1% of tumours there. Unless its origin can be seen to be from salivary tissue rather than from surface epithelium, such tumours are not likely to be distinguishable from the usual type of squamous cell carcinoma, and indeed the distinction is not likely to be of clinical significance.

Basal cell carcinoma is a skin tumour and does not arise in the oral mucosa. However, other tumours such as adenoid cystic carcinomas of salivary glands may have a basaloid appearance (Chapter 12).

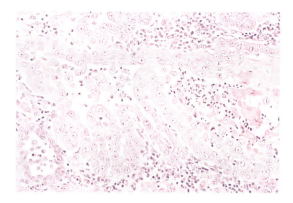

Figure 10.13   Adenoid squamous carcinoma. The pseudo-glandular appearance in squamous cell carcinoma is due to malignant acantholysis. This is more frequently seen in lip tumours

Merkel cell carcinoma

Merkel cells are neuroendocrine cells which have synaptic associations with intra-epidermal and dermal nerve endings, but their function is unknown. Merkel cell carcinomas are rare but aggressive tumours which mainly affect sun-damaged skin in elderly patients with a mean age of 75 years. Approximately 40% of these tumours arise in the skin of the head and neck region and most of the remainder in the skin of the limbs. A few examples have been reported in the oral cavity. Vigneswaram *et al.* (1992), in their review, found 12 oral examples of which 11 were in males. Consistent with predilection of these tumours for areas vulnerable to actinic damage, 10 were in the lips while 1 was in the buccal mucosa and the other in the mucobuccal fold. Another example, reported by Hayter *et al.* (1991), arose from just beneath the buccal mucosa in a man of 73.

Clinically, oral Merkel cell carcinomas form small, painless nodules which grow rapidly, may ulcerate and may become painful.

Microscopy

Merkel cell carcinomas usually consist of uniform cells with little cytoplasm, but large round basophilic nuclei with one or two small nucleoli and

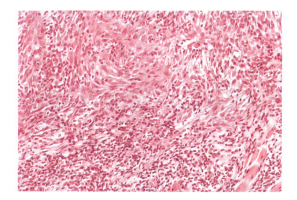

Figure 10.12   Spindle cell squamous carcinoma showing sheets of spindle-shaped cells resembling a sarcoma

prominent nuclear membranes. When in sheets, these cells have a lymphoma-like appearance. Otherwise they may form trabeculae, whorls or strands of cells spreading between collagen fibres and do not initially involve the surface epithelium. Intermediate and small cell Merkel cell carcinomas with worse prognoses have also been described.

Differentiation from other small cell tumours, particularly metastases, may be difficult. Immunocytochemistry shows a characteristic staining with the epithelial marker CAM 5.2 and with other low molecular weight, but not high molecular weight keratin antibodies, and Vigneswaram *et al.* (1992) suggest this type of keratin staining, together with globular paranuclear staining with antibody to neurofilament proteins, is unique to Merkel cells. Approximately 50% of these tumours are also positive for neuron-specific enolase or chromogranin, but in cases of doubt electron microscopy may be required.

Ultrastructurally, Merkel cells contain dense membrane-bound neurosecretory granules and paranuclear whorls of intermediate filaments.

Behaviour and management

Eight of the 12 oral examples reviewed by Vigneswaram *et al.* (1992) metastasized to lymph nodes or distant sites and 3 patients died from their tumours within 1–11 months. The periods of follow-up of most of the remaining reported cases were short.

The treatment of choice appears to be as wide surgical excision as possible, followed by radiotherapy to which these tumours are sensitive. Prophylactic irradiation of the regional nodes is also advised. Vigneswaram *et al.* (1992) quote a recommended dose of 50 Gy in 25 fractions and with this regimen their patient was disease-free after a year. Complete clinical remission has also been reported with chemotherapy by Wynne and Kearsley (1988). Nevertheless, the aggressiveness of these tumours is shown by the patient reported by Hayter *et al.* (1991) who, after surgery and radiotherapy (50 Gy), developed a metastasis and pathological fracture in the upper arm. Despite radiotherapy to the humerus and a course of chemotherapy, multiple metastases were found in many sites after the patient died from other causes 8 months after the initial diagnosis.

Carcinoma of the maxillary antrum

Carcinoma of the antrum is so uncommon as not to have justified an individual entry in national cancer statistics, but is included with nose, nasal cavities, middle ear and other sinuses. Even these together account for only about one-third as many cases as cancer of the mouth. A few (about 15%) of these rare carcinomas spread through the floor of the antrum to appear as oral tumours. They are, with rare exceptions, squamous cell carcinomas, often well differentiated and therefore not distinguishable from carcinomas arising from the oral mucosa. Confirmation of the diagnosis depends on finding the antral mass and destruction of the antral floor. Wide excision and radiotherapy are the usual lines of treatment.

References

Abbey, L.M., Page, D.G. and Sawyer, D.R. (1980) The clinical and histopathologic features of a series of 464 oral squamous cell papillomas. *Oral Surgery, Oral Medicine and Oral Pathology,* **49,** 419–427

Anderson, D.L. (1971) Cause and prevention of lip cancer. *Journal of the Canadian Dental Association,* **37,** 138–142

Anneroth, G., Batsakis, J. and Luna, M. (1987) Review of the literature and recommended system of malignancy grading in oral squamous cell carcinomas. *Scandinavian Journal of Dental Research,* **95,** 229–249

Ator, G.A., Abemayor, E., Lufkin, R.B. *et al.* (1990) Evaluation of mandibular tumor invasion with magnetic resonance imaging. *Archives of Otolaryngology and Head and Neck Surgery,* **116,** 454–459

Bahadur, S. (1984) Mandibular involvement in oral cancer. *Journal of Laryngology and Otology,* **110,** 564–565

Barsh, L.I. (1966) Molluscum contagiosum of the oral mucosa. *Oral Surgery, Oral Medicine and Oral Pathology,* **22;** 42–46

Belamarie, J. (1969) Malignant tumors in Chinese. *International Journal of Cancer,* **4,** 560–573

Binnie, W.H. (1976) Epidemiology and etiology of oral cancer in Britain. *Proceedings of the Royal Society of Medicine,* **69,** 734–740

Binnie, W.H., Cawson, R.A., Hill, G.B. *et al.* (1972) *Oral Cancer in England and Wales,* Her Majesty's Stationery Office, London

Bouquot, J.E., Weiland, L.H. and Kurland, L.T. (1988) Leukoplakia and carcinoma in situ synchronously associated with invasive oral oropharyngeal carcinoma in Rochester, Minn., 1935–1984. *Oral Surgery, Oral Medicine and Oral Pathology,* **65,** 199–207

Brodsky, L., Siddiqui, S.Y. and Stanievich, J.F. (1987) Massive oropharyngeal papillomatosis causing obstructive sleep apnea in a child. *Archives of Otolaryngology and Head and Neck Surgery,* **113,** 882–884

Bryne, M. (1991) Prognostic value of various molecular and cellular factors in oral squamous cell carcinomas: a review. *Journal of Oral and Pathological Medicine,* **20,** 413–420

Bryne, M., Koppang, H.S., Lilleng, R. *et al.* (1989) New malignancy grading is a better prognostic indicator than Broders' grading in oral squamous cell carcinomas. *Journal of Oral and Pathological Medicine,* **18,** 432–437

Caniff, J.P., Harvey, W. and Harris, M. (1986) Oral submucous fibrosis: its pathogenesis and management. *British Dental Journal,* **160,** 429–434

Cawson, R.A. (1966) Chronic oral candidiasis and leukoplakia. *Oral Surgery, Oral Medicine and Oral Pathology,* **22,** 582–591

Cawson, R.A. (1973) Induction of epithelial hyperplasia by *Candida albicans. British Journal of Dermatology,* **89,** 497–503

Cawson, R.A. and Binnie, W.H. (1980) Candida leukoplakia and carcinoma: a possible relationship. In *Oral Premalignancy* (eds Mackenzie, I.C., Dabelsteen, E. and Squier, C.A.), Proceedings of the first Dows Symposium, University of Iowa, pp. 59–66

Cawson, R.A. and Rajasingham, K.C. (1972) Ultrastructural features of the invasive phase of *Candida albicans. British Journal of Dermatology,* **87,** 535–543

Close, L.G., Brown, P.M., Vuitch, M.F. *et al.* (1989) Microvascular invasion and survival in cancer of the oral cavity and oropharynx. *Archives of Laryngology and Head and Neck Surgery,* **115,** 1304–1309

Close, L.G., Burns, D.K., Reisch, J. *et al.* (1987) Microvascular invasion in cancer of the oral cavity and oropharynx. *Archives of Laryngology and Head and Neck Surgery,* **113,** 1191–1195

Crile, G. (1906) Excision of cancer of the head and neck with special reference to the plan of dissection based on 132 operations. *Journal of the American Medical Association,* **47,** 1780–1784

Devlin, M.F., Barrie, R. and Ward-Booth, R.P. (1992) Cowden's disease: a rare but important manifestation of oral papillomatosis. *British Journal of Oral and Maxillofacial Surgery,* **30,** 335–336

Dorn, H.F. and Cutler, S.J. (1959) *Morbidity from Cancer in the United States,* 1–11 Public Health Monographs, No. 56, Washington, DC

Evans, S.J.W., Langdon, J.D., Rapidis, A.D. *et al.* (1982) Prognostic significance of STNMP and velocity of tumor growth in oral cancer. *Cancer,* **49,** 773–776

Eversole, L.R. and Sorenson, H.W. (1974) Oral florid papillomatosis in Down's syndrome. *Oral Surgery, Oral Medicine and Oral Pathology,* **37,** 202–207

Gilbert, S., Tzadik, A. and Leonard, G. (1986) Mandibular involvement by oral squamous cell carcinoma. *Laryngoscope,* **96,** 96–101

Graham, S., Dayal, H. and Rohrer, T. (1977) Dentition, diet, tobacco and alcohol in the epidemiology of oral cancer. *Journal of the National Cancer Institute,* **59,** 1611–1618

Habel, G., O'Regan, B., Eissing, A. *et al.* (1991) Intra-oral keratoacanthoma: an eruptive variant and review of the literature. *British Dental Journal,* **170,** 336–339

Hayter, J.P., Jacques, K. and James, K.A. (1991) Merkel cell tumour of the cheek. *British Journal of Oral and Maxillofacial Surgery,* **29,** 114–116

Hirayama, T. (1966) An epidemiological study of oral and pharyngeal cancer in Central and South East Asia. *Bulletin of the World Health Organisation,* **34,** 41–47

Hoffman, N.D., Sanghvi, L.D. and Wynder, E.L. (1974) Comparative chemical analysis of Indian bidi and American cigarette smoke. *International Journal of Cancer,* **14,** 49–53

Hogewind, W.F.C., van der Waal, I., van der Kwast, W.A. *et al.* (1989) The association of white lesions with oral squamous cell carcinoma. A retrospective study of 212 patients. *International Journal of Oral and Maxillofacial Surgery,* **18,** 163–164

Jaftarey, J. and Zaidi, S.H.M. (1976) Carcinoma of the oral cavity and oropharynx in Karachi (Pakistan). An appraisal. *Tropical Doctor,* **6,** 63–67

Keller, A.Z. Cirrhosis of the liver, alcoholism and heavy smoking associated with cancer of the mouth and pharynx. *Cancer,* **20,** 1015–1022

Kennedy, A.W. and Hart, W.R. (1982) Multiple squamous-cell carcinomas in Fanconi's anemia. *Cancer,* **50,** 811–814

Kramer, I.R.H., El-Labban, N. and Lee, K.W. (1978) The clinical features and risk of malignant transformation in sublingual keratosis. *British Dental Journal,* **144,** 171–176

Langdon, J.D., Rapidis, A.D., Harvey, R.W. *et al.* (1977) STNMP – a new classification for oral cancer. *British Journal of Oral Surgery,* **15,** 49–54

Larrson, A., Axell, T. and Andersson, G. (1991) Reversibility of snuff dippers' lesion in Swedish moist snuff users: a clinical and histologic follow-up study. *Journal of Oral and Pathological Medicine,* **20,** 258–264

Lemon, F.R., Walden, R.T. and Woods, R.W. (1964) Cancer of the lung and mouth in Seventh-Day Adventists. Preliminary report on a population study. Cancer, **17,** 486–497

Lindqvist, C. and Teppo, L. (1978) Epidemiological evaluation of sunlight as a risk factor of lip cancer. *British Journal of Cancer,* **37,** 983–989

Link, M.J.O., Kaugars, G.E. and Burns, J.C. (1992) Comparison of oral carcinomas in smokeless tobacco users and nonusers. *Journal of Oral and Maxillofacial Surgery,* **50,** 452–455

Lukinmaa, P.-L., Hietanen, J., Soderholm, A.-L. *et al.* (1992) The histologic pattern of bone invasion by squamous cell carcinoma of the mandibular region. *British Journal of Oral and Maxillofacial Surgery,* **30,** 2–7

Luna, M.A. (1983) Oral communication quoted by Goepfert H. in Are we making any progress? *Archives of Otolaryngology,* **110,** 563

Martinez, I. (1969) Factors associated with cancer of the oesophagus, mouth and pharynx in Puerto Rico. *Journal of the National Cancer Institute,* **42,** 1069–1073

Mehta, F.S., Pindborg, J.J., Daftary, D.K. *et al.* (1969) Oral leukoplakia among Indian villagers. The association with smoking habits. *British Dental Journal,* **127,** 73–77

Millesi, W., Prayer, L., Helmer, M. *et al.* (1990) Diagnostic imaging of tumor invasion of the mandible. *International Journal of Oral and Maxillofacial Surgery,* **19,** 294–298

Moore, C., Flynn, M.B. and Greenberg, R.A. (1986) Evaluation of size in prognosis of oral cancer. *Cancer,* **58,** 156–162

Murti, P.R., Bhonsle, R.B., Pindborg, J.J. *et al.* (1985) Malignant transformation rate in oral submucous fibrosis over a 17-year period. *Community Dentistry and Oral Epidemiology,* **13,** 340–341

O'Brien, P.H., Carlson, R., Steuber, E.H. *et al.* (1971) Distant metastases in epidermoid cell carcinoma of the head and neck. *Cancer,* **27,** 304–307

Ogden, G.R., Kiddie, R.A., Lunny, D.P. *et al.* (1992) Assessment of p53 protein expression in normal, benign and malignant oral mucosa. *Journal of Pathology,* **166,** 389–394

Ogus, H.D. and Bennett, M.H. (1978–79) Carcinoma of the dorsum of the tongue: a rarity or misdiagnosis. *British Journal of Oral Surgery,* **16,** 115–124

Pindborg, J.J., Kiaer, J., Gupta, P.C. *et al.* (1967) Studies in oral leukoplakia, prevalence of leukoplakia among 10,000 persons in Lucknow, India, with special reference to use of tobacco and betel nut. *Bulletin of the World Health Organisation,* **37,** 109–124

Pindborg, J.J., Roed-Petersen, B. and Renstrup, G. (1972) Role of smoking in floor of the mouth leukoplakias. *Journal of Oral Pathology,* **1,** 22–29

Praetorius-Clausen, F. (1973) Geographical aspects of oral focal epithelial hyperplasia. *Pathologia et Microbiologia,* **39,** 204–213

Protzel, M., Giardina, A.C. and Albano, E.H. (1964) The effect of liver imbalance on the development of oral tumors in mice following the application of benzypyrene in tobacco tar. *Oral Surgery, Oral Medicine and Oral Pathology,* **18,** 622–635

Rapidis, A.D., Langdon, J.D., Patel, M.F. *et al.* (1976) Clinical classification and staging in oral cancer. *Journal of Maxillofacial Surgery,* **4,** 219–224

Rapidis, A.D., Langdon, J.D., Patel, M.F. *et al.* (1977) STNMP: a new system for the clinico-pathological classification and identification of intra-oral carcinomata. *Cancer,* **39,** 204–209

Reil, B., Podlesch, I. and Pallade, E. (1975) Diagnostic and therapeutic regime for reducing mortality after resection of tumours in the head and neck. *Journal of Maxillofacial Surgery,* **3,** 54–60

Renstrup, G., Smulow, J.B. and Glickman, I. (1962) Effect of chronic mechanical irritation on chemically-induced carcinogenesis in the hamster cheek pouch. *Journal of the American Dental Association,* **64,** 770–775

Rich, A.M. and Radden, B.G. (1984) Prognostic indicators for oral squamous cell carcinoma: a comparison between the TNM and STNMP systems. *British Journal of Oral and Maxillofacial Surgery,* **22,** 30–36

Shah, J.P. (1990) Patterns of cervical lymph node metastasis from squamous carcinomas of the upper aerodigestive tract. *American Journal of Surgery,* **160,** 405–409

Shear, M. and Pindborg, J.J. (1980) Verrucous hyperplasia of the oral mucosa. *Cancer,* **46,** 1855–1862

Stafford, N., Waldron, J., Davies, D. *et al.* (1992) Complications following fast neutron therapy for head and neck cancer. *Journal of Laryngology and Otolaryngology,* **106,** 144–146

Stell, P.M. (1990) Adjuvant chemotherapy in head and neck cancer (Editorial). *Clinical Otolaryngology,* **15,** 193–195

Stell, P.M. (1992) Prognosis in mouth cancer: host factors. *Journal of Laryngology and Otolaryngology,* **106,** 399–402

Swart, J.G.N., Lekkas, C. and Allard, R.H.B. (1985) Oral manifestations in Cowden's syndrome. Report of four cases. *Oral Surgery, Oral Medicine and Oral Pathology,* **59,** 264–268

Tytor, M. and Olofsson, J. (1992) Prognostic factors in oral cavity carcinomas. *Acta Oto-laryngologica (Stockholm),* Suppl. 492, 75–78

Tytor, M., Olofsson, J., Ledin, T. *et al.* (1990) Squamous cell carcinoma of the oral cavity. A review of the 176 cases with application of malignancy grading and DNA measurements. *Clinical Otolaryngology,* **15,** 235–252

Vigneswaram, N., Muller, S., Lense, E. *et al.* (1992) Merkel cell carcinoma of the labial mucosa. An immunohistochemical and ultrastructural study with a review of the literature on Merkel cell carcinomas. *Oral Surgery, Oral Medicine and Oral Pathology,* **74,** 193–200

Vikram, B. (1984) Changing pattern of failure in advanced head and neck cancer. *Archives of Otolaryngology,* **110,** 564–565

Waterhouse, J., Muir, C., Correa, P. *et al.* (eds) (1976) *Cancer Incidence in Five Continents,* International Agency for Research on Cancer, Lyon

Winn, D.M. and Blot, W.J. (1985) Second cancer following cancers of the buccal cavity and pharynx in Connecticut, 1935–1982. *National Cancer Institute Monograph,* **68,** 25–48

Wynder, E.L., Bross, I.J. and Feldman, R.M. (1957) A study of the etiological factors in cancer of the mouth. *Cancer,* **10,** 1300–1323

Wynne, C. and Kearsley, J. (1988) Merkel cell tumor: a chemosensitive skin cancer. *Cancer,* **62,** 28–31

11

Non-neoplastic diseases of salivary glands

Investigation
Investigations will be discussed in relation to specific disorders and those more appropriate to neoplasms are discussed in the following chapter. However, it must be emphasized that chronic inflammatory swellings of the major salivary glands, in particular, sometimes cannot be distinguished from neoplasms clinically. Nevertheless, biopsy of the parotid glands is contraindicated because of the frequency of pleomorphic adenomas which can be seeded into the surrounding tissues to produce multiple recurrences. There are also the risks of damaging branches of the facial nerve or of producing a parotid fistula.

For imaging techniques, see Chapters 1 and 12.

Congenital salivary fistulae These are sometimes seen in association with branchial clefts.

Aberrant salivary tissue This is common in the cervical lymph nodes (where it should not be mistaken for a metastasis) and may be found in the middle ear cleft. Stafne's bone cavity is another example.

Accessory ducts and lobes These are so common as to form normal variations rather than anomalies. A distinct accessory duct and lobe in the parotid is present in as many as 50% of patients.

Cysts Cysts of salivary glands can be developmental or, more frequently, acquired. Both types are discussed below.

Developmental disorders

Aplasia/agenesis Complete absence of one or more salivary glands is very rare, but occasionally the parotid gland are absent. Absence of all major salivary glands is even more rare.

Duct atresia This is also rare, but usually affects the submandibular duct in the floor of the mouth. Absence of the duct results in retention cysts of the submandibular and sublingual glands.

Salivary gland hypoplasia This can be a feature of the Melkersson–Rosenthal syndrome. The hypoplasia possibly may be secondary to atrophy of parasympathetic nerves thought to be implicated in this syndrome.

Infections and other inflammatory diseases

Acute bacterial sialadenitis

Ascending infection usually affects the parotid gland. The parotid duct is of larger calibre than the submandibular duct and the opening of the duct at the parotid papilla, unlike that of the submandibular gland, is not guarded by a sphincter-like mechanism.

Ascending parotitis was more common in the past when debilitated and dehydrated surgical patients were at risk from infection ascending from the oral cavity as a result of inadequate salivary flow and probably also oral sepsis. This is now unusual and the single most common pre-disposing cause is chronic failure of salivary flow usually as a result of Sjögren's syndrome (Figure 11.1) or radiation damage, or occasionally a consequence of tricyclic antidepressant treatment. It can also occasionally affect healthy persons for no obvious reason.

Clinically, the parotid gland is hot, red, tender and swollen. Frequently, pyrexia and lymphaden-opathy are associated. If neglected, fluctuation will result from parotid abscess formation.

Staphylococcus aureus is the most common causative microbe; viridans streptococcal infection is less frequent and it may be difficult to exclude it as a contaminant. A wide variety of other bacteria has been incriminated, such as Gram-negative bacilli and anaerobes. In 23 cases reported by Brook (1992), anaerobes were isolated in 20 patients, but often in association with aerobes. Parotitis is occasionally a nosocomial infection or, in the past particularly, secondary to septicaemia.

Microscopy

Vasodilatation is followed by increasing infiltration by neutrophils into the ducts and parenchyma from blood vessels. Colonies of bacteria may be seen, particularly in the ducts, which become dilated and filled with neutrophils. Ducts and then acinar tissue are progressively destroyed, leading to formation of micro-abscesses. If neglected or if host defences are impaired, destruction progresses to gross abscess formation and destruction of large areas of the gland (Figure 11.2). With subsidence of the infection, healing by fibrosis follows.

Management

Antibiotics should be given as soon as pus has been obtained for culture and sensitivity testing. To prevent contamination from the mouth, pus should be milked from the duct after the mucosa round its orifice has been wiped dry with a sterile swab. Since staphylococci are so frequent a cause, flucloxacillin is usually the first choice, but changed if the microbiological findings dictate. Metronidazole can be added because of the frequency of anaerobic infections. Other investigations in the acute stage are a full blood picture and the temperature. A sialogram should never be taken in the acute phase, as this drives more organisms into the gland parenchyma and could result in bacteraemia or septicaemia. Early treatment with antibiotics, fluids to correct any dehydration and stimulation of salivary flow with tart drinks (lemon juice) is usually effective.

A comprehensive report by Raad and Sabbagh (1990) of 29 cases and review of earlier reports, from 1911 to 1969, comprised in all 722 cases.

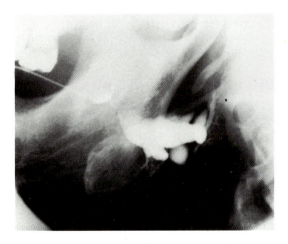

Figure 11.1 Chronic parotid abscess cavity. In this patient with Sjögren's syndrome, suppurative infection has led to a large area of gland destruction. Contrast medium has failed to penetrate beyond the cavity as a result of destruction of the duct system by the lymphoproliferation. Bilateral parotidectomy had to be carried out

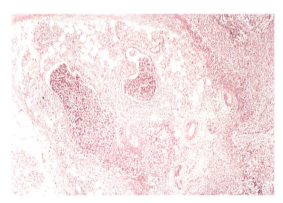

Figure 11.2 Acute suppurative parotitis. Surviving acini are difficult to discern. There is widespread inflammatory infiltration and, most conspicuously, ducts are distended by inflammatory cells

The earlier cases frequently required drainage and had a mortality of 10–50%. By contrast, none of the more recent cases required surgery but responded to fluids and antibiotics alone.

However, if an abscess forms it must be drained, with care not to damage branches of the facial nerve. Sharp dissection should therefore be confined to the skin and blunt sinus forceps used to perforate the parotid fascia and the abscess cavity.

Once the acute phase has resolved, a sialogram is useful to assess the functional state of the gland, and for this purpose the emptying film is essential. Sialography at this stage helps also to flush out the gland, and the iodized medium may possibly have some local disinfectant activity. In general, the parotid recovers well from acute infection, whereas the submandibular gland usually goes on to chronic sialadenitis which ultimately necessitates its excision.

Chronic bacterial sialadenitis

The submandibular are more frequently affected than the parotid glands. The serous parotid secretion and wider parotid duct probably allows infection to clear mechanically, whereas the more viscid mixed secretion and narrower duct of the submandibular gland predisposes to chronic infection. Chronic sialadenitis often follows an acute infective episode or is associated with chronic obstruction.

Clinically, the inflamed gland may form a painless tumour-like firm mass (a Küttner 'tumour'), but chronic sialadenitis is frequently also a chance finding on microscopy.

Microscopy
The main features are varying degrees of loss of acini, duct dilatation and a chronic inflammatory infiltrate, usually predominantly lymphocytic, with widespread interstitial fibrosis in the later stages. Squamous metaplasia and calculus formation may be seen in the dilated ducts (Figures 11.3 and 11.4).

Management
Sialography shows varying degrees of sialectasis and acinar atrophy, sometimes with dystrophic

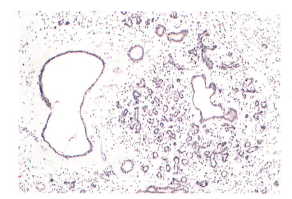

Figure 11.3   Obstructive sialadenitis. Duct dilatation, acinar atrophy and interstitial fibrosis and inflammation are shown

calcification in the gland itself. Again, the emptying film is essential, as this demonstrates the functional status of the gland. Often it also shows obstruction due to a calculus or stricture. In the case of the submandibular gland, the only effective treatment is excision. For the parotid, a superficial lobectomy with tying-off of the parotid duct is usually sufficient. Any functioning remnants of the deep lobe atrophy spontaneously.

Recurrent parotitis

This puzzling condition is seen in children starting at about 6 years of age and recurring usually

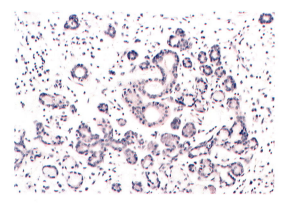

Figure 11.4   Obstructive sialadenitis. Higher power view shows extensive loss of secretory units

only until adolescence. Boys are affected twice as often as girls. Occasionally, younger children and frequently adults are also affected. The history is usually of recurrent unilateral or bilateral parotid pain and swelling ('recurrent mumps'), particularly at mealtimes. Heat, redness, fluctuation and pyrexia are absent. Sialography in the acute phase shows widespread punctate sialectasis with a snowstorm appearance (Figure 11.5).

An association with Epstein–Barr virus has been reported by Akaboshi *et al.* (1983), in that children with recurrent parotitis often show a considerably higher incidence of antibody to EBV than controls, but this has not been generally confirmed. However, the histological findings suggest that obstruction, probably secondary to formation or transport of abnormal secretion, is probably a major factor in the aetiology.

Microscopy

Mild dilatation of ducts containing inspissated mucus and desquamated epithelial cells, but no significant inflammation in the early stages, may be seen. Oedema and swelling of acinar cells is followed by periductal inflammation and patchy destruction of the lobular structure. Ultimately fibrosis, dilatation of the proximal ducts and degeneration of the duct epithelium, which frequently undergoes metaplastic change, progresses until some lobules consist only of proliferated ducts and fibro-fatty tissue.

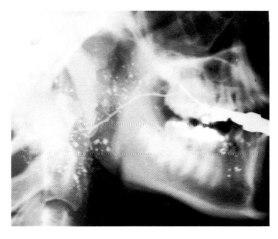

Figure 11.5   Childhood recurrent parotitis. The snowstorm appearance is typical

Management

Although there is no evidence of a bacterial cause, the episodes are usually treated with an antibiotic and resolve progressively in 5–10 days. Six or more months may elapse between attacks. It is not known if the sialographic changes resolve at puberty, but recurrent parotitis starting in childhood is usually self-limiting.

In adults, by contrast, persistent recurrent parotitis can be troublesome and difficult to treat, as indicated by the range of measures that have been recommended. These have ranged from duct ligation to low-dose radiotherapy or, if all else fails, parotidectomy. The only reliable treatment is to perform a superficial lobectomy with tying off of the main duct as far distally as possible.

Granulomatous infections and sarcoidosis

Tuberculosis, syphilis or toxoplasmosis can involve the salivary glands, but rarely do so. However, the incidence of tuberculosis is beginning to rise in several countries and O'Connell *et al.* (1993) reported 6 cases of parotid swelling among 187 new cases of mycobacterial infections admitted to their hospital during the previous 3 years. These appeared clinically to be parotid gland tumours and diagnosis was only made after excision or enucleation. Fine-needle aspiration biopsy was unhelpful in 2 out of the 3 cases where it was used, all the patients had normal chest radiographs and all who were Mantoux tested showed weakly or strongly positive reactions. Diagnosis of mycobacterial infection of the parotid gland is, therefore, only likely to be made postoperatively by microscopy.

Sarcoidosis (Chapter 14) has a predilection for salivary tissue. It causes either diffuse enlargement, often involving all the major salivary glands, or it may affect a single gland, sometimes with rapid growth mimicking a tumour. The diagnosis is usually suggested by microscopy of an excised gland showing typical granuloma formation, and confirmed by finding hilar lymphadenopathy or other signs of sarcoidosis, or a positive Kveim test. Usually there is a mumps-like salivary gland swelling, and this is occasionally the presenting feature of systemic sarcoidosis.

Less commonly, Heerfordt's syndrome (parotid swelling, uveitis and cranial nerve palsies, and fever) can develop. Facial palsy is the usual neurological complication. Rarely, sarcoidosis may give rise to a localized pseudo-tumour within a single parotid gland.

The labial salivary glands are involved histologically in a high proportion of cases of systemic sarcoidosis. When there are other suggestive features, particularly hilar lymphadenopathy and widespread pulmonary infiltration, labial gland biopsy may provide valuable confirmation of the diagnosis by avoiding more invasive procedures.

Microscopically, sarcoidosis is characterized by discrete non-caseating granulomas which may be surrounded by a dense lymphocytic infiltrate (Figures 11.6 and 11.7). It should be noted, however, that granuloma formation in salivary glands is often due to other causes, which are not necessarily identifiable (Chapters 12 and 14).

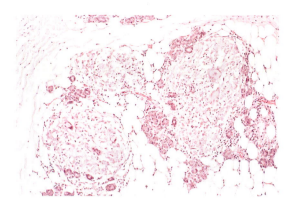

Figure 11.7 Sarcoidosis of the parotid gland. Higher power view of a non-caseating granuloma with associated multinucleated giant cells

Viral sialadenitis

Sialadenitis caused by the mumps virus is the most common cause of acute parotitis. Mumps is usually a disease of childhood, but can affect any non-immune adult. The parotid is involved in 70% of cases and the swelling may be unilateral or bilateral. The submandibular glands may also be involved. Immunity following a first attack is absolute and lifelong, so that patients claiming to have recurrent mumps probably suffer from recurrent non-specific parotitis. If there is any

doubt about the diagnosis, it can be confirmed by a complement fixation test soon after the onset of the illness. The S (soluble) mumps antibody develops within a few days, then disappears after convalescence.

Microscopy

There is interstitial inflammation of the gland which is infiltrated predominantly by lymphocytes and plasma cells. Vacuolation of acinar cells, and small haemorrhages are widespread (Figure 11.8), but destruction of acini is probably less than appears microscopically, as full functional recovery of the glands typically follows.

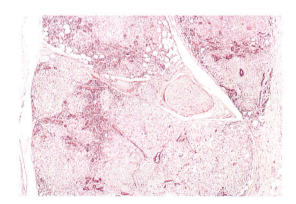

Figure 11.6 Sarcoidosis of the parotid gland showing many discrete and confluent non-caseating granulomas

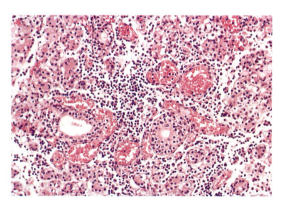

Figure 11.8 Mumps. Intense vascular hyperaemia, cytoplasmic vacuolation and interstitial lymphocytic infiltration are shown

Management

There is no specific treatment, and serious complications such as encephalitis or sensory nerve deafness are rare. Nevertheless, because of these risks, mumps vaccination with triple vaccine is strongly recommended for children.

Other viral infections of salivary glands

Congenital cytomegalovirus infection (salivary gland inclusion disease) gives rise to a characteristic picture with owl's eye viral inclusion bodies larger than the duct cells (Figure 11.9). However, salivary gland involvement is of little clinical significance in comparison with the congenital defects.

Acute parotitis may be caused by viruses such as Coxsackie, Echo, or Epstein–Barr or choriomeningitis viruses, but rarely in comparison with mumps. Chronic parotitis is a common feature, particularly of childhood AIDS, but its cause is as yet unclear.

Post-irradiation sialadenitis

All patients undergoing radiotherapy develop acute sialadenitis when the irradiated field includes the parotid or submandibular glands. Xerostomia and tender swelling of the glands develop within

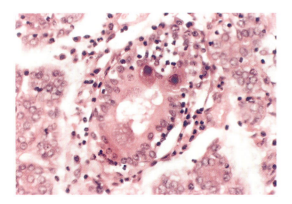

Figure 11.9 Cytomegalovirus infection. The typical owl's eye inclusion bodies in duct cells are shown

24 hours, but the symptoms resolve spontaneously within about 3 days. During the acute phase there is a sharp rise in salivary amylase both in the serum and urine. More important are the chronic effects described later.

Sialadenitis of minor glands

The minor salivary glands may be involved in a variety of systemic diseases, particularly sarcoidosis and Sjögren's syndrome, as discussed later. So-called stomatitis nicotina affects the palate of pipe smokers or those who practise reverse smoking. In this condition, the inflamed duct orifices stand out as red dots or small swellings within the white hyperkeratinized mucosa (Chapter 9). Necrotizing sialometaplasia by contrast gives rise to a tumour-like swelling.

Necrotizing sialometaplasia

This lesion is seen most commonly in the minor glands of the palate. It is of unknown cause, though thought to result in part from cigarette smoking. It is far more frequent in the USA than in Britain.

Middle-aged males are predominantly affected. Typically, the patient develops a relatively painless ulcerated swelling on the hard palate midway between the midline and gingival margin, often in the first molar region. The base of the ulcer is often on the underlying bone and the margins are irregular and heaped-up or everted. The ulcer, which may be 15–20 mm in diameter, clinically resembles a squamous cell carcinoma for which it has, in the past, also been mistaken on microscopy (Figures 11.10 and 11.11).

Microscopy

There is chronic inflammation of minor salivary tissue and necrosis of acini. The duct tissue undergoes squamous metaplasia and proliferates to produce a pseudo-epitheliomatous appearance

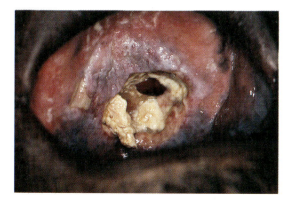

Figure 11.10   Necrotizing sialometaplasia. There is a cratered ulcer with a keratotic halo on the palate

(Figures 11.12 and 11.13). These lesions are often excised for diagnosis, but usually heal spontaneously over 8–10 weeks. An acrylic cover plate is sometimes needed to protect the healing area, particularly at meal times.

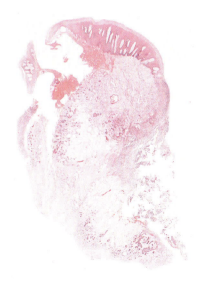

Figure 11.12   Necrotizing sialometaplasia. Low-power view shows the ulcer base with proliferating, pseudo-epitheliomatous islands of squamous epithelium

Allergic sialadenitis

Some foods, chloramphenicol, oxytetracycline, pollens and heavy metals have been reported to produce allergic parotitis. Eosinophilia in saliva and the peripheral blood are suggestive, but otherwise allergic sialadenitis is a questionable entity. Antihistamines are not reliably effective, and there is little reason why they should be expected to be. Iodides in contrast media are a recognized but rare cause of salivary gland swelling. However, this appears to be an inflammatory reaction to the concentration of iodide in the salivary gland rather than an allergic reaction, and is not prevented by prophylactic administration of corticosteroids (Berman and Delaney, 1992).

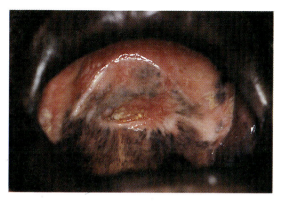

Figure 11.11   Necrotizing sialometaplasia. Spontaneous healing took place within 2 months

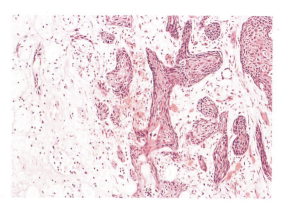

Figure 11.13   Necrotizing sialometaplasia. High-power view shows regenerating ducts in inflamed tissue closely resembling squamous carcinoma

Obstruction and trauma

Obstruction to salivary flow is frequently caused by calculi and can lead to chronic sialadenitis. Another consequence of obstruction is the formation of mucoceles.

Papillary obstruction

Trauma to the parotid papilla as a result of cheek biting, abrasion from a rough tooth or denture flange, or occasionally an aphthous ulcer, can cause inflammatory oedema. This may be sufficient to obstruct salivary flow. Typically, the patient complains of acute pain and swelling of the affected gland at mealtimes or other gustatory stimuli, but it resolves slowly over the ensuing 2 hours. Removal of the source of irritation relieves the symptoms permanently.

Chronic trauma from similar causes can eventually result in a stricture and stenosis of the parotid papilla. When established, this condition is best treated surgically by papillotomy. A probe is inserted through the duct opening and an incision made through the wall of the papilla down on to the probe. Once laid open, the papilla should not be sutured. Occasionally, after this procedure, some patients, particularly woodwind and brass instrument players, complain of swelling as a result of inflation of the parotid. Ascending infection does not appear to follow.

The submandibular papilla, although having a smaller orifice than that of the parotid, rarely becomes obstructed other than by a calculus impacting at the opening (see below). Occasionally, a child traumatizes the submandibular papilla by falling while holding a pencil or other object in the mouth. When the submandibular papilla becomes stenosed, a new opening of the submandibular duct into the floor of the mouth should be created proximal to the site of the papillary obstruction.

Stricture

Salivary duct strictures are usually secondary to ulceration of the duct wall from calculi and mostly affect the submandibular duct. Any trauma –

accidental or surgical – to the floor of the mouth may result in stricture formation (Figure 11.14). Congenital submandibular duct strictures are rare.

Masseteric or buccinator hyperplasia is a rare cause of stricture of the parotid duct which becomes chronically irritated and fibrosed where it curves around the anterior border of the thickened masseter or perforates the buccinator muscle. Attempts may be made to dilate salivary strictures with graded bougies but often, for submandibular duct strictures, it is easier to bring the duct directly into the floor of the mouth proximal to the site of the stricture and make a new opening.

Tumours

Occasionally, benign parotid tumours can compress a duct and produce more rapid enlargement of the gland. Malignant parotid tumours may also cause duct obstruction by infiltrating the duct wall and blocking the lumen.

Calculi (sialolithiasis)

Radiopaque calculi consist predominantly of calcium phosphate and carbonate which crystallize

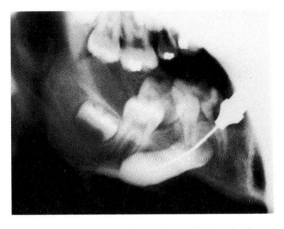

Figure 11.14   Stricture of the submandibular gland duct. The needle had been inserted proximal to the stricture into the dilated part of the duct. Beyond this dilatation, degeneration of the salivary ducts has prevented entry of contrast material

round an organic nidus – usually cellular debris or casts from the duct walls. Microscopically, calculi have a lamellated or radial structure and the duct walls may undergo squamous metaplasia.

Submandibular calculi

The majority of calculi form within the ducts. The more viscid, mixed submandibular secretion probably predisposes to stasis and crystallization of mineral salts. Most submandibular calculi are radiopaque and show up on plain radiographs. They frequently impact at the junction of the main duct and deep lobe of the submandibular gland where the duct bends around the posterior border of the mylohyoid muscle. The other common site of impaction is in the distal third of the submandibular duct often just behind the papilla.

The typical presentation of a submandibular calculus is acute pain and swelling at mealtimes. Nevertheless, many submandibular calculi are asymptomatic or produce chronic obstruction with progressive atrophy and fibrosis of the affected gland. Eventually, infection in the damaged gland brings the patient to seek help.

Management
Radiopaque submandibular calculi are readily recognized on plain radiographs (Figure 11.15). If stones are in an accessible part of the duct (distal to the point at which the lingual nerve crosses the duct), they should be removed surgically through the floor of the mouth before sialography. A sialogram should not be taken as it can flush the calculus towards the gland where it may not be accessible through the floor of the mouth.

Surgical removal of submandibular stones in an accessible part of the duct (distal two-thirds) is straightforward and can be undertaken under local analgesia. A stay suture inserted around the duct proximal to the calculus prevents subsequent manipulation from milking the stone backwards towards the gland. A linear incision is made along the submandibular duct, to expose the calculus which is then readily teased out. The duct proximal and distal to the site of impaction is then gently irrigated to remove any gravel. The incision in the duct is left open, as closure invariably results in stricture formation.

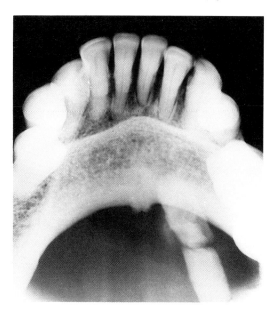

Figure 11.15 Large stone in the submandibular gland duct

After removal of the calculus, sialography should be undertaken to assess any damage within the gland. Anything more than mild sialectasis with minimal delay in emptying indicates permanent damage. In a fit patient, surgical removal of the affected gland is advisable, as the gland is otherwise liable to become chronically infected and the site of recurrent calculi. Unlike the parotid, the submandibular gland has a poor capacity for recovery.

For a calculus in the proximal third of the duct or within the submandibular gland, excision of the gland from an external approach is advocated, with due care to avoid branches of the facial, lingual and hypoglossal nerves.

Parotid calculi

Only about 20% of parotid calculi are radiopaque. They rarely cause acute pain and swelling at mealtimes and many are probably flushed out spontaneously by the salivary flow and sometimes noticed by patients as gritty particles.

Most patients with larger, impacted parotid calculi have chronic diffuse swelling of the gland and discomfort, usually at the start of a meal.

Sialography is then required to show the calculus and its site. The great majority of parotid calculi are lodged at the junction of the main duct and the two primary divisions, and have a staghorn shape.

On the rare occasions when parotid calculi impact near the duct papilla, it is often sufficient gently to dilate the parotid papilla and encourage salivary flow to flush out the calculus. Surgical removal of a staghorn calculus is indicated, as the parotid has such good powers of recovery after obstruction.

The surface marking of the parotid duct on the cheek is readily identified and constant. A conventional pre-auricular parotidectomy incision is used, but care must be taken to avoid the buccal branch of the facial nerve which is frequently running close to and parallel with the duct.

Piezoelectric shock wave lithotripsy offers an alternative to the surgical removal of salivary gland calculi. Iro *et al.* (1992) report its successful use, without anaesthesia or sedation, in 81% of parotid gland and 40% of submandibular gland calculi in 51 patients. The only adverse effects were localized petechiae after 13% of treatments and transient swelling of the gland immediately after treatment in 3%.

Mucoceles

Mucoceles usually result from damage to the duct or obstruction to the drainage of a minor salivary gland. The common sites are the lower lip, particularly in class 2, division 2 malocclusions, and the retromolar pad and cheek from occlusal trauma from erupting upper wisdom teeth. Rarely, mucoceles form in the palate following trauma from sharp bones or crusts.

Microscopy
Mucoceles are usually mucous extravasation cysts rather than retention cysts. In their early stages, pools of extravasated mucus surrounded by an inflammatory reaction can be seen in the submucosal connective tissue. These pools coalesce to produce a macroscopic cyst with a wall of compressed but cellular connective tissue and the inflammatory reaction progressively subsides (Figure 11.16). Occasionally, such cysts form

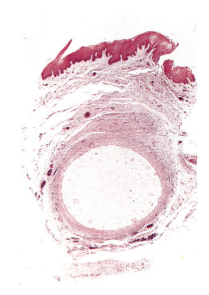

Figure 11.16   Deeply located extravasation mucocele

immediately beneath the epithelium to produce a pemphigoid-like bulla (Figure 11.17).

Occasionally, obstruction causes the duct to become distended, resulting in a true retention cyst lined by duct epithelium, sometimes containing mucous cells (Figure 11.18).

Treatment
Mucoceles, if untreated, eventually burst and discharge spontaneously. As the overlying epithelium

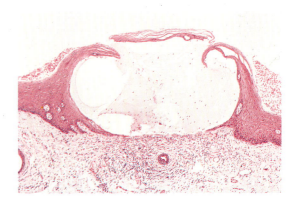

Figure 11.17   Superficial mucocele presenting as a blister which could easily be mistaken for a mucocutaneous disease. There is a duct from a minor gland below the blister and serial sectioning often shows this opens directly into the mucocele

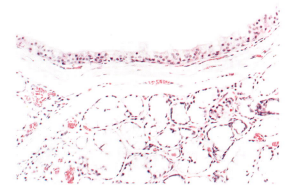

Figure 11.18 Retention mucocele. The cyst is lined by columnar epithelium with some mucous cells

In the case of plunging ranula, Mizuno and Yamaguchi (1993) recommend transoral drainage in addition.

Other salivary cysts

Congenital cysts are occasionally seen and lympho-epithelial (branchial cleft) cysts can extend into the parotid area.

Benign lymphoepithelial parotid cysts, often bilateral, can be found on CT scanning, and in association with cervical lymphadenopathy are strongly suggestive of HIV infection, as discussed later.

heals, the secretion accumulates again and the mucocele recurs. Surgery is, therefore, indicated. A linear incision is made just through the overlying mucosa and the lesion is excised *in toto* together with the underlying minor gland of origin. Occasionally, mucoceles recur after surgery either because the affected glandular tissue has not been completely excised or operation has caused further trauma or scarring which blocks adjacent glands. In this situation, cryosurgery or diathermy is often curative.

Ranula

Occasionally, damage to the duct of the sublingual gland causes the formation of a mucous extra-vasation cyst appearing as a tense bluish swelling in the anterior floor of the mouth just to one side of the midline. Such a ranula is submucosal but lies entirely above the mylohyoid muscle. It may reach 3 or 4 cm in diameter and cause speech disturbance.

A deep ranula lies entirely within the submental space or it may be plunging and hourglass in shape, lying partly superficial and partly deep to the mylohyoid. As the cyst expands, it passes through a developmental dehiscence in the mylohyoid muscle. The lining of an extensive ranula is difficult to excise and usually ruptures during surgery. However, this is unimportant as permanent cure is achieved by excision of the affected sublingual gland with little regard to the ranula itself.

Sjögren's syndrome

Sjögren's syndrome is a common, chronic connective tissue disorder characterized by dry mouth and dry eyes due to infiltration of salivary and lacrimal glands by T and B lymphocytes, and acinar destruction. Primary Sjögren's syndrome (sicca syndrome) consists of dry mouth and dry eyes in the absence of any other connective tissue disease. The glandular destruction tends to be severe and is more often associated with lymphomatous change. Secondary Sjögren's syndrome is the well-known triad of dry eyes, dry mouth and a connective tissue disorder, usually rheumatoid arthritis. The sicca symptoms are frequently less severe than in the primary type.

Clinical features

Women, usually of middle age or older, are predominantly affected. Paradoxically, the majority do not complain of dry mouth, but rather of its effects, such as disturbed taste sensation, the need to take fluids with dry food, or soreness of the mucosa. Speech may be impaired as a result of the tongue sticking to the palate. Rarely, the mucosa is dry and parchment-like, but more frequently appears normal, though there may be no obvious flow of saliva from the parotid ducts or frothing in the floor of the mouth. In established cases, the tongue becomes partially depapillated and develops a lobulated surface. Redness and soreness of the mucosa is due to candidal infection. Intermittent salivary gland enlargement is seen in approximately 20% of patients, and persistent enlargement in 4%. In secondary Sjögren's syndrome, rheumatoid arthritis, the most common connective tissue disease, is most frequently associated. Sjögren's syndrome can also be associated with widespread changes of varying severity in many organ systems either as a result of associated autoimmune diseases or secondary to exocrine gland dysfunction (Table 11.1). Depressed lacrimal secretion (keratoconjunctivitis sicca) is particularly important but may be asymptomatic.

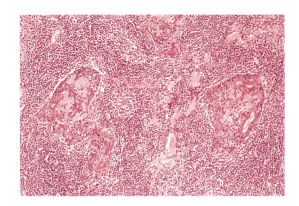

Figure 11.19   Epimyoepithelial islands in a dense mass of small lymphocytes in end-stage Sjögren's syndrome

Microscopy

Sjögren's syndrome is characterized by lympho-plasmacytic infiltration of salivary tissue; this is initially periductal but leads to progressive destruction of acini, which are replaced by the lymphoid infiltrate. Persistence and proliferation of duct epithelium gives rise to so-called epimyoepithelial islands (Figure 11.19) which may contain hyaline material (Figure 11.20). This lymphoproliferation, unlike a lymphoma, is polyclonal and respects the lobular septa. The same microscopic picture is typical of benign lymphoepithelial lesions.

Labial salivary glands show similar changes and have a close correlation with those in the parotid

glands but rarely show epimyoepithelial islands (Figure 11.21). Labial glands are a more convenient site for biopsy, to avoid risk of damage to branches of the facial nerve or parotid fistula. However, in assessing labial gland biopsies, non-specific sialadenitis must be excluded. This is characterized by scattered, rather than periductal infiltrates, variable numbers of neutrophils, acinar damage and ductal dilatation.

It is also important to assess several labial salivary gland lobules, as the greater the number of lymphocytic foci found, the greater the accuracy of diagnosis. If there are more than 5 foci per 4 mm^2 the accuracy of diagnosis is 95%.

Table 11.1   Disorders of other organ systems that may be associated with secondary Sjögren's syndrome

---

Cutaneous: Rashes of lupus erythematosus or dermatomyositis

Respiratory: Nasal crusting, or chronic bronchitis and dyspnoea associated with bronchiectasis

Gastrointestinal: Hepatomegaly associated with primary biliary cirrhosis, chronic active hepatitis or cryptogenic cirrhosis. Acute or chronic pancreatitis. Pernicious anaemia

Renal: Renal tubular acidosis, nephrogenic diabetes insipidus, nephrocalcinosis or other renal tubular dysfunctions

Musculoskeletal: Rheumatoid arthritis. Polymyositis or myasthenia gravis. Sensory and/or motor neuropathy and cranial nerve palsies

---

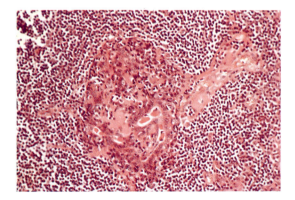

Figure 11.20   Sjögren's syndrome. Higher power view of an epimyoepithelial island with extensive deposits of hyaline material

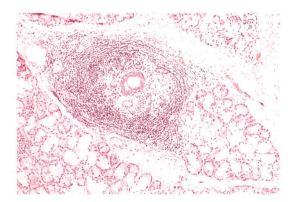

Figure 11.21 Sjögren's syndrome in a labial gland biopsy showing focal periductal lymphocytic sialadenitis

Management

If the mouth is not obviously dry on clinical examination, depressed salivary function should be confirmed by measuring the total, unstimulated flow rate. Other causes of xerostomia (Table 11.2) should be excluded. However, it must be emphasized that though the patient may have a dry mouth, investigation of lacrimal function is more important, as keratoconjunctivitis sicca can damage or destroy sight and is therefore more disabling than the oral effects of the disease. The Schirmer test is a measure of tear secretion. A healthy eye should wet more than 15 mm of the standard filter strip in 5 min. A more reliable assessment is made by staining the cornea with 1% rose bengal dye and examination with a slit lamp to show punctate or filamentary keratitis if the cornea is dry.

There is usually a raised erythrocyte sedimentation rate and frequently mild anaemia and leucopenia. Fifty per cent of patients have polyclonal hypergammaglobulinaemia. Autoantibodies, particularly rheumatoid factor and rheumatoid arthritis precipitin (RAP), are found in 90% and 75%, respectively, of cases of secondary Sjögren's syndrome, but in only 50% and 5%, respectively, in primary disease. SS-A antibodies are more specific and found in 5–10% of cases of the primary disease, but in 50–80% of cases of secondary disease. SS-B antibodies are found in up to 75% of cases of primary disease, but in 5% or less of secondary disease. Gastric parietal cell, thyroid microsomal, thyroglobulin and smooth muscle autoantibodies may also be detected.

Table 11.2 Causes of xerostomia

Organic
  Sjögren's syndrome
  Irradiation
  Mumps (transient)
  HIV infection
  Sarcoidosis
  Amyloid
  Iron deposition (haemochromatosis, thalassaemia)
  Hypercholesterolaemia type V

Functional
  Dehydration
  Water deprivation or excessive loss
  Haemorrhage
  Persistent diarrhoea and/or vomiting
  Diuretic overdosage

Drugs with antimuscarinic effects
  Atropine, ipratropium, hyoscine and other analogues
  Tricyclic and some other antidepressants
  Antihistamines
  Antiemetics (including antihistamines and
    phenothiazines)
  Neuroleptics, particularly phenothiazines
  Some antihypertensives, especially ganglion blockers
    and clonidine

Drugs with sympathomimetic actions
  'Cold cures' containing ephedrine, etc.
  Decongestants containing sympathomimetics
  Bronchodilators containing sympathomimetics
  Appetite suppressants, particularly amphetamines

Psychogenic
  Anxiety states and depression

A labial minor salivary gland biopsy, readily performed under local anaesthesia, will usually confirm the diagnosis by showing focal lymphocytic infiltration (Figures 11.22 and 11.23).

Diagnosis, therefore, depends on confirmation of depressed salivary output and exclusion of other causes of xerostomia, and in the case of secondary Sjögren's syndrome the association with another connective tissue disease. Labial salivary gland biopsy and the autoantibody profile are probably the most reliable confirmatory investigations. Sialography of the parotid glands usually shows varying degrees of sialectasis and duct atrophy as glandular destruction progresses, but is less useful.

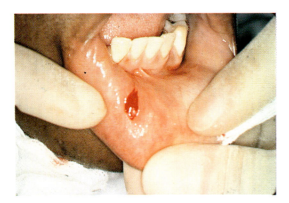

Figure 11.22   Labial salivary gland biopsy showing the double semilunar incision

Treatment is largely palliative. Immunosuppressive therapy has not been shown to be effective, as salivary gland destruction is usually too far advanced. Such treatment may increase the risk of malignant change. Treatment with hydroxychloroquine may cause a decline in autoantibody production, but does not improve salivary or lacrimal secretion.

Frequent use of lubricant eye drops is necessary when lacrimal secretion fails: fulguration of the nasolacrimal ducts also helps to conserve any secretion, but paradoxically may lead to epiphora. For the dry mouth, frequent sips of water while eating and frequent rinsing with saliva substitute are the main aids. Meticulous oral hygiene is essential and, for dentate patients, restriction of

dietary sugar, topical fluoride and chlorhexidine mouthwashes help to control caries. Candidal infection may be troublesome, particularly for those wearing dentures, and topical antifungal agents should be given.

Any underlying connective tissue disorder is treated as appropriate and all patients must be carefully followed up because of the increased risk of lymphoma.

Complications
These include:

● ocular damage from xerophthalmia
● those resulting from xerostomia (oral and salivary gland infections)
● those resulting from any associated connective tissue disease
● lymphomas of salivary glands or other sites.

Lymphomatous change may be preceded by a fall in serum immunoglobulin levels and may be suggested clinically by persistence or, particularly, late onset of salivary gland swelling. Approximately 5% of patients with Sjögren's syndrome develop lymphomas; this may represent more than a 40-fold increase in risk compared with normal. However, early lymphomatous change in Sjögren's syndrome may be difficult to recognize microscopically, as discussed later.

Functional xerostomia

In the differential diagnosis of xerostomia, organic diseases of the salivary glands, discussed earlier, must be distinguished from conditions where the glandular tissue is normal but salivary secretion is depressed as a result of dehydration or interference with the neurohumoral control.

An important difference between organic and functional causes of xerostomia is that the latter tend to be only temporary unless caused by long term drug treatment.

Functional causes of xerostomia are summarized in Table 11.2.

It is important to re-emphasize that patients with objectively confirmed depression of salivary flow, as in Sjögren's syndrome, relatively rarely complain of dryness of the mouth itself, but often of its

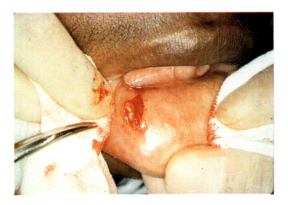

Figure 11.23   Labial salivary gland biopsy showing a lobule of minor salivary gland protruding through the incision

secondary effects such as disturbed taste sensation, or soreness resulting from candidal infection.

In anxiety states, excessive sympathetic activity can frequently depress salivary flow rates. Most people have experienced the dry mouth induced by anxiety before such occasions as examinations or public speaking. In a few, such as actors, this may become so great an occupational problem that treatment with a beta-blocker may have to be considered.

Other patients may complain of dry mouth as an essentially delusional symptom and salivary flow measurements do not confirm any reduction in secretion. Salivary flow studies may, therefore, be useful in helping to identify patients with psychiatric disorders presenting with this somatic symptom.

Despite statements to the contrary, there is no evidence that either benzodiazepines ('minor tranquillizers') or beta-blockers cause dry mouth.

HIV-associated salivary gland disease

Chronic parotitis in children is said by Prose (1990) to be virtually pathognomonic of HIV infection. In adults, swelling due to lymphocytic infiltration, often with cyst formation, of salivary glands and in some cases xerostomia are also well-recognized abnormalities. In some cases, the parotid swellings are bilateral, cystic and may be massive. Unlike patients with Sjögren's syndrome, most patients with HIV-associated sialadenitis are males in a considerably younger age group. An autoantibody picture typical of Sjögren's syndrome is also not associated with the sicca syndrome of HIV infection: SS-A or SS-B antibodies are not detectable and rheumatoid or antinuclear factors are no more frequent than in a healthy population. Another important difference is that in Sjögren's syndrome the infiltrate is mainly of CD4 lymphocytes, but in HIV infection there is typically dense CD8 lymphocytic infiltration.

Smith *et al.* (1988) have reported typical Sjögren-like changes (benign lymphoepithelial lesions), but associated with microcyst formation, in parotid glands from males at high risk from AIDS. All patients had generalized lymphadenopathy concurrent with painless parotid swellings, which

had developed over periods of one or more years, but none reported dryness of the mouth or eyes.

Holliday *et al.* (1988) have also reported, painless facial swelling due to benign lymphoepithelial parotid cysts in patients with HIV infection. These were bilateral in most cases and visible in CT scans.

Microscopy

The lymphoplasmacytic infiltrate and formation of epimyoepithelial islands is essentially the same as that seen in Sjögren's syndrome and may also be found in labial salivary glands biopsies. However, there may be gross or microscopic cyst formation (Figure 11.24). Major cysts are lined by cuboidal and squamous epithelium overlying nodules of hyperplastic lymphoid tissue. Cervical lymphadenopathy due to follicular hyperplasia (Chapter 14) is usually associated.

Parotid swelling with changes typical of benign lymphoepithelial lesion, particularly with cyst formation, in an adult male below the age group at risk from Sjögren's syndrome, is therefore strongly suggestive of HIV infection. However, dryness of the mouth or eyes is not always associated, and an autoantibody picture typical of Sjögren's syndrome is not found. Typical differences between Sjögren's syndrome and HIV-associated salivary gland disease are summarized in Table 11.3. Other salivary gland lesions associated with HIV infection include parotid swellings due to involvement of intra- or paraparotid lymphoid

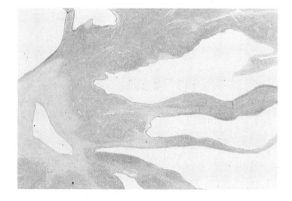

Figure 11.24 Cystic lymphoepithelial lesion associated with HIV infection. Large cystic cavities extend between the lymphoepithelial infiltration which has replaced the gland parenchyma

Table 11.3 Typical differences between Sjögren's syndrome and HIV-associated salivary gland disease

	Sjögren's syndrome	*HIV-associated salivary gland disease*
Sex	Up to 90% females	Predominantly males
Age	Mostly over 50	Usually 20–40
Lymphadenopathy	–	+ + +
Xerostomia/ xerophthalmia	++	Variable
Salivary gland cysts	–	+
Autoantibodies	RF, RAP, SS-A, SS-B*, etc.	None characteristic of Sjögren's syndrome
Lymphocytic infiltrate	CD4	CD8 (but microscopy otherwise similar*)
HLA	DR3/DR4	DR5

*See text.

tissues in the lymphoproliferative process of this disease, or a salivary gland lymphoma.

Irradiation damage

Salivary glands are sensitive to ionizing radiation. The acute self-limiting reaction has been described earlier, but long-term irreversible changes follow exposure to 16 Gy or more of irradiation. This destroys salivary acini and causes obliterative endarteritis.

Microscopy
Progressive atrophy of gland acini leads to fibrosis: ischaemic damage due to obliterative endarteritis persists indefinitely. In severe cases, little of the gland may remain, apart from the remnants of ducts and obliterated blood vessels in a dense fibrous matrix.

Management
Symptomatic management of the dry mouth is the same as for Sjögren's syndrome and care should be taken to relieve this distressing symptom as far

as possible. If enough salivary tissue is destroyed, the resulting xerostomia will lead to severe caries in any remaining teeth, and other oral infections if precautions are not taken. The consequences of any such dental disease are likely to be considerably more serious for the irradiated patient because of the risk of osteoradionecrosis if subsequent dental extractions are undertaken. Protection and preservation of the teeth are therefore particularly important in the patient who has therapeutic irradiation. Preventive measures are liberal use of artificial saliva, minimal sugar consumption, meticulous oral hygiene, regular application of fluorides and treatment of any infections secondary to the xerostomia. Acute candidosis (thrush) is common in such patients, but responds well to a course of miconazole gel.

Mikulicz's disease and Mikulicz's syndrome

These terms are an unnecessary source of confusion and are referred to here only for clarification. Mikulicz's disease is an alternative clinical term for benign lymphoepithelial lesion of the parotid glands, particularly when bilateral.

Mikulicz's syndrome refers to the much less common clinical condition of bilateral enlargement of the parotid, other salivary and lacrimal glands by definable disorders such as sarcoidosis, lymphoma or sialosis.

Sialosis (sialadenosis)

Sialosis is an uncommon condition consisting of bilateral, soft, painless enlargement of the parotids and occasionally of other glands. The pathogenesis is unknown, but sialosis seems particularly likely to develop in association with a variety of diseases (Table 11.4).

Microscopically, the acinar cells become swollen and there is loss of cytoplasmic granulation. The striated ducts may atrophy, fatty infiltration may increase and interstitial oedema may develop (Figure 11.25). In some cases, there is extensive fatty replacement of acinar tissue, but inflammation is notably absent.

There is no reliably effective treatment. The underlying condition should be controlled if possible, but regression of the salivary gland enlargement does not necessarily follow.

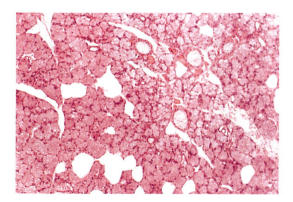

Figure 11.25 Sialosis. Distended serous cells and compressed striated ducts are shown

Table 11.4 Sialosis: associated conditions and possible causes

Hormonal
  Ovarian insufficiency
  Hypothyroidism
  Acromegaly
  Diabetes mellitus

Metabolic
  Cirrhosis
  Alcoholism (with or without cirrhosis)
  Chronic pancreatitis
  Chronic renal failure
  Malnutrition

Drug-associated

References

Akaboshi, I., Katsuki, T., Jamamoto, J. *et al.* (1983) Unique pattern of Epstein–Barr virus specific antibodies in recurrent parotitis. *Lancet*, **ii**, 1049–1050

Berman, H.L. and Delancy, V. (1992) Iodide mumps due to low-osmolality contrast material. *American Journal of Roentgenology*, **159**, 1099–1100

Brook, I. (1992) Diagnosis and management of parotitis. *Archives of Otolaryngology and Head and Neck Surgery*, **118**, 469–471

Holliday, R.A., Cohen, W.A., Schinella, R.A. *et al.* (1988) Benign lymphoepithelial parotid cysts and hyperplastic cervical lymphadenopathy in AIDS-risk patients: a new CT appearance. *Radiology*, **168**, 439–441

Iro, H., Schneider, H.Th., Födra, C. *et al.* (1992) Shockwave lithotripsy of salivary duct stones. *Lancet*, **339**, 1333–1336

Mizuno, A. and Yamaguchi, K. (1993) The plunging ranula. *International Journal of Oral and Maxillofacial Surgery*, **22**, 113–115

O'Connell, J.E., George, M.K., Speculand, G.B. *et al.* (1993) Mycobacterial infection of the parotid gland: an unusual cause of parotid swelling. *Journal of Laryngology and Otology*, **107**, 560–564

Prose, N.S. (1990) HIV infection in children. *Journal of the American Academy of Dermatology*, **22**, 1223–1231

Raad, I.I., Sabbagh, M.F. and Caranasos, G.J. (1990) Acute bacterial sialadenitis: a study of 29 cases and review. *Review of Infectious Diseases*, **12**, 591–601

Smith, F.B., Rajdeo, H., Panesar, N. *et al.* (1988) Benign lymphoepithelial lesion of the parotid gland in intravenous drug users. *Archives of Pathology and Laboratory Medicine*, **112**, 742–745

12

Tumours of salivary glands

A great variety of neoplasms can form in the salivary gland tissues. The classification of Thackray and Sobin (1972) (Table 12.1) is still widely used, but inevitably has been overtaken by the recognition of new types of tumours. A modified classification broadly based on changes proposed by the WHO Collaborating Center for Salivary Gland Tumors is therefore shown in Table 12.2, but even so it is not always easy to fit a particular tumour into one of these many categories. Non-neoplastic diseases have been discussed in the previous chapter, but in the parotid gland particularly it is not always possible to distinguish them from neoplasms preoperatively.

Age, site and sex distribution in relation to tumour type

In the British Salivary Gland Tumour Panel series of more than 3500 unselected tumours, there is a wide age distribution, but the peak incidence for benign tumours is in the sixth decade and, for malignant tumours, the seventh. Thus in the third decade, nearly 95% of tumours are benign, but by the seventh decade and after, 30% of tumours are malignant. Overall, women are only slightly more frequently affected, until the eighth and ninth decades, when women are almost twice as frequently affected as men. This, however, must be related to a female predominance of 2 to 1 at these ages in the general population. For certain tumour types there is also a female predominance, as discussed later.

Over 70% of salivary gland tumours are in the parotid, 11% are in the submandibular glands, and the remainder are distributed as shown in Table 12.3. However, in relative terms, malignant tumours are more frequent in the minor salivary glands; thus only 16% of parotid tumours but 78% of sublingual gland and 46% of minor gland tumours are malignant.

As to minor glands (approximately 14% of all salivary gland tumours), 54% are in the palate, 20% in the lips and 10% in the buccal mucosa.

Table 12.1 Classification of salivary gland tumours (After Thackray and Sobin, 1972)

EPITHELIAL

A. Adenomas
1. Pleomorphic adenoma (mixed tumour)
2. Monomorphic adenoma
   (a) Adenolymphoma (Warthin's tumour)
   (b) (Oxyphilic adenoma (oncocytoma)
   (c) Other monomorphic adenomas

B. Mucoepidermoid tumour
C. Acinic cell tumour
D. Carcinomas
1. Adenoid cystic carcinoma
2. Adenocarcinoma
3. Squamous cell carcinoma
4. Undifferentiated carcinomas
5. Carcinoma in pleomorphic adenoma

NON-EPITHELIAL

Haemangioma
Lymphangioma
Neurofibroma
Lipoma
Others including malignant variants of the above
Lymphoma

Table 12.2 Modified histopathological classification of salivary gland tumours

I. ADENOMAS
    Pleomorphic adenoma
    Myoepithelioma
    Warthin's tumour (adenolymphoma)
    Oncocytoma
    Duct adenomas
        Basal cell adenoma and membranous variant
        Canalicular adenoma
    Sebaceous adenoma and sebaceous lymphadenoma
    Duct papillomas
        Inverted duct papilloma
        Intraduct papilloma
        Sialadenoma papilliferum
    Papillary cystadenoma

II. CARCINOMAS
    Mucoepidermoid carcinoma
    Acinic cell carcinoma
    Adenoid cystic carcinoma
        Cribriform/tubular
        Solid
    Adenocarcinoma (not otherwise specified)
    Papillary cystadenocarcinoma
    Mucinous adenocarcinoma
    Carcinoma in pleomorphic adenoma
        Intracapsular (non-invasive)
        Invasive
        Carcinosarcoma
        Metastasizing pleomorphic adenoma
    Polymorphous low-grade (terminal duct) adenocarcinoma
    Epithelial-myoepithelial carcinoma
    Salivary duct carcinoma
    Basal cell (basaloid) carcinoma
    Sebaceous carcinoma
        Sebaceous carcinoma with lymphoid stroma
    Oncocytic carcinoma
    Squamous cell carcinoma
    Adenosquamous carcinoma
    Undifferentiated carcinoma
        Small cell and neuroendocrine carcinomas
    Undifferentiated carcinoma with lymphoid stroma
    Other carcinomas

III. MESENCHYMAL TUMOURS
    Angiomas
    Lipomas
    Neural tumours
    Other benign mesenchymal tumours and hamartomas
    Sarcomas

IV. MALIGNANT LYMPHOMAS

V. SECONDARY TUMOURS

VI. UNCLASSIFIED TUMOURS

VII. TUMOUR-LIKE DISORDERS
    Sialosis (sialadenosis)
    Oncocytosis
    Necrotizing sialometaplasia (salivary gland infarction)
    Benign lymphoepithelial lesion
    Salivary gland cysts
    HIV-related cysts and other disorders
    Kuttner tumour (chronic submandibular sialadenitis)

General clinical features

Though usually painless, a painful salivary gland swelling is strongly suggestive of malignancy. However, non-malignant parotid swellings such as infections, some Warthin's tumours and a few cases of Sjögren's syndrome can also be painful, and there are no reliable clinical indicators of malignancy. However, rapid growth, pain, lymphadenopathy and, in the case of the parotid gland, facial palsy are strongly suggestive and are likely to indicate a poor prognosis.

Within the mouth, salivary gland tumours may be firm or rubbery, and may feel lobulated. If benign, they are mobile on deeper tissues; the overlying mucosa is normal, unless traumatized, but sometimes appears bluish. Growth of some adenomas can be exceedingly slow.

Imaging techniques

Despite the advances in imaging techniques, they will not as yet distinguish neoplastic from inflammatory disease, nor benign from malignant tumours in all cases.

Sialography This is useful only for chronic inflammatory disease and is of little value in tumour diagnosis.

Computerized tomography CT scanning distinguishes well between glandular and adjacent soft tissue. It also allows examination in the transverse plane (Figure 12.1). The density of a gland varies considerably; it is always greater than that of fat but less than that of muscle. Most benign tumours have well-defined borders, while those with irregular or indistinct margins suggest malignancy. The latter may be confirmed by extension into the infratemporal fossa or base of skull, or metastatic

Table 12.3   Distribution of tumours in minor and major salivary glands

	Palate (%)	Lips (%)	Buccal mucosa (%)	Total minor glands (%)	Total major glands (%)
ADENOMAS					
Pleomorphic adenoma	47	44	37	43	63
Other adenomas	6	30	13	11	7
CARCINOMAS					
Mucoepidermoid carcinoma	9	–	8	9	2
Acinic cell carcinoma	1	4	–	2	2
Adenoid cystic carcinoma	12	9	13	13	4
Adenocarcinomas	12	9	18	12	3
Squamous cell carcinoma	1	–	3	1	1
Undifferentiated carcinoma	1	3	3	2	2
Pleomorphic adenoma	8	3	5	7	4

Notes: 1. Percentages rounded up to whole figures.
2. A few tumours in the tongue, pharynx, tonsil, retromolar fossa, alveolar ridge, maxillary tuberosity and ethmoid have been omitted, as there was often only a single tumour in each of these sites.

deposits. Multiple lesions suggest malignant lymphoma, Warthin's tumour or metastases.

CT may help to predict the relationship of a mass to the facial nerve. Such information is of preoperative value, as removal of a lesion which distorts the anatomy at the foramen, or has a

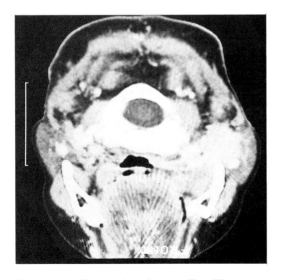

Figure 12.1   Pleomorphic adenoma. This CT scan shows the typical lobulated appearance. Calcification or bone formation sometimes provides a useful hint that a salivary gland tumour is a pleomorphic adenoma but this example is unusually opaque

significant component deep to the nerve, is likely to be demanding. Deep-lobe tumours are as easy to visualize as superficial tumours, and their extent is precisely shown.

CT scanning is also valuable for distinguishing intrinsic from extrinsic parotid disease and may help to distinguish deep-lobe parotid from lateral pharyngeal (minor gland) tumours. Parapharyngeal tumours are usually separated from the gland by a layer of normal fat. If this layer is absent, the mass is probably a deep-lobe parotid tumour. However, large deep-lobe tumours obliterate this plane and make diagnosis difficult.

Intravenous contrast medium may help to demonstrate the relationship of tumours to major vessels and vascular malformations. Jugulotympanic paraganglionomas, being highly vascular, are enhanced dramatically by contrast medium. Rarely, a paraganglionoma may mimic deep-lobe salivary gland tumours of the parotid clinically.

Unfortunately, extensive dental restorations cause disruptive artefacts which can significantly detract from the quality of CT scans.

Magnetic resonance imaging   MRI is as sensitive as CT for detection of salivary gland tumours. Both T_1 and T_2 images show the margins of the lesion with equal clarity, but T_2 sequences may define tumour composition better. Paramagnetic contrast materials may improve this aspect of MR imaging even further. Unlike CT, MR images are not distorted by dental restorations.

There is little to choose between CT and MRI for the diagnosis of salivary gland disease and the ultimate choice is mainly influenced by the type of scanners available, cost and personal preference. The indications for CT or MRI can be summarized as follows:

Parotid glands
● masses confined to the deep lobe
● tumours with involvement of both the deep and superficial lobes (dumb-bell tumours)
● tumours causing facial weakness, other neural deficit or signs of malignancy
● congenital masses.

Submandibular glands
● tumours with neural deficit or fixation to the mandible.

Minor glands
● tumours of the palate with suspected involvement of the nose or maxillary antra
● any tumours with clinically ill defined margins.

Neither CT nor MRI should be expected to be completely reliable and the main purpose of imaging is for detecting masses within the salivary glands and providing surgically useful images of the extent of disease. Sensitivity rates approaching 100% are claimed for both modalities, but image quality is influenced mainly by the generation of scanner or protocol adopted.

Ultrasound The value of ultrasound in parotid disease is limited. The superficial portion of the gland is readily accessible to ultrasound examination, but the deep part is obscured by the ramus of the mandible.

The normal gland is homogeneous and gives fine, medium-range echoes. Its borders, although not sharply delineated, are easily visualized. Useful adjacent landmarks are the mandible (linear and strongly echogenic), and the masseter and sterno-mastoid muscles which are echo-poor compared with the parotid gland.

Ultrasound cannot characterize a focal lesion, but various ultrasonic characteristics may suggest the nature of the mass. It has the advantages of being non-invasive, inexpensive and relatively quick, and is useful if CT or MRI are not available.

Surgical management of parotid gland tumours

Pleomorphic adenomas are the most common tumours and readily recur but cannot be identified clinically. In view of the major risk of tumour cells disseminating during incisional biopsy of parotid gland tumours, fine-needle aspiration biopsy (Chapter 1) should therefore be used wherever possible.

Superficial parotidectomy should be carried out for all clinically benign superficial lobe tumours. Total parotidectomy is required for deep lobe and dumb-bell tumours. Deep lobe tumours should never be approached from the pharyngeal aspect as the risk of recurrence is high. The facial nerve should be preserved wherever possible.

The prognosis for many malignant parotid tumours is poor. Radical parotidectomy with sacrifice of the facial nerve may not improve survival significantly, but it greatly worsens morbidity. If not macroscopically invaded by tumour, the facial nerve should therefore be preserved during parotidectomy. This should be followed by radiotherapy.

Anatomical considerations The superficial lobe of the parotid gland rests on the masseter muscle. The deep part extends behind the mandible posterior to the pterygoid muscles. Medially lie the lateral pharyngeal space, internal carotid artery and internal jugular vein. The facial nerve leaves the skull at the stylomastoid foramen and enters the posterior surface of the gland between the digastric and sternocleidomastoid muscles. It lies lateral to the retromandibular vein before dividing into its major branches over the ramus of the mandible. The gland is divided into superficial and deep lobes joined by an isthmus. The facial nerve lies in a connective tissue plane between these two lobes.

Successful parotid surgery depends upon taking into account two major anatomical features, namely:

1. The two lobes united by an isthmus.
2. The facial nerve and its branches, is surrounded by these lobes, but invested in loose connective tissue. The facial nerve, except when invaded by tumour, is separable from the substance of the parotid parenchyma.

Despite competent surgery, permanent facial nerve weakness may be expected after approximately 1–2% of parotidectomies. Disturbances of facial nerve function can follow 30% of parotidectomies but are usually of short duration.

Frey's syndrome may develop in a high proportion of patients undergoing parotidectomy, but its onset is usually delayed for about 2 years. Rare complications after parotid surgery include sialocele or salivary fistula.

Surgical management of submandibular gland tumours

All submandibular salivary tumours should be treated by total gland excision. For obviously malignant tumours, this forms part of a radical neck dissection and postoperative radiotherapy is also advocated.

Surgical management of minor salivary gland tumours

Biopsy is usually carried out before surgery. Treatment is by wide local excision, including palatal fenestration for tumours in this site if there is evidence of bony involvement.

Radiotherapy Salivary tumours are often considered to be radioresistant. This is not necessarily true; regression after radiotherapy is usually slow, but this reflects the slow cell turnover time of the majority of these tumours, rather than the inability of radiation to effect a cure, and there are many reports of long-term local control of large inoperable tumours by radiotherapy. Nevertheless, the cure rate for radiotherapy seems to be lower than for squamous cell carcinoma of the oral mucosa, and therefore the primary treatment should be surgical wherever possible.

Radiotherapy may be given postoperatively wherever there is doubt about complete excision, but should only be given for malignant tumours. It should be given prophylactically after excision of any malignant salivary tumour. However, reliable information on the response of particular types of salivary gland tumour to radiation is scanty.

A wide margin around the tumour should be irradiated. This is frequently recommended, particularly for adenoid cystic carcinomas, though there is little evidence that it improves survival. A dose close to the limits of normal tissue tolerance is necessary.

Chemotherapy There appears to be little place for chemotherapy in the treatment of salivary gland

carcinomas, and as yet it seems to be no more than a treatment of last resort. Lymphomas, by contrast, respond well to radiotherapy or chemotherapy, or both.

Benign epithelial tumours

Pleomorphic adenoma

Pleomorphic adenomas account for 63% of parotid, 60% of submandibular and 43% of minor gland tumours. By contrast, they are rarely seen in the sublingual gland. Almost any age can be affected, but the peak incidence is in the fourth and fifth decades. There is a slight female predominance.

Microscopy

The main components are duct cells, often producing a multiplicity of duct-like structures, and sheets of epithelial or myoepithelial cells. The latter are not reliably identifiable by light microscopy as they may be small, dark and nondescript, spindle shaped or resemble plasma cells. Squamous metaplasia of epithelial cells is common (Figure 12.2). The result is a mixed and variable picture of epithelial and myoepithelial cells together with

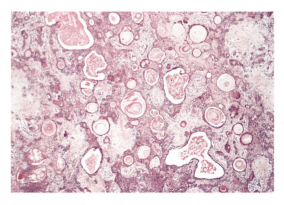

Figure 12.2 Pleomorphic adenoma with squamous metaplasia and inspissated secretion resembling corpora amylacea

mucoid or myxomatous tissue, which may form the bulk of the tumour. Cartilage or, less frequently, true bone formation may be seen (Figure 12.3). This stroma forms 80% of the mass in approximately 50% of tumours. There is no proven correlation between these varied appearances and clinical behaviour, but recurrence may be more common with stroma-rich (mucoid) variants and carcinomatous change is most frequent in highly cellular tumours.

The mixed microscopic pictures are well known, but widespread misapprehensions persist about the capsule and have led to attempts to enucleate parotid gland tumours. Encapsulation may appear complete (Figure 12.4) in the plane of section but the tumour, despite being benign, can bulge through or invade the capsule (Figures 12.5 and 12.6). Focal infiltration of the capsule is common and subcapsular clefts can provide false planes of cleavage. Whole organ sectioning of excised parotid pleomorphic adenomas by Lam *et al.* (1990) showed that in all cases the capsule was infiltrated by tumour and that in a third of the cases the capsule was incomplete, with tumour in direct contact with salivary tissue. Apparently isolated islands of tumour can also occasionally form outgrowths of the main mass and be joined to it by only a thin neck.

Dysplasia in pleomorphic adenoma

The appearance, within the tumour, of areas of epithelial atypia despite absence of evidence of

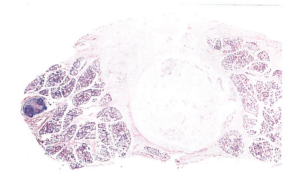

Figure 12.4 Pleomorphic adenoma. Low-power view shows a sharply demarcated tumour in the parotid gland which includes an intraparotid lymph node on the left

invasion (also sometimes termed intracapsular carcinoma or 'carcinoma-in-situ') inevitably causes concern. If it is possible to be confident that this change is confined within the substance of the tumour, then it can be treated like other pleomorphic adenomas by parotidectomy or wide excision of other glands. However, follow-up must be rigorous.

Spread, response to treatment and recurrence
Pleomorphic adenomas expand and grow in localized areas of proliferation to form irregular nodular masses. Major difficulties in the management of pleomorphic adenomas include the following:

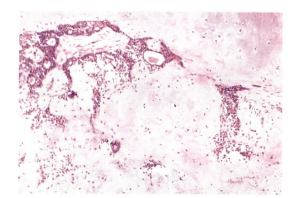

Figure 12.3 Pleomorphic adenoma. Duct-like epithelial structures and chondroid areas are shown

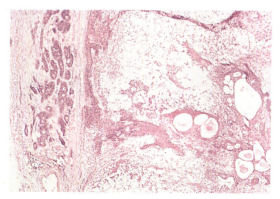

Figure 12.5 Predominantly mucoid/myxoid pleomorphic adenoma. Capsulation is extremely variable

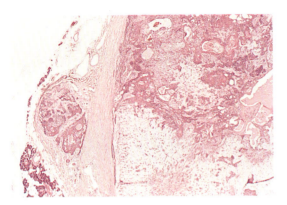

Figure 12.6 Pleomorphic adenoma. Tumour has extended through the capsule

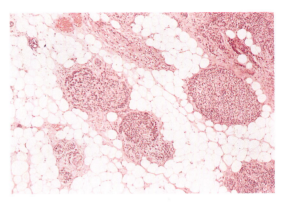

Figure 12.7 Recurrent pleomorphic adenoma. Nodules of tumour have spread into surrounding fat

● removal of tumours from the parotid gland without damage to the facial nerve is technically demanding
● biopsy of parotid gland tumours is not feasible because of their ability to seed in the line of incision to produce multiple recurrences
● the capsule is often incomplete and its integrity cannot be assumed if there is an unwise attempt at enucleation
● mucinous tumours can readily burst to produce multiple seedlings if enucleation is attempted
● removal of recurrences, which are typically multifocal, becomes more difficult with each attempt and the end result can be innumerable nodules of tumour, spreading in the neck far beyond the original site (Figure 12.7); treatment of recurrences increases the risk of having to resect the facial nerve or they may prove to be unmanageable
● the chances of malignant change are greater in recurrences, increase with each subsequent recurrence and may be increased further if radiotherapy is used.

In short, the ability of seeded tumour cells to proliferate outside the original margins and particularly in the incision scar, after incisional biopsy or incomplete excision, is well established. Malignant change is also more frequent in scarred areas. Recurrences may not become apparent for 10 or even 20 years and this can give a false sense of the completeness of excision and encourage dangerously conservative treatment policy. High reported cure rates after enucleation are based on inadequate duration of follow-up.

These considerations make it clear that incisional biopsy and so-called enucleation are contra-indicated and that it is essential to remove pleomorphic adenomas completely by total or subtotal parotidectomy at the first operation.

Irradiation as a supplement to surgery may increase the chances of or accelerate malignant change. If reoperation is necessary, post-irradiation scarring and ischaemia greatly increase the difficulties. Nevertheless, radiotherapy is widely used if the tumour ruptures during surgery.

Myoepithelioma

Myoepithelial tumours are rare and, in effect, a variant of pleomorphic adenoma. The term *myoepithelioma* is frequently used for tumours where myoepithelial cells are predominant but some elements of a pleomorphic adenoma are present.

Microscopy

Spindle cell myoepitheliomas, the most common type, are highly cellular and consist of elongated, slender spindle cells forming interlacing streams with little stroma. They, therefore, resemble mesenchymal tumours such as neurofibroma (Figure 12.8). Occasionally, immunocytochemistry is required to detect the typical double staining of myoepithelial cells with epithelial (keratin) markers

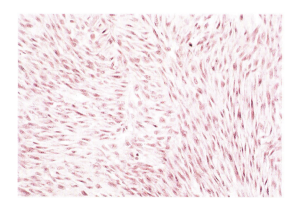

Figure 12.8 Myoepithelioma. Spindle cell variant resembling a mesenchymal tumour

as well as mesenchymal markers, particularly S-100 protein, vimentin and smooth muscle actin.

Aggressive behaviour may not be entirely predictable from the microscopic appearances but mitotic activity and cellular pleomorphism are highly suspicious.

Plasmacytoid myoepitheliomas consist of elliptical or rounded cells, with hyaline, basophilic cytoplasm and eccentrically placed nuclei, in an abundant, loose and myxoid stroma (Figure 12.9). This variant does not appear to have any potential for aggressive behaviour. It is also unlikely for the resemblance to plasma cells to be so close as to be mistaken for solitary extramedullary plasmacytomas (Chapter 5).

Warthin's tumour (adenolymphoma, cystadenolymphoma)

These tumours are completely benign, and carcinomatous or lymphomatous change is extraordinarily rare. Strangely, there has been in the past a heavy predominance of males with this tumour, but a male to female ratio of 10 to 1 has fallen to only 1.6 to 1 in the most recent series. The age affected is between 50 and 70 years. In the parotid glands, Warthin's tumour forms 14% of neoplasms, while other types of monomorphic adenoma – mainly the canalicular variant in the upper lip – form 11% of tumours of the minor glands.

Clinically, Warthin's tumour only affects the parotid glands and the authenticity of some of those reported in other glands is questionable. They usually produce soft painless swellings but sometimes there can be pain or rapid expansion, probably as a result of the partly cystic nature of most of them. Occasionally the tumour is bilateral or multifocal in a single gland.

Microscopy

Warthin's tumours have a thin capsule and consist of tall, columnar, finely granular, eosinophilic epithelial cells (Figure 12.10) surrounding lymphoid tissue which frequently forms germinal follicles. The epithelium typically forms papillary projections into cystic spaces (Figure 12.11). The amount of

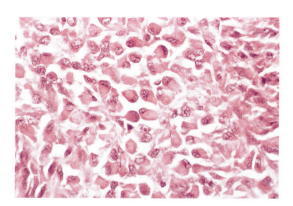

Figure 12.9 Myoepithelioma. Plasmacytoid (hyaline cell) variant

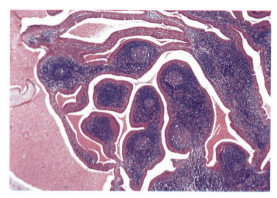

Figure 12.10 Warthin's tumour. The papillary projections of oncocytic epithelium cover cellular lymphoid stroma with germinal centres

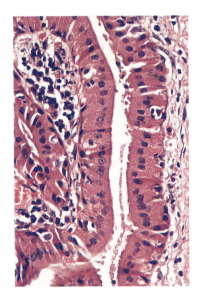

Figure 12.11   Warthin's tumour. Higher magnification shows intensely oncocytic double-layered epithelium with palisading of the luminal cells

epithelium and lymphoid stroma is highly variable and either may predominate.

Occasionally, part of the tumour can undergo apparently spontaneous necrosis (infarction) and epithelioid granulomas resembling those of tuberculosis may form. Taxy (1992) has also described squamous and mucinous metaplasia in foci of necrosis, giving rise to appearances resembling squamous or mucoepidermoid carcinoma. However, Warthin's tumour can also occasionally be concurrent with other salivary gland tumours.

Treatment

Excision is curative but incomplete excision can lead to recurrence. Alternatively, recurrence may result from the tumour being multifocal.

Oncocytoma (oxyphilic adenoma)

Oncocytomas form less than 0.5% of epithelial salivary gland tumours. They particularly affect those in the seventh or eighth decades and are more frequent in women. The parotid glands are the usual site.

Microscopically, oncocytomas consist of distinctive, uniform, plump cells with abundant, granular eosinophilic cytoplasm, separated by fine fibrous septa (Figure 12.12). Occasionally, transition of oncocytes to clear cells can be seen. Oncocytomas consisting only of clear cells are a recognized entity but exceedingly rare.

Oncocytomas are benign and excision is curative. Reports of recurrences may be due to incomplete removal or failure to recognize either an oncocytic adenocarcinoma or oncocytic change in a carcinoma.

Multifocal nodular oncocytic hyperplasia

Foci with a structure resembling that of oncocytomas may be seen, but they are small (up to 1 cm across), multiple and interspersed by normal salivary tissue. It is possible that oncocytomas arise by confluence of these foci. Clear cells are most frequently seen in these foci, which may thus mimic a clear cell tumour infiltrating the gland.

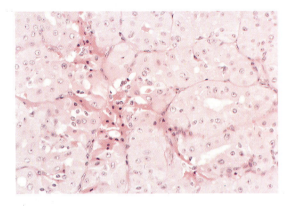

Figure 12.12   Oncocytoma. Large pale granular cells (light cells) and smaller numbers of compressed cells with intensely eosinophilic cytoplasm and pyknotic nuclei (dark cells) are shown

Oncocytosis

Oncocytic change, which is occasionally extensive, can be seen as an age change in normal duct tissue and in other tumours such as pleomorphic adenomas or, more important, in adenocarcinomas. Since oncocytomas are benign, it is important to differentiate them from oncocytic change in other tumours which are far more difficult to manage. Palmer *et al.* (1990) have shown that the majority of oncocytomas had been incorrectly categorized. Many were the result of oncocytic change in other tumours or oncocytosis.

Duct adenomas

Seventy-five per cent of this group are found in the parotid glands, 22% in the minor glands, where the lip is a site of predilection, but very few in other glands. Duct adenomas constitute about 20% of all adenomas. Duct adenomas comprise basal cell (tubular, trabecular and membranous types) and canalicular types which form slow-growing, well-circumscribed swellings.

Tubular adenomas consist of tubules, containing eosinophilic secretions. The tubules have a lining of small, dark epithelial cells and an outer layer of myoepithelial cells which may also form strands extending between the tubules; alternatively they may be few and inconspicuous (Figure 12.13). The stroma is usually scanty and unremarkable, but a rare variant shows myoepithelial stromal proliferation.

Trabecular adenomas consist of a monotonous pattern of cords, uniform in width, of darkly staining cells in a sparse, featureless stroma (Figure 12.14). Rarely, a trabecular adenoma shows oncocytic change and may mimic an oncocytoma.

Membranous basal cell adenomas are rare. They have a thick, eosinophilic, PAS-positive hyaline layer surrounding the epithelium which may contain lumens and hyaline material. They are usually multilobular and may be incompletely encapsulated. They can also contain foci of normal salivary tissue to add to the impression of invasiveness and enhance their similarities to an adenoid cystic carcinoma.

Membranous basal cell adenomas most frequently affect the parotid glands and then may be associated with multiple similar (turban) tumours of the scalp. They are sometimes, therefore, termed dermal analogue tumours of the parotid. They may rarely undergo malignant change.

Canalicular adenomas, unlike tubular adenomas, lack myoepithelial cells surrounding the duct-like structures or cords of columnar or cuboidal epithelial cells. Cyst formation may be prominent (Figure 12.15), while degeneration of the stroma may leave it virtually structureless, and often only ghosts of blood vessels remain.

Treatment

Excision is normally curative. The chief risk with duct adenomas is that of confusing some of them with adenoid cystic carcinomas or basal cell adenocarcinomas. A thorough search of many

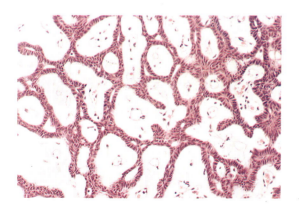

Figure 12.13   Tubular-trabecular basal cell adenoma

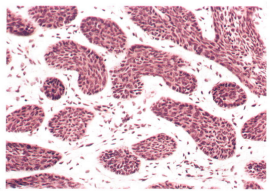

Figure 12.14   Solid basal cell adenoma

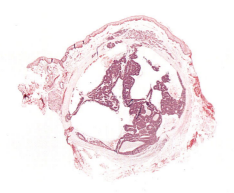

Figure 12.15   Canalicular adenoma of the lip. These tumours often present as cysts

fields may occasionally be necessary to confirm absence of invasion. If the biopsy is small it may be impossible to make the necessary distinction. Canalicular adenomas in the upper lip, in particular, have been mistaken for adenoid cystic carcinomas.

Clear cell adenoma

In the past, benign clear cell tumours have been described but their existence is doubtful. Most clear cell tumours are malignant, despite a cytologically benign appearance.

Papillary cystadenoma

The papillary cystadenoma is probably also not an entity and such tumours are well-differentiated papillary cystic adenocarcinomas. However, the fact that they may take between 10 and 20 years to recur has led to the belief that they were benign.

Sebaceous lymphadenoma and sebaceous adenoma

Both of these tumours are rare. The sebaceous lymphadenoma resembles Warthin's tumour but with sebaceous cells, forming solid masses and

sebaceous cysts in place of the oncocytic cells. The pure sebaceous adenoma is particularly rare and consists of solid masses of sebaceous tissue in a fibrous stroma. Sebaceous elements can rarely also be seen in pleomorphic adenomas.

Duct papillomas

Sialadenoma papilliferum

Most of these rare tumours have been in the minor glands, usually at the region of the junction of hard and soft palates. Unlike other salivary gland tumours, they form painless exophytic growths that resemble papillomas of the oral mucosa but grow from the orifice of a minor gland. The mean age of incidence is 59, but almost any age can be affected.

Microscopically, the superficial part closely resembles a squamous cell papilloma and consists of stratified squamous epithelium thrown up into papillae with a fibrovascular core. More deeply, this epithelium merges with proliferating, dilated duct-like structures and, frequently, microcysts with papillary projections into their cavities.

Local excision appears to be curative.

Inverted duct papilloma

Inverted duct papillomas of salivary glands are exceedingly rare; Clark *et al.* (1990) found only 5 earlier reports.

Clinically, patients have been adults between the ages of 33 and 66 years, in whom the tumours formed smooth discrete masses 1–1.5 cm in diameter in various sites within the oral cavity, with no features to suggest the diagnosis.

Microscopically, inverted duct papilloma frequently forms just within the orifice of a gland and its epithelium may be continuous with that of the surface mucosa. The tumour consists of thick papillae covered by basal or squamous cells and may contain a few goblet or columnar cells. The papillary overgrowth fills the duct lumen and also bulges into, but does not infiltrate, the lamina propria. Microcysts lined by squamous or columnar epithelium occasionally form.

Excision appears to be curative and there is no evidence of a similar propensity for recurrence to inverted papillomas of the nasal cavity.

Intraduct papilloma

Intraduct papilloma is even more rare than other duct papillomas. It differs from the inverted duct papilloma in its origin more deeply in the salivary gland duct.

Microscopically, it consists of fibrovascular papillae covered by columnar or cuboidal epithelium, forming a mass which distends the duct lumen to form a cyst-like cavity. Unlike inverted duct papillomas, the tumour does not extend into the duct wall but obstruction by the tumour can give rise to secondary duct dilatation proximally. Excision is curative.

Carcinomas of salivary glands

Mucoepidermoid carcinoma

These form 1.5% of parotid tumours, nearly 9% of tumours of the minor glands but are virtually never found in the sublingual glands. Most mucoepidermoid carcinomas are in the parotid (49%) or minor glands (47%). Almost any age can be affected, but the peak incidence is in the fifth decade.

Clinically, most mucoepidermoid carcinomas are usually indistinguishable from benign tumours and rarely cause facial weakness or pain. Intra-oral mucoepidermoid carcinomas may appear more vascular and may grow faster than benign tumours.

Microscopically, mucoepidermoid carcinomas consist mainly of two distinct but contiguous cell types. These are epidermoid (squamous) cells and large, pale, faintly granular mucous cells (Figures 12.16 and 12.17). Microcyst formation is common and, as with ameloblastomas, mucoepidermoid carcinomas can occasionally consist of a large

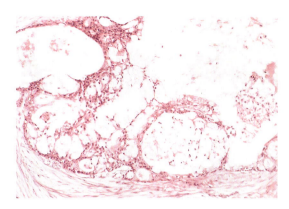

Figure 12.16 Mucoepidermoid carcinoma. A well-differentiated tumour with prominent mucous cells and cyst formation

monolocular cyst with the tumour forming only a mural thickening. Careful assessment of the nature of the lining of salivary gland cysts is, therefore, essential.

In a survey of 143 intra-oral mucoepidermoid carcinomas, Auclair *et al.* (1992) found that a short history, production of symptoms and location in the tongue or floor of the mouth, in association with microscopic criteria of malignancy, were indicative of a poor prognosis. These latter features comprised a small intracystic component, high mitotic activity, neural invasion, necrosis and anaplasia. Six out of 10 of their patients with high scores on these points died from their disease. However, even a benign cytological appearance

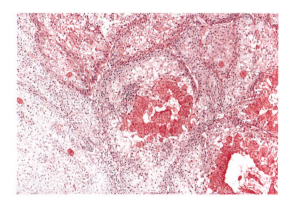

Figure 12.17 Mucoepidermoid carcinoma. The mucous cells become particularly conspicuous with specific stains (PAS stain)

does not guarantee benign behaviour. Even cytologically benign-looking tumours can sometimes metastasize.

Treatment

Even in the absence of microscopic evidence of invasion, all mucoepidermoid carcinomas should be regarded as potentially malignant and excised completely. Higher grade tumours should probably be treated like squamous cell carcinomas, but their response to radiotherapy is less predictable. Radiotherapy should only be used to supplement excision.

A retrospective analysis of 749 reported cases (Hickman *et al.*, 1984) showed that an estimated 5-year survival rate for mucoepidermoid carcinomas was 70.7% and the 10-year survival rate was 50%. Their prognosis appears, therefore, to confirm that overall they are of relatively low-grade malignancy.

Acinic cell carcinoma

Acinic cell carcinomas usually have a characteristic and benign histological appearance, but nevertheless their behaviour is unpredictable.

Over 85% of acinic cell carcinomas are found in the parotid glands where they comprise about 3% of all tumours. Most of the remainder are found in the minor glands, but rarely in the sublingual or submandibular glands. Almost any age can be affected, but the peak incidence is in the seventh decade and there is a female preponderance of almost 2 to 1.

Clinically, acinic cell carcinomas are frequently indistinguishable from adenomas, but 17% of poorly differentiated specimens have been reported by Seifert *et al.* (1986) to cause facial palsy.

Microscopically, acinic cell carcinomas usually present an almost uniform picture of large, granular basophilic cells, closely resembling normal serous cells in sheets or in acinar configurations (Figures 12.18 and 12.19). There are usually many clear round spaces thought to result from entrapped secretion. Sometimes these spaces may be so numerous as to give the tumour a microcystic or

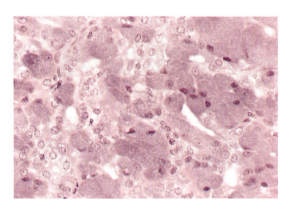

Figure 12.18 Acinic cell carcinoma. This well-differentiated example shows granular, basophilic cells that closely resemble normal serous cells

lacy pattern. There may also be clear cells which are occasionally numerous or, rarely, predominant.

The tumour usually appears well circumscribed, but even cytologically benign tumours can sometimes be invasive. Occasionally, poorly differentiated acinic cell carcinomas are seen. They are more likely to cause facial nerve paralysis and have a poorer prognosis.

On the basis of only 101 reported cases suitable for analysis, Hickman *et al.* (1984) estimated the 5-year survival rate for acinic cell carcinomas to be 82.2% and the 10-year survival rate 67.6%.

In view of the fact that even cytologically benign acinic cell carcinomas can occasionally metastasize, treatment (as with mucoepidermoid carcinomas) should be by parotidectomy, or wide excision of

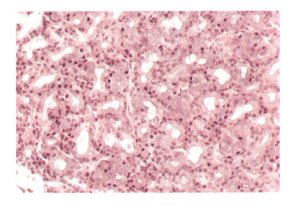

Figure 12.19 Acinic cell carcinoma. Basophilic cells have formed acinar structures

other glands. If poorly differentiated, excision should be followed by radiotherapy.

Adenoid cystic carcinoma (cylindroma)

Adenoid cystic carcinomas form 30% of parotid, 30% of submandibular and 40% of minor gland tumours, but only 1% of sublingual gland tumours. Unlike most other salivary gland tumours, 70% of adenoid cystic carcinomas affect the submandibular or minor salivary glands.

Clinically, the peak age for adenoid cystic carcinoma is in the sixth decade. The features are similar to those of other salivary gland tumours, but facial palsy is particularly frequent, especially with the solid type.

Microscopically, small darkly staining cells of uniform appearance comprise both duct-lining and myoepithelial-like cells. They are typically arranged in well-circumscribed, rounded groups surrounding more or less circular spaces to give a cribriform (Swiss cheese) pattern (Figure 12.20). A few of these tumours have a tubular pattern. Hyaline material often forms in the connective tissue surrounding the islands of tumour and in the microcystic spaces. This mucoid material may form in such large quantities as to spread the tumour cells into a lace-like pattern or form coalescing nodules with thin, widely separated strands of tumour cells. At the opposite extreme

there may be solid sheets of tumour cells with a solid (basaloid) pattern and, sometimes, areas of necrosis (Figure 12.21). Such an appearance is associated with the worst prognosis. However, in all these variants it is often possible to find more typical cribriform areas.

Adenoid cystic carcinoma, though slow growing, has a characteristically infiltrative pattern of growth. Perineural and intraneural invasion is typical of, though not unique to, this tumour (Figures 12.22 and 12.23). It can, therefore, spread along bony canals and the distance of spread may be far greater than suggested by the radiographic area of bone destruction. Growth tends to be slow but inexorable and metastatic spread is usually late. Metastases are usually in regional lymph nodes and the lungs, but their growth may also be slow and allow survival for many more years. Excision of isolated metastases may be beneficial.

Hickman *et al.* (1984), from reports of 1065 cases of adenoid cystic carcinomas, estimated the 5-year survival rate to be 62.4% and the 10-year survival rate 38.9%. Seifert *et al.* (1986) gives a 5-year recurrence or metastasis rate of 36% for the cribriform type and of 70% for the solid type with areas of necrosis. Their 8-year survival rate was 67% for the cribriform type and 32% for the solid type. Overall, they report 5- and 12-year survival rates of 76% and 33%.

Treatment

There is no definitive protocol of management for adenoid cystic carcinoma. For example, Blanck *et al.*

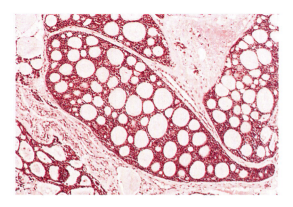

Figure 12.20 Adenoid cystic carcinoma. The characteristic cylindromatous or 'Swiss cheese' pattern is shown

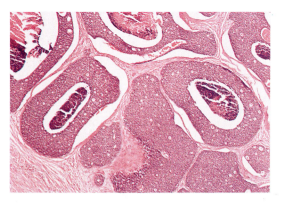

Figure 12.21 Adenoid cystic carcinoma, solid type. This type, with tumour islands showing central necrosis, is likely to have the worst prognosis

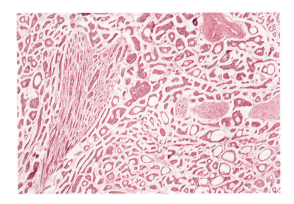

Figure 12.22   Adenoid cystic carcinoma. Islets and strands of tumour have been spread widely by hyaline production. There is extensive intraneural infiltration and nerve fibres have become incorporated into adjacent areas

(1967) reported 5- and 12-year survival rates of 73% and 39% for 35 patients, even though only 3 of them underwent parotidectomy. Another reflection of the difficulties in establishing a protocol for treatment is the remarkable degree of spread of reported survival rates which range from 0% at 10 years to 75% at up to 14 years. Even though spread of this tumour is relentlessly infiltrative, the present consensus is that supra-radical surgery is not indicated and mutilating surgery cannot be justified. Its value is unproven and Seifert *et al.* (1986) suggest that it may even worsen the prognosis. Since there is even less room for manoeuvre in treating adenoid cystic carcinoma of intra-oral glands, the prognosis may be worse than for the parotid gland. Quite frequently the postoperative history is one of limited local recurrences, each of which responds to local treatment, over the course of years. Adenoid cystic carcinomas should probably, therefore, be treated by radical resection (parotidectomy or its equivalent), with as wide a margin as is anatomically possible, but compatible with reasonable rehabilitation. In the case of the parotid gland, sacrifice of branches of the facial nerve invaded by tumour may be unavoidable. Radiotherapy should also be given. Though Seifert *et al.* (1986) could not confirm that it prolonged survival, the consensus is that the best control is probably achieved by 'simple' radical surgery followed by radiotherapy.

Adenocarcinomas

Adenocarcinomas (not otherwise specified) show neoplastic duct or tubule formation microscopically, but lack any evidence of origin from a pleomorphic adenoma. Two variants, papillary cystic and mucinous adenocarcinomas, are recognized.

Adenocarcinomas probably form less than 5% of salivary gland tumours. Approximately 48% of these are in the parotid, 10% in the submandibular, and 21% in minor salivary glands; fewer than 1% are in the sublingual glands. Males are usually in the seventh decade and appear to be affected almost twice as frequently as females.

Microscopically, adenocarcinomas consist of duct-like (tubular) structures. The cells may show significant atypia, although the tubules are well formed or the cytology may be relatively bland but tubules are poorly formed. Invasion and destruction of surrounding tissues and, sometimes, perineural invasion may be seen.

Management

The behaviour and prognosis of adenocarcinomas depend mainly on the degree of differentiation. Microscopically, solid (undifferentiated) types tend to have the worst prognosis. However, lymph node metastasis and bloodstream spread is frequent with most types, though the rapidity with which this happens varies widely. Inevitably the prognosis is also strongly affected by the extent of the primary tumour at operation. The overall 5-year survival rate is thought to be approximately 40%.

Papillary cystadenocarcinoma frequently affects the palate and is rare in other glands. Folds of epithelium project as papillary ingrowths into irregular cyst spaces. This epithelium appears cytologically completely bland and such tumours, which may also shell out readily at operation, have been wrongly categorized in the past as papillary cystadenomas. However, despite wide excision and even radiotherapy, these tumours are on record as metastasizing and causing the death of patients 15–30 years later.

Mucinous adenocarcinoma is another rare variant resembling its mucin-producing counterpart in the breast. Mucous cells and microcysts may cause it to simulate, to some degree, a mucoepidermoid carcinoma.

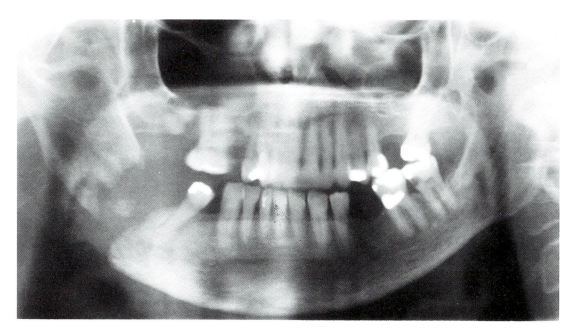

Figure 12.23   Adenoid cystic carcinoma. This tumour in its inexorable advance had invaded the mandible and caused a pathological fracture

Treatment is by parotidectomy, if necessary with sacrifice of the facial nerve, or wide excision of other glands followed by radiotherapy.

Polymorphous low-grade adenocarcinoma (terminal duct carcinoma)

Patients are usually aged between 50 and 75 years. Minor glands, particularly of the palate, are affected and the tumour typically forms a firm, painless swelling which may later ulcerate.

Microscopically, cytologically uniform, bland-looking cells are in a variety of configurations. The main microscopic patterns are:

- solid lobules surrounded by fibrous tissue
- cribriform areas containing hyaline stromal material
- duct-like structures (Figure 12.24)
- fascicles of cells sometimes in concentric (target-oid) arrangement

- papillary or papillary cystic structures (Figure 12.25).

The stroma is hyaline or mucinous (Figure 12.26) and fibrous or hyaline bands often separate different areas of the tumour. An unusual feature is the survival of relatively large areas of normal gland tissue or fat within the tumour.

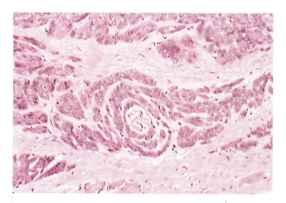

Figure 12.24   Polymorphous low-grade adenocarcinoma. Small duct-like structures and conspicuous perineural whorling or targeting can be seen

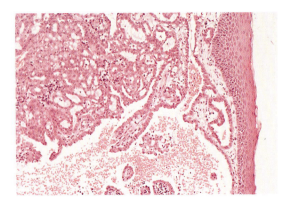

Figure 12.25   Polymorphous low-grade adenocarcinoma. Papillary cystic area

Management

These tumours are locally invasive, but appear only rarely to metastasize. Local excision has been followed by recurrences, so that excision should be complete.

Salivary duct carcinoma

This highly malignant tumour consists microscopically of eosinophilic cells in cribriform or papillary configurations, or is solid with central necrosis in the comedo type (Figure 12.27). It grows and spreads rapidly. Ruiz *et al.* (1993), for example, reported 9 cases. Five died of the disease, and the outcome was unaffected by the aggressiveness of the surgery or irradiation.

Clear cell tumours

All clear cell tumours (apart from the rare clear cell oncocytoma) should be regarded as at least potentially malignant and treated accordingly. The main types of clear cell tumours are as follows:

● clear cell oncocytoma
● clear cell mucoepidermoid or acinic cell carcinomas
● epithelial-myoepithelial (intercalated duct) carcinoma
● metastatic renal cell carcinoma.

Of these, only the clear cell variant of oncocytoma is benign, while metastatic renal carcinoma inevitably has the worst prognosis. Oncocytoma and mucoepidermoid and acinic cell carcinomas have been described earlier and the behaviour of their clear cell variants does not differ from their more common conventional counterparts. Renal cell carcinoma is discussed later with other clear cell tumours.

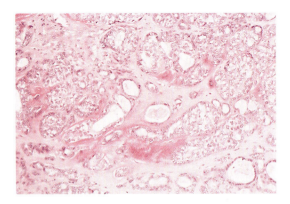

Figure 12.26   Polymorphous low-grade adenocarcinoma. Discrete lobules of pale-staining, cytologically bland cells can be seen

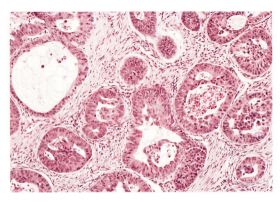

Figure 12.27   Duct carcinoma. Papillary ingrowths and comedo-type necrosis can be seen

Epithelial-myoepithelial carcinoma

Clinically, the mean age of affected patients appears to be about 60 years and the peak incidence is in the seventh and eighth decades. Women have been affected in the ratio of 2 to 1. Over 80% of these tumours have been in the parotid glands and usually caused otherwise asymptomatic swellings. However, a minority have caused pain or facial weakness.

Microscopy

The growth is typically multinodular and though the tumour appears circumscribed, encapsulation is incomplete. The tumour consists of duct-like structures or larger spaces which sometimes contain eosinophilic, PAS-positive material. Alternatively, the cells may be predominantly in an organoid or thecal pattern with a well-defined basal membrane which may be thickened and hyaline.

Small dark cells line the duct-like spaces and are surrounded by large glass-clear cells which usually predominate (Figure 12.28). The clear cells are considerably larger, of rounded polygonal shape and usually contain glycogen (Figure 12.29).

The patterns and numbers of clear cells can vary between individual tumours or within a single example. In some areas there may only be solid sheets of clear cells. In others, there are cyst-like spaces into which there are papillary projections of tumour cells. Mitoses are rarely found, but there

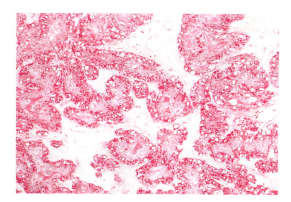

Figure 12.29 Epithelial-myoepithelial carcinoma. The glycogen-rich peripheral cells have stained positively with PAS stain

may be perineural infiltration or intravascular growth.

Electron microscopy and immunocytochemistry have confirmed that the dark cells are epithelial but that the clear cells are myoepithelial. Positive staining for S-100 protein, vimentin, myosin and keratins may, therefore, be useful in confirming the nature of the clear cells. Additionally, Jones *et al.* (1992) have reported that the outer layer of the myoepithelial cells reacts positively for alpha smooth muscle actin.

Behaviour and prognosis

These tumours have recurred in a significant number of the reported cases and some patients have died with metastases to lymph nodes, lung or kidney. Seifert *et al.* (1986) suggest that the 5-year survival rate is 65%.

Management

Despite the relatively bland microscopic picture, the behaviour of epithelial-myoepithelial carcinomas suggests that radical parotidectomy or *en bloc* resection of other glands is indicated.

Metastatic renal cell carcinoma (hypernephroma)

When any feature suggests that a clear cell tumour of a salivary gland is a secondary deposit, the

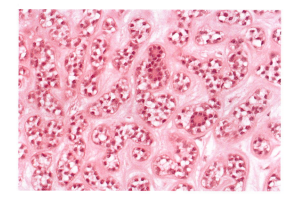

Figure 12.28 Epithelial-myoepithelial carcinoma. The duct-like structures consist of dark-staining lining cells and outer, clear myoepithelial cells

kidney is the only important source. Metastases are frequently the first sign of a renal cell carcinoma. If renal symptoms are absent, microscopic haematuria alone may be found in 60% of patients and about 50% of patients have non-specific systemic symptoms such as fever, fatigue or loss of weight. Gross haematuria, pain in the loin and a renal mass are late in appearance and present in only 10% of patients.

Microscopy

Renal cell carcinoma consists of solid masses of clear cells with small eccentric nuclei in an organoid or trabecular arrangement (Figure 12.30). The blood vessels are typically dilated, form scattered sinusoids and may leave foci of haemorrhage and deposits of haemosiderin. Granular cells may also be present and, in some cases, predominate.

Differentiation from epithelial-myoepithelial carcinomas microscopically can sometimes be very difficult. Ellis and Gnepp (1988) suggest that a helpful distinguishing feature is that epithelial-myoepithelial carcinoma has small blood vessels running between the groups of tumour cells, but renal cell carcinomas have large sinusoids. In unblocked material, the presence of fat is typical of renal carcinomas but not invariably present.

If doubt remains, intravenous urography and if necessary a CT or ultrasound scan should be carried out. Excision of a primary renal cell carcinoma and a metastasis has occasionally proved curative.

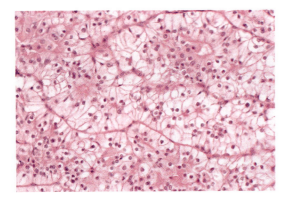

Figure 12.30 Metastasis of renal cell carcinoma of the parotid gland showing the clear cells

Basal cell adenocarcinoma

These tumours are predominantly found in the parotid or submandibular glands and the mean age affected is approximately 60 years.

Microscopy

Multiple nodules of small dark cells with scanty cytoplasm are frequently surrounded by larger, eosinophilic or amphophilic cells, but the latter are rarely palisaded. A distinct perinodular, hyalinized basal membrane and hyaline intranodular droplets are frequently present.

Basal cell carcinomas closely resemble basal cell adenomas, particularly the membranous variant, and diagnosis depends on finding cellular or nuclear pleomorphism, mitotic activity, foci of necrosis or, particularly, evidence of infiltration which may be perineural or intravascular, even in cytologically benign-looking tumours. Some examples may have cribriform areas simulating an adenoid cystic carcinoma.

Management

From the limited data available, basal cell adenocarcinomas appear to be of low-grade malignancy. Recurrence or metastasis after wide excision is relatively uncommon, but occasionally metastases may appear more than a decade later. Total conservative parotidectomy (and its equivalent for other glands), therefore, seems to be the minimal requirement.

Squamous cell (epidermoid) carcinoma

Despite the frequency of squamous metaplasia in pleomorphic adenomas, squamous cell carcinomas of salivary glands are rare. They account for only 1–3% of salivary gland tumours. They are a disease of the elderly: men are more than twice as frequently affected as women at a mean age of 70 (range 50–90 years). Nearly 70% of these tumours are in the parotid glands.

Clinically, squamous cell carcinomas do not seem to have any distinctive features, though they may be particularly firm on palpation and readily ulcerate. Facial palsy may also develop and metastasis to regional nodes is rapid. In the mouth, squamous cell carcinomas of minor salivary glands may not be distinguishable from those arising from the mucosa.

Microscopy

These tumours do not differ from squamous cell carcinomas from other sites and range from well-differentiated, keratinizing tumours to poorly differentiated examples without keratinization. However, it is essential to determine whether they are primary salivary gland tumours, metastases from elsewhere (when the prognosis is particularly bad) or have spread from a mucosal or skin tumour. It may occasionally be difficult to distinguish them from high-grade mucoepidermoid carcinomas and to be certain that mucous cells are absent.

Management

The reported survival rates of such rare tumours are not very helpful in predicting the response to treatment, but Seifert *et al.* (1986) quote a 5-year survival rate of 40%. Treatment is by radical excision, neck dissection and radiotherapy.

Undifferentiated carcinomas

Undifferentiated carcinomas are rare and of similar frequency to squamous cell carcinomas. Sixty-three per cent of these tumours are in the parotid glands, while 22% are in the submandibular glands.

Microscopy

A variety of appearances can be seen, but typically there are sheets of small cells which may be more or less spheroidal or spindle shaped, have a basaloid appearance or can closely resemble an oat cell carcinoma of the lung. The cells have large nuclei and the cytoplasm is scanty and poorly defined. Nuclear pleomorphism and mitotic activity may be prominent. The centres of cell masses may undergo necrosis. Neuroendocrine differentiation is

sometimes detectable by means of such stains as Grimeleus's in the first instance, but appears not to affect the prognosis. Large cell undifferentiated carcinomas may also be seen occasionally.

Management

Metastasis from a distant site must be excluded as the prognosis is likely to be hopeless. Even with primary salivary gland tumours, rapid spread of undifferentiated carcinomas, particularly to regional lymph nodes, is to be expected, while distant metastases are likely to be the chief cause of death.

Radical excision of the gland and neck dissection should be followed by radiotherapy. The 5-year survival rate is approximately 25% (Seifert *et al.*, 1986).

Undifferentiated carcinoma with lymphoid stroma (lymphoepithelial carcinoma; malignant lymphoepithelial lesion)

This neoplasm is common in some Eskimo races and Southern Chinese, but very rare in those of European origin. Men are more frequently affected.

Microscopy

Ill-defined islands of poorly differentiated epithelium, which often appears syncytial, are buried in a dense stroma of lymphocytes. This appearance is identical to that of one type of nasopharyngeal carcinoma which is even more common in these racial groups, so that occasionally a salivary gland tumour is a metastasis from the nasopharynx. Better differentiated, low-grade tumours may also be seen.

Management

The frequency of metastases is so high that, in addition to radical excision, there is some argument for neck dissection even in the absence of palpable nodes, unless the tumour is unusually well differentiated. Radiotherapy must be used if complete excision is not possible, but its value is questionable.

Carcinoma in pleomorphic adenoma

Malignant change in a pleomorphic adenoma is more common in long-standing tumours (more than 10 years) or in multinodular recurrences. Thackray and Lucas (1974) suggest that up to 25% of pleomorphic adenomas may undergo malignant change if left untreated for a decade or more. As a consequence, carcinoma in pleomorphic adenoma is typically a tumour of older persons with a mean age of 63 (range 25–83 years). The incidence is between 5% and 6% of epithelial tumours, but this may be an underestimate because of cases where the carcinomatous component has obliterated the adenoma.

Clinically, malignant change in pleomorphic adenoma is suggested by a sudden acceleration of growth or the onset of pain or facial palsy after years of gradual or episodic growth.

Microscopy

Both pleomorphic adenoma and carcinoma can be seen contiguously (Figure 12.31). The malignant component may form only a small part of the tumour; alternatively, the original adenoma may be difficult to find. However, ghost-like areas of cartilage tend to resist destruction and can provide a marker of a pre-existent pleomorphic adenoma.

The malignant component is most often an adenocarcinoma or undifferentiated carcinoma or, less frequently, other types of carcinoma.

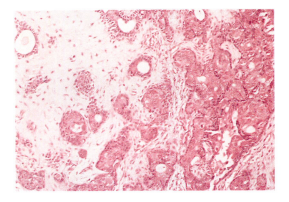

Figure 12.31   Carcinoma in pleomorphic adenoma. Carcinomatous cellular proliferation is present on the right

As noted earlier, carcinoma in pleomorphic adenoma must be distinguished from atypia without invasive activity within the substance of a pleomorphic adenoma.

Management

The importance of recognizing carcinoma in pleomorphic adenoma histologically is that the prognosis appears to be poorer than for similar carcinomas arising *de novo*. Metastasis to lymph nodes was reported in nearly 60% of cases by Seifert *et al.* (1986) and later to distant sites. Treatment depends on the type of carcinoma and its extent, and is usually by radical excision in the first instance.

On the basis of analysis of 383 reported cases, the 5-year survival rate appears to be 55.7% and the 10-year rate 31% (Hickman *et al.*, 1984).

Carcinosarcoma is a very rare variant in which both the epithelial and mesenchymal elements of a pleomorphic adenoma have undergone malignant transformation. Bleiweiss *et al.* (1992) reviewed earlier reports and described the findings in a submandibular gland carcinosarcoma, which combined an adenocarcinoma with an osteogenic sarcoma. Both carcinomatous and sarcomatous elements can, therefore, be seen adjacently in the same tumour. The prognosis is poor.

Metastasizing mixed tumour

Rarely, a cytologically benign pleomorphic adenoma proves to be invasive or metastasizes, or both. The metastases reproduce the benign cytology of the primary. Such tumours are rare and frequently not distinguished from carcinomas in pleomorphic adenomas in reports. Wenig *et al.* (1992) have reported the findings in 11 cases and reviewed the findings in 34 case reports. Metastases appeared from 6 to 52 years after the primary tumour was first treated. Metastases either coincided with local recurrences or followed them by 5 to 29 years. No histological variable or flow cytometry was successful in identifying criteria for predicting metastasis.

Since the potential for metastasis is unpredictable, initial treatment has to be the same as that for a pleomorphic adenoma.

Other rare carcinomas of salivary glands

These include malignant oncocytomas, sebaceous carcinomas and sebaceous carcinomas with lymphoid stroma.

Non-epithelial tumours and tumour-like lesions of salivary glands

Almost any variety of tumour can develop from mesenchymal components of salivary glands, but in them, lymphomas are the most common non-epithelial tumours. Overall, less than 5% of salivary gland tumours are non-epithelial.

Benign lymphoepithelial lesion

Benign lymphoepithelial lesion (BLL) gives rise, clinically, to a tumour-like mass and is usually treated as a tumour. However, the histological features of BLL are the same as those of Sjögren's syndrome and it is questionable whether they are distinct entities. However, in patients with tumour-like parotid swelling, the possibility of autoimmune disease is rarely considered, especially as remarkably few patients with proven xerostomia complain spontaneously of dry mouth. Nevertheless, Ostberg (1983) has shown by postoperative investigation that over 80% of patients with BLL have symptoms or other abnormalities consistent with Sjögren's syndrome.

Clinical aspects
The diagnosis of BLL is rarely made preoperatively but should be suspected in:

- women of 50 years or over, with firm, smooth, diffuse parotid gland swellings which are not fixed superficially or deeply
- bilateral parotid swellings, though unilateral swelling is more common
- patients with rheumatoid arthritis or any other connective tissue disease
- patients with dry mouth or eyes, though neither may be clinically obvious.

Pain is present in approximately 40% of patients.

Microscopy
Benign lymphoepithelial lesion is characterized by lymphocytic infiltration of the gland with destruction of acini, but preservation of some duct tissue which becomes transformed into so-called epimyoepithelial islands. The final picture is one of sheets of lymphocytes among which are scattered epimyoepithelial islands. The interlobular septa and capsule are preserved. However, careful examination should be made for early lymphomatous change, as discussed below.

Management
Since the diagnosis is rarely made preoperatively, parotidectomy is usually carried out. Once the diagnosis has been made, the patient should be investigated for Sjögren's syndrome and, if it is present, treated appropriately. Prolonged follow-up is essential because of the risks of development of salivary gland or extra-salivary lymphoma later.

Parotidectomy is also appropriate treatment of BLL or of persistently painful, swollen glands in Sjögren's syndrome, as it allows full examination for possible lymphomatous change. Irradiation or cytotoxic/immunosuppressive drug treatment increase the risk of lymphomatous change and are contraindicated.

Lymphoma

Primary lymphomas of salivary glands are uncommon. They most frequently arise in intra- or periglandular lymphoid tissue and are frequently a result of disseminated disease. CT scanning or other staging procedures are, therefore, essential.

Occasionally, destruction of the nodal architecture makes it appear that the tumour has arisen in the gland parenchyma, but even in such cases, the possibility that it is a secondary deposit needs to be excluded.

Clinically, lymphomas of salivary glands most frequently develop in the parotids which have a significant content of lymphoid tissue. The submandibular gland accounts for 15–20% of cases and the remainder are in the minor glands, particularly of the palate. Lymphomas produce firm swellings usually of rapid growth and a history of little more than 6 months' duration. Pain and facial nerve palsy develop early in a minority. Fixation to deep or superficial structures and involvement of regional lymph nodes are also uncommon early, but frequently develop later if the tumour is neglected. Most patients are aged between 50 and 70 years and women are more frequently affected in the ratio of 2 to 1. In younger males especially, the possibility of HIV infection must be excluded. Exceptionally rarely, a lymphoma may develop in the lymphoid tissue of a Warthin's tumour.

Microscopy

Most lymphomas of salivary glands are non-Hodgkin's type. The salivary tissue is replaced to a greater or lesser extent by sheets of lymphocytes either diffusely or in a follicular pattern. The degree of maturation and differentiation is also variable, but are the same as lymphomas in other sites (Chapter 14).

Signs of malignancy, namely, destruction of interlobular septa and capsule, and invasion of surrounding tissues, may be evident. Typing of lymphomas and sometimes even recognition of these tumours is difficult, and wherever possible should be referred for a specialist opinion.

Lymphoma in benign lymphoepithelial lesion and Sjögren's syndrome

The incidence of lymphoma in BLL or Sjögren's syndrome may be 20% or more. Takahashi *et al.* (1992) found that in 32 salivary gland lymphomas the initial diagnosis had been myoepithelial

sialadenitis in 9 cases. Lymphoma is typically a complication of long-standing disease and is, therefore, more likely to be seen in the elderly, particularly women. There is also a greater risk of lymphoma in patients with connective tissue diseases, particularly rheumatoid arthritis.

Lymphoma may be difficult to recognize in the lymphoproliferation characteristic of these diseases. It is indicated by cytological features of malignancy, signs of invasion, destruction of adjacent tissues, and evidence of intracytoplasmic monoclonal immunoglobulin production by immunostaining. Most are B cell lymphomas but almost any type of lymphoma may develop. Persistence of epimyoepithelial islands or of germinal centres does not exclude the diagnosis of lymphoma.

Management

Histological typing and staging must be carried out as for a lymphoma in any other site. From the limited published data it appears that salivary gland lymphomas are usually stage I or II. Treatment is determined by extent of the disease as well as by the histological subtype. Though the prognosis might be expected to be affected by the stage at presentation, this has not been confirmed in all reported series (Gleeson *et al.*, 1986).

Excision is likely to have been carried out in the first instance, but typing and staging will determine the need for radiotherapy or chemotherapy or both.

Among 36 cases from the British tumour panel material, the median survival was only 49 months. Other reports have indicated considerably better survival rates, but overall the numbers are so small, and the variables affecting prognosis so many, that generalizations are not useful.

Hodgkin's disease

Primary Hodgkin's disease of salivary glands is very rare. The figures are sometimes inflated by inclusion of disease of juxtaglandular cervical lymph nodes, but the gland parenchyma is rarely involved. However, the mass may occasionally be mistaken for a salivary gland tumour, particularly of the submandibular gland, but in many cases the disease has already disseminated. Unlike non-Hodgkin's lymphomas, Hodgkin's disease has a peak in the third and fourth decades, and males predominate in the ratio of 4 to 1.

Microscopy

Lymphocyte-predominant, nodular sclerosing and mixed types appear to be virtually equally frequent, but lymphocyte-depleted disease to be rare.

Management

Histological typing and staging investigation should be carried out. The findings should determine whether treatment is by radiotherapy or combination chemotherapy and is by currently accepted protocols.

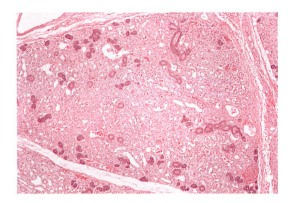

Figure 12.32 Juvenile haemangioma of the parotid gland. Widespread formation of vasoformative tissue and capillaries has replaced the gland parenchyma, leaving only duct tissue

Salivary gland tumours in infancy and childhood

Only 3.5–5% of salivary gland tumours are in infants or children, but a major problem in their surgical management is the difficulty of avoiding damage to the developing facial nerve.

Haemangioma of the parotid gland

Juvenile haemangioma may be evident at birth, is usually seen before the age of 10 and is exceedingly rare in adults. It gives rise to a soft, sometimes bluish, enlargement of the gland.

Microscopy

Only isolated remnants of glandular tissue, particularly ducts, can be seen in the vascular tissue, which is usually capillary in type (Figure 12.32).

Management

Progress of these lesions is variable – some may grow or even spread into adjacent tissue for a time, but may regress spontaneously. However, the extent of the vascular proliferation may occasionally be so gross as to produce an arteriovenous shunt which can, rarely, give rise to high output circulatory failure.

If the tumour shows no signs of regressing, treatment should be delayed until the age of at least 5 years to lessen the risk of damaging the delicate, developing facial nerve. Excision, if it cannot be avoided, should be curative. Alternatives, such as injection of sclerosing agents or irradiation as primary treatment or to reduce the bulk of the tumour preoperatively, are likely to cause complications which outweigh any possible benefits.

Epithelial salivary gland tumours in children

Epithelial salivary gland tumours in the young are considerably more frequently malignant than in adults. The parotid glands are most often affected and Callender *et al.* (1992) report that 21 out of 29 epithelial salivary gland tumours in children were malignant. Shikhani and Johns (1988) found that pleomorphic adenomas formed 87% of the benign tumours, but the recurrence rate was between 20% and 40% when enucleation was carried out. Two of the recurrent tumours developed into highly aggressive carcinomas. Of the malignant tumours, mucoepidermoid carcinomas appear to be the most common type. Two of the 29 patients reported by Callender *et al.* (1992) died from their tumours.

In view of the high recurrence rate of pleomorphic adenomas and the high incidence of malignant tumours, radical parotidectomy seems to be necessary for epithelial salivary gland tumours in children. However, the chances of damaging the facial nerve are high, particularly in younger children, and even superficial parotidectomy of pleomorphic adenomas has a high chance of being followed by recurrence.

Embryoma (sialoblastoma)

Embryomas are congenital or neonatal salivary gland tumours and can be benign, but 25% may be malignant. Rarely, they are so large as to cause difficulties in delivery.

Microscopy

Embryomas consist essentially of tissue resembling embryonic salivary gland epithelia in a loose mesenchymal stroma. The appearances are varied, but typically consist of small dark cells with scanty cytoplasm forming duct-like structures, trabeculae or occasionally a cribriform pattern and may, therefore, resemble a basal cell adenoma or adenoid cystic carcinoma. Like other embryonic epithelia, this tissue is able to grow infiltratively even when benign. Malignant embryomas may be recognized by greater atypia, but more objectively by invasion of such structures as nerves or blood vessels, and foci of necrosis.

Treatment is clearly difficult and depends on the histological findings. In the case of malignant embryomas, interstitial irradiation may have to be considered.

Other mesenchymal tumours of salivary glands

As mentioned earlier, mesenchymal tumours other than juvenile haemangiomas are rare in salivary glands. Neural tumours are the most common single type, but any other may occasionally be seen. These tumours do not differ from their counterparts in other sites and are considered in more detail in Chapter 13.

Because of the rarity of mesenchymal tumours in salivary glands, it is not clear whether their behaviour differs from that of histologically similar tumours elsewhere, and no practical comments can be made. However, in the case of sarcomas, despite the fact that unusually small tumours are likely to be recognized in salivary glands, the outcome is worse than that for sarcomas in general. The difficulties of surgery, particularly in the parotid region, may contribute to this poor prognosis.

As mentioned earlier, a myoepithelioma may occasionally be mistaken microscopically for a mesenchymal tumour, but if necessary can be identified by immunohistochemistry.

Metastatic tumours in salivary glands

Metastases to salivary glands are rare. The most frequent metastases are from skin tumours, particularly melanomas and epidermoid carcinomas, but are usually in juxtaglandular nodes as are many other metastases which appear as salivary gland tumours. Frequently, the possibility of a salivary gland tumour being a metastasis may be suspected, but metastatic renal cell carcinoma occasionally presents special problems, as noted earlier.

In the case of melanomas, as with other metastases, the prognosis is poor and the diagnosis is likely to be made only after parotidectomy, but Ball and Thomas (1990) state that parotidectomy and elective neck dissection provide valuable loco-regional palliation, though the long-term prognosis remains poor.

Juxtaglandular tumours

Tumours of adjacent tissues occasionally involve or appear to involve salivary glands. An example is lymphomas in juxtaglandular lymph nodes, as discussed earlier.

Skin tumours can extend into the parotid gland especially, but are likely to be recognized as such. Rarely, a jugulotympanic paraganglioma can mimic a parotid gland tumour. A mandibular or masseteric tumour can also involve the parotid region. All of these possibilities are exceedingly rare, but should be borne in mind when a salivary gland tumour has unusual features.

Intraosseous salivary gland tumours

Rarely, salivary gland tumours form within the jaw from foci of ectopic tissue such as the Stafne bone cavity (Chapter 3) and are most frequently near this site in the region of the angle of the mandible. They do not differ microscopically from their soft tissue counterparts and most have been mucoepidermoid carcinomas. Benign tumours are exceptionally rare.

Radiographically, intraosseous salivary gland tumours present a variety of appearances, such as uni- or multilocular cyst-like areas of radiolucency whose nature is only recognizable after biopsy or excision. More malignant tumours are likely to show peripheral bone destruction and be less sharply circumscribed.

Management

If histology shows a malignant tumour, the possibility that it is a metastasis may be considered, but only because adenocarcinomas of other organs can occasionally resemble salivary gland tumours microscopically.

Treatment of intraosseous mucoepidermoid carcinomas or more malignant tumours should be wide excision and, if necessary, grafting. Rare benign intraosseous tumours have been enucleated satisfactorily.

References

Auclair, P.L., Goode, R.K. and Ellis, G.L. (1992) Mucoepidermoid carcinoma of intraoral salivary glands. Evaluation and application of grading criteria in 143 cases. *Cancer,* **69,** 2021–2030

Ball, A.B.S. and Thomas, J.M. (1990) Management of parotid metastases from cutaneous melanoma of the head and neck. *Journal of Laryngology and Otology,* **104,** 350–351

Blanck, C., Eneroth, C.-M., Jacobsson, F. *et al.* (1967) Adenoid cystic carcinoma of the parotid gland. *Acta Radiologica Therapeutics, Physiology, Biology,* **6,** 177–196

Bleiweiss, I.J., Huvos, A.J., Lara, J. *et al.* (1992) Carcinosarcoma of the submandibular gland: immunohistochemical findings. *Cancer,* **69,** 2031–2035

Callender, D.L., Frankenthaler, R.A., Luna, M.A. *et al.* (1992) Salivary gland neoplasms in children. *Archives of Otolaryngology and Head and Neck Surgery,* **118,** 472–476

Clark, D.B., Priddy, R.W. and Swanson, A.E. (1990) Oral inverted ductal papilloma. *Oral Surgery, Oral Medicine and Oral Pathology,* **69,** 487–490

Ellis, G.L. and Gnepp, D.R. (1988) Unusual salivary gland tumors. In *Pathology of the Head and Neck* (ed. Gnepp, D.R.), Livingstone, New York, pp. 627–631

Gleeson, M.J., Bennett, M.H. and Cawson, R.A. (1986) Lymphomas of salivary glands. *Cancer,* **58,** 699–704

Hickman, R.E., Cawson, R.A. and Duffy, S.W. (1984) The prognosis of specific types of salivary gland tumors. *Cancer,* **54,** 1620–1624

Jones, H., Moshtael, F. and Simpson, R.H.W. (1992) Immunoreactivity of alpha smooth muscle actin in salivary gland tumours: a comparison with S-100 protein. *Journal of Clinical Pathology,* **45,** 938–940

Lam, K.H., Wei, W.I., Ho, H.C. *et al.* (1990) Whole organ sectioning of mixed parotid tumours. *American Journal of Surgery,* **160,** 377–381

Ostberg, Y. (1983) The clinical picture of benign lymphoepithelial lesion. *Clinical Otolaryngology,* **8,** 381–390

Palmer, T.J., Gleeson, M.J., Eveson, J.W. *et al.* (1990) Oncocytic adenomas and oncocytic hyperplasia of salivary glands: a clinicopathological study of 26 cases. *Histopathology,* **161,** 487–493

Ruiz, C.C., Romero, M.P. and Pérez, M.M. (1993) Salivary duct carcinoma. A report of nine cases. *Journal of Oral and Maxillofacial Surgery,* **51,** 641–646

Seifert, G., Miehlke, A., Haubrich, J. *et al.* (1986) *Diseases of the Salivary Glands,* Georg Thieme, Stuttgart

Shikhani, A.H. and Johns, M.E. (1988) Tumors of the major salivary glands in children. *Head and Neck Surgery,* **10,** 257–263

Takahashi, H., Cheng, J., Fujita, S. *et al.* (1992) Primary malignant lymphoma of salivary gland: a tumor of mucosa-associated lymphoid tissue. *Journal of Oral Pathology and Medicine,* **21,** 318–325

Taxy, J.B. (1992) Necrotizing squamous/mucinous metaplasia in oncocytic salivary gland tumors. A potential diagnostic problem. *American Journal of Clinical Pathology,* **97,** 40–45

Thackray, A.C. and Lucas, R.B. (1974) Tumors of the major salivary glands. In *Atlas of Tumor Pathology,* Second Series – Fascicle 10, Armed Forces Institute of Pathology, Washington

Thackray, A.C. and Sobin, L.H. (1972) *Histological Typing of Salivary Gland Tumours,* World Health Organisation, Geneva

Wenig, B.M., Hitchcock, C.L., Ellis, G.L. *et al.* (1992) Metastasizing mixed tumour of salivary glands. A clinicopathologic study and flow cytometric analysis. *American Journal of Surgical Pathology,* **16,** 845–858

13

Tumours and tumour-like lesions of mesenchymal tissues

Fibromas and fibrous nodules

The current view is that true fibromas of the mouth are exceedingly rare and in any case cannot necessarily be distinguished with certainty from non-neoplastic fibrous hyperplastic lesions. Rarely, fibromas may be confused with neurofibromas or, more important, with well-differentiated fibrosarcomas. From the practical viewpoint, however, the vast majority of fibrous swellings in the mouth are benign.

Fibrous epulis, denture-induced hyperplasia and other fibrous nodules

These hyperplastic fibrous nodules are the most common tumour-like swellings in the mouth. They are traditionally regarded as resulting from low-grade trauma, but in practice a source of irritation is by no means always found or may be no more severe than in other parts of the mouth.

Clinically, these lesions all form pinkish nodules unless the surface has been injured and has ulcerated. Fibrous epulides form on the gingival margin, typically, in relation to anterior teeth, denture-induced hyperplasias form under the flanges of dentures or sometimes in the vault of the palate, while fibrous ('fibroepithelial') polyps form on the buccal mucosa, edges of the tongue or other sites.

Microscopically, these nodules consist of irregularly interlacing bundles of collagenous fibrous tissue in continuity with the corium and without any capsule or pseudo-capsule (Figure 13.1). The epithelium is usually mildly acanthotic. The area of an epulis in contact with gingival plaque is usually inflamed. Nodules related to dentures, however, may show no inflammation unless ulcerated or superficially infected by *C. albicans*. Bilateral, symmetrical fibrous overgrowths of the maxillary tuberosities are structurally similar.

Dystrophic calcification, osteoid or bone formation is common in fibrous epulides (Figure 13.2).

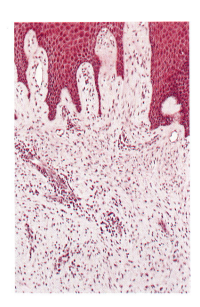

Figure 13.1 Hyperplastic fibrous nodule

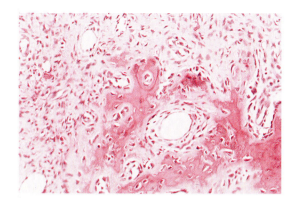

Figure 13.2   Fibrous epulis. This cellular fibrous overgrowth contains an area of osseous metaplasia

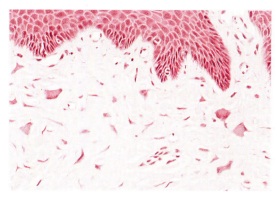

Figure 13.3   Giant cell fibroma showing collagen bundles and characteristic stellate giant fibroblasts

Management

The growth potential of these lesions is not known for certain, as few are left untreated. However, patients' histories often suggest that some of these lumps can remain stationary for several years. Excision is necessary to confirm the diagnosis and is usually curative, but recurrence can follow, particularly if any irritant such as a badly fitting denture, rough restoration or calculus has not been removed.

Small denture-induced lesions may sometimes regress if the denture is trimmed adequately, but excision is required to confirm the diagnosis.

Giant cell fibroma

The giant cell fibroma is a common minor histological variant with distinctive microscopic and clinical characteristics.

Clinically, nearly 60% develop in the first three decades and nearly 60% are in women with an average age of 26 years. The single most common site (50%) is on the lower gingiva; other sites together account almost equally for most of the remainder.

Unlike the more common fibrous lesions the giant cell fibroma is typically pedunculated. About 60% have a warty or nodular surface and may be mistaken clinically for a papilloma.

Microscopically, the giant cell fibroma has a distinctive pattern of arcuate or sinuous bundles

of collagenous connective tissue which surround but are clearly separated from stellate, rather than multinucleate, giant cells (Figure 13.3). The nuclei of the giant cells are large and vesicular while the cytoplasm may have prominent dendritic processes and contain melanin granules. Blood vessels, particularly capillaries, are prominent. These features are therefore quite different from the typical giant cell epulis (see below).

Management

The giant cell fibroma is benign and excision is usually curative.

Pyogenic granuloma and pregnancy epulis

Oral pyogenic granulomas usually develop on the gingival margins and less frequently at other sites. They are considerably less common than fibrous overgrowths and there is no evidence to suggest that they are a stage in the development of the latter or are merely inflamed fibrous nodules but, rather, vascular overgrowths. Clinically they form red, soft nodules.

Microscopically, pyogenic granulomas consist of a loose, oedematous and mucinous stroma containing larger, thin-walled blood vessels and are typically infiltrated throughout by leucocytes (Figures 13.4 and 13.5). The blood vessels are so

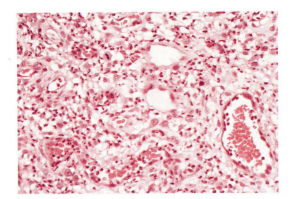

Figure 13.4   Pyogenic granuloma showing newly-formed blood vessels in inflamed oedematous stroma

numerous that the alternative term for cutaneous pyogenic granulomas is 'granuloma telangiectaticum' and Enziger and Weiss (1995) categorize them as polypoid capillary haemangiomas. Their thin epithelial covering is frequently ulcerated and there is then a more intense inflammatory infiltrate and fibrinous exudate on the surface.

Management
Excision is typically curative.

Pregnancy epulis

There is an enhanced tendency to develop a proliferative gingivitis and gingival pyogenic

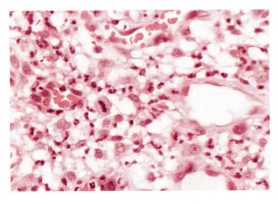

Figure 13.5   Pyogenic granuloma showing mitoses in regenerating tissue

granulomas during pregnancy, particularly in the last two trimesters. Like pyogenic granulomas in non-pregnant persons, inflammation may be minimal or absent but vascular proliferation is occasionally so active as to suggest a neoplasm. Nevertheless the behaviour is benign.

Management
Gingival hyperplasia of pregnancy should be treated by meticulous oral hygiene. A pregnancy epulis persisting after parturition should be excised. As these lesions are often a cause of anxiety to the pregnant patient, it may be necessary to excise them during pregnancy if reassurance fails.

Giant cell epulis

This lesion (at one time given the inept and ponderous title of 'peripheral reparative giant cell granuloma') is of unknown aetiology, but since it often develops in relation to teeth which have deciduous predecessors, it may result from proliferation of the giant cells responsible for their resorption.

Clinically, giant cell epulides are more common in relation to the upper teeth, particularly in the second and third decades, and are rare after 25 years of age. It is equally common in males and females. It is smooth surfaced and sessile: it may be purplish red and soft, but may be indistinguishable clinically from a fibrous epulis.

Microscopically, a giant cell epulis is attached to and appears to arise from the periodontal ligament; it consists of closely set multinucleate giant cells in a vascular stroma of plump spindle cells separated from its epithelial covering by a connective tissue corium. Some specimens contain no more than a small focus of giant cells within a fibrous mass, and are probably regressing.

The giant cell component of giant cell epulis is not histologically distinguishable either from a giant cell granuloma of the jaw or a bone lesion of hyperparathyroidism (Chapter 6) when either of these have eroded through the bone and extended under the mucosa. However, both of these conditions are associated with an underlying area of radiolucency and appear as broad-based mucosal swellings.

Management

Thorough excision, including curettage of the base, is necessary to avoid recurrence, which is relatively common. Occasionally it is necessary to extract adjacent teeth. However, these lesions are completely benign and do not metastasize.

Neoplastic epulides

Epulis is a useful clinical term defining the site of a lesion but it has no specific histological connotation. Most epulides are fibrous and benign, but occasionally malignant tumours, particularly metastatic tumours, can produce lesions clinically mimicking a simple (non-neoplastic) epulis. Rare though this may be, it makes it mandatory to biopsy all such lesions including denture 'granulomas'.

Nasopharyngeal (juvenile) angiofibroma

This uncommon tumour occasionally involves the oral cavity. With rare exceptions it affects males, usually during adolescence, and is exceptionally rare before the age of 10 years. This age and sex distribution suggests a hormonal influence as reviewed by Weprin and Siemers (1991). Nasopharyngeal angiofibroma typically forms a soft polypoid mass in the nasal cavity or sinuses. It grows both expansively and by infiltration peripherally. Typical early signs are nasal obstruction, infection and bleeding (epistaxes) which can rarely be life-threatening. Erosion of the palate can produce an intra-oral swelling or there may be bulging of the face, with loss of the nasolabial fold, which brings the patient to seek attention.

Radiographically, typical features are a soft tissue mass in the nasopharynx, causing bulging of the posterior wall of the antrum. The bony margins are usually clearly defined, but may occasionally be eroded.

Microscopically, angiofibromas typically consist mainly of cellular fibrous tissue containing cleft-like or wider vascular spaces (Figure 13.6). The latter are lined by a single layer or endothelium

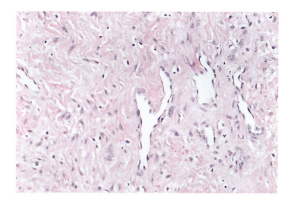

Figure 13.6 Nasopharyngeal angiofibroma. The wide, irregularly shaped, thin-walled vascular spaces in a moderately cellular fibrous stroma are typical

with a thin or incomplete muscle layer; an elastic lamina is typically lacking.

The microscopic appearances often do not adequately indicate this tumour's potential for torrential bleeding. CT scanning and angiography are, therefore, essential investigations to show the extent and vascularity of the tumour.

Management

If an angiofibroma is suspected clinically, biopsy should only be carried out after admission to hospital and in anticipation of severe bleeding. However, the decision is difficult in that the clinical or radiographic features may simulate a malignant tumour, but the risk of dangerous haemorrhage makes the surgeon reluctant to confirm this by biopsy.

Angiofibromas usually behave aggressively and invade surrounding tissues. The Le Fort I downfracture and other access osteotomies are useful in gaining access, but because of the risk of otherwise uncontrollable haemorrhage, bilateral control of the external carotid arteries before formal excision is essential. Preoperative embolization has been recommended by Siniluoto *et al.* (1993) who found that it reduced blood loss to a third of that in their previous cases. There were also fewer recurrences, presumably because the control of bleeding allowed more complete excision. Cryosurgery and/or radiotherapy are other options but unless excision or destruction of the tumour is complete, the risk of recurrence is high. The hazards of irradiation in the young must be borne in mind and there is a possibility of inducing sarcomatous change. In addition, it is not universally accepted that irradiation will cause the fibrous component to regress, but in over 75% of cases it is likely to control symptoms and cause the tumour to shrink after a single course of 30–35 Gy.

The level of risk from surgery is probably similar to that from irradiation, but if surgery is chosen, it should only be undertaken with a clear appreciation of the hazards.

In contrast to the dangers of treatment, Weprin and Siemers (1991) reported spontaneous regression of an untreated juvenile angiofibroma over a 12-year period, in a boy whose parents refused consent to surgery. Weprin and Siemers (1991) also reviewed earlier reports of spontaneous regression of these tumours after incomplete excision. Whenever possible, therefore, an expectant approach to the management of these tumours should be considered.

Spindle cell and pseudo-mesenchymal tumours of salivary glands

Occasionally pleomorphic adenomas consist predominantly of spindle (myoepithelial) cells (Chapter 12). Rarely, also, malignant myoepithelial tumours (malignant myoepithelioma, myoepithelial carcinoma) can have a sarcomatous appearance. Differential diagnosis from true mesenchymal tumours of salivary glands may depend on finding recognizable epithelial elements but, if this fails, the myoepithelial cells should be identifiable by immunostaining for keratin, actin and vimentin.

Fibromatoses

Fibromatoses are proliferative lesions of connective tissue which infiltrate surrounding tissues, have a strong tendency to recur, but are non-neoplastic and do not metastasize. Their aetiology is uncertain and they do not appear to be reactive in nature.

The more common superficial fibromatoses such as Dupuytren's contracture or Peyronie's disease have specific site distributions, while the deep fibromatoses (desmoids) affect the abdomen, particularly after childbirth. The extra-abdominal fibromatoses far more frequently involve the limbs or chest wall and an analysis by Enzinger and Weiss (1995) of 376 extra-abdominal fibromatoses (seen over a period of 20 years at the Armed Forces Institute of Pathology) found only 35 cases affecting the head or neck region. Of these, only 7 cases involved the head.

Fibromatoses mainly affect adults, and infantile fibromatosis is rare. In younger patients, fibroblastic proliferation may be more active; fibromatoses may, therefore, appear even more alarming microscopically than in adults, and be interpreted as sarcomas. Nevertheless, infantile fibromatoses in many sites have, overall, less tendency to recur or may rarely regress spontaneously.

Vally and Altini (1990) were able to find reports of 28 cases in the oral or periotal tissues and to add three new examples. They were also able to add 9 new cases of the intraosseous counterpart, desmoplastic fibroma of the jaws, and found 51 earlier reports.

Of 27 oral or perioral fibromatoses, Vally and Altini (1990) found that the great majority (16) developed within the first 9 years of life, 8 appeared between the ages of 10 and 19 years and only 3 between 20 and 29: the mean age at diagnosis was 8.3 years. The most common site was in the paramandibular region and radiographically there was superficial erosion of the underlying bone of the jaw in 16 cases. All showed similar histological features and these workers considered that there was no valid distinction between the so-called adult and infantile aggressive types of fibromatoses.

Clinical features

Fibromatoses typically form relatively slowly growing, usually painless, poorly circumscribed, tumour-like masses. Later, if the growth has involved nerve fibres, it can cause pain. Rarely fibromatoses can be multifocal.

In addition to those few arising in the mouth, fibromatoses originating in the neck can spread to the jaw or floor of the mouth.

Microscopy

Fibromatoses consist of proliferating fibrous tissue which ranges in appearance from mature fibrous tissue with abundant collagen to highly cellular lesions consisting of tumour-like fibroblasts alone. The collagen fibres in the more fibrous specimens tend to form short bundles which lack the streaming patterns, and are less well defined than those of fibrosarcomas. These appearances can vary from one specimen to another and also within a single specimen.

The nuclei of the fibroblasts may contain two or three nucleoli, but tend to be small and uniform in size. Mitoses may be seen in the more cellular areas, but are never atypical. Within the fibrous tissue, the blood vessels often form slit or cleft-like spaces. Inflammation is typically slight or absent but, when present due to superimposed infection, can alter the microscopic appearances.

Particularly characteristic of these lesions is their tumour-like infiltration of surrounding tissues including nerve and muscles fibres and occasionally bone. Despite this property and the cellular appearances, fibromatoses do not metastasize. The current belief is that previously reported metastases were of fibrosarcomas rather than fibromatoses. Evidence for the value of microscopy for predicting behaviour is conflicting.

Management

Surgical control of fibromatoses in the oral or perioral area is difficult because of the close proximity of vital structures, their infiltrative nature and the consequent limited room for manoeuvre.

The current consensus is that the treatment should be as wide an excision as possible, but since fibromatoses are not truly malignant, mutilating operations should be avoided. Nevertheless, recurrence rates range from 25% to 65%, depending on the aggressiveness of the lesion and the completeness of excision. At the other extreme, such lesions have occasionally regressed spontaneously, particularly in infants.

In view of the limited opportunities for total excision of oral or perioral fibromatoses, the likelihood of recurrence must be accepted. Unfortunately, little alternative to such treatment has been offered. The value of megavoltage irradiation has not been widely confirmed and, as always with such treatment, the possibility of inducing malignant

change cannot be dismissed. Vally and Altini (1990), in their review of oral and para-oral fibromatoses, found a recurrence rate of 22%. None of these lesions metastasized or, unlike fibromatoses in other sites, had a fatal outcome despite their proximity to vital structures.

In all cases, prolonged follow-up is necessary. Rarely, recurrences have appeared as long as 10 years after initial treatment. It therefore may be unwise to interpret treatment as being curative unless there is a disease-free period of at least 3 years after excision.

Myofibromatosis

This rare lesion was termed *infantile myofibromatosis* by Chung and Enzinger (1981), but can occasionally affect adults. Speight *et al.* (1991) have described 3 cases (one in an adult) and reviewed earlier reports of oral and perioral cases.

Clinically, myofibromatosis is usually solitary but can occasionally be multifocal and fatal by involving vital structures. Solitary lesions in the oral cavity typically form painless lumps.

Microscopically, myofibromatosis has considerably more varied appearances than fibromatosis but like the latter has no clear margin and infiltrates muscle. There are two cell types. The configurations include spindle cells with eosinophilic cytoplasm and long, blunt-ended nuclei, in diffuse sheets or in streaming, fascicular patterns, sometimes interlacing or in whorls. Small cells are rounded or polygonal and have large nuclei relative to the amount of cytoplasm which is weakly eosinophilic. The small cells form foci in areas of spindle cells, but elsewhere can be close-packed and surround slit-like or dilated blood vessels to give a haemangiopericytoma-like appearance. There are occasional normal mitoses. Speight *et al.* (1991) noted myofibromatous cells within the lumen of veins, and degenerating or reactive muscle fibres within the lesion, as a result of infiltration of adjacent tissue. They also noted that many of the cells were PTAH positive and some showed conspicuous longitudinal striations. Immunocytochemistry showed all the cells to be strongly positive for vimentin and smooth muscle actin. The ultrastructural features were also typical of myofibroblasts.

These varied appearances have led to mis-diagnoses of myofibromatosis as neural tumours, leiomyomas, leiomyosarcomas or haemangiopericytomas in the past.

Management

Excision appears to be the treatment of choice, but may have to be repeated. Enzinger and Weiss (1988) consider myofibromatosis to be a hamartoma of myofibroblasts and, if so, this should discourage mutilating surgery.

Gingival fibromatosis

Enzinger and Weiss used to include gingival fibromatosis among the fibroproliferative diseases. However, gingival fibromatosis is obviously not a fibromatosis of the type described earlier. It can be familial or acquired, usually as a result of treatment with phenytoin, or less often with cyclosporin, nifedipine or other calcium channel blockers.

Familial gingival fibromatosis (typically an autosomal dominant trait) is generalized, and may completely bury the teeth (pseudo-anodontia) and can affect the deciduous dentition. Unlike drug-induced gingival hyperplasia, the fibrous overgrowth extends uniformly along the alveolar ridge. Thickening of the facial features until they may resemble acromegaly, hypertrichosis and sometimes epilepsy, or, rarely, mental defect may be associated. Despite the deep false pocketing, there may be little gingival inflammation. Drug-induced gingival fibromatosis tends to be associated with poor oral hygiene, and particularly affects the interdental papillae, which become bulbous and separated from each other by pseudo-clefts. Typically, the gingival stippling is enhanced, giving the tissue an orange-peel texture.

Microscopically, fibrous gingival hyperplasia is characterized by dense collagenous fibrous tissue, often with elongation of the rete ridges of the overlying epithelium (Figure 13.7). The appearances of the drug-induced and familial types are similar.

Meticulous oral hygiene may control this hyperplasia to some extent, but is unlikely to cause it to resolve. Gingivectomy may be justifiable, particularly for cosmetic reasons, but in the familial type

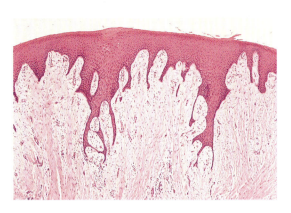

Figure 13.7 Fibrous overgrowth of gingiva with hyperplasia of the epithelium overlying sparsely cellular non-inflamed fibrous tissue

should preferably be delayed until after puberty, when regrowth of the fibrous tissue is likely to be slower. Gingivectomy may then be necessary and may have to be repeated at intervals.

In all such cases, the fibrous nature of these lesions should be distinguished from the gingival swelling of acute leukaemia.

Diffuse fibrous hyperplasias

Systemic sclerosis (scleroderma) and oral submucous fibrosis have been discussed in Chapter 7.

Fasciites

Fasciites are benign proliferative lesions of fibroblasts. Their aetiology is unknown, but they are thought to be reactive rather than neoplastic, even though any stimulus is unlikely to be identifiable. Despite their name, fasciites are not inflammatory and do not necessarily arise from fascial tissue.

In the body as a whole, fasciites are said by Enziger and Weiss (1995) to be more common than any other tumour or tumour-like lesion of fibrous tissue. However, such statements, probably take no account of the innumerable fibrous epulides and other fibrous nodules in the mouth.

Fasciites tend to affect the limbs and are rare in the region of the mouth. Barnes (1985) found that among 225 reported cases of nodular fasciitis, 11 were in the mouth and a further 4 had been described as being in the 'jaw and cheek'.

Fasciitis presents the paradox of rapid tumour-like growth and, often also, microscopic appearances which have frequently been mistaken for sarcomas ('pseudosarcomatous fasciitis'), but are considerably less aggressive than the fibromatoses and have little or no tendency to recur after limited excision.

The two chief types of fasciitis most relevant to the mouth are nodular and proliferative fasciitis.

Nodular fasciitis

In keeping with the tumour-like microscopic features, nodular fasciitis produces a rapidly growing localized mass, typically reaching a few centimetres in diameter in 1–3 weeks.

Young adults between the ages of 20 and 35 years are predominantly affected and, in this group, the upper extremity is the most frequent site. Though nodular fasciitis is uncommon in children, the head and neck region is said· to be relatively more commonly affected in them.

Microscopy

Fasciites are poorly circumscribed and consist essentially of short irregular interlacing bundles of fibrous tissue characteristically forming feathery patterns as a result of abundant mucopolysaccharide ground substance, but small amounts of mature collagen. The fibroblast nuclei are plump, vesiculated and with large nucleoli (Figures 13.8 and 13.9). Mitoses are common, but usually normal. Lymphocytes and erythrocytes are often scattered in the fibrous tissue.

Parosteal fasciitis

This rare variant originates from periosteum and may result in destruction of cortical bone and

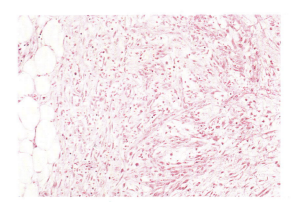

Figure 13.8 Nodular fasciitis showing interlacing bundles of fibroblasts and intermingled chronic inflammatory cells extending into the surrounding fat

reactive subperiosteal new bone formation. Microscopically, the appearances are those of nodular fasciitis and therefore distinguishable from sclerosing periostitis.

Proliferative fasciitis

Proliferative fasciitis differs from nodular fasciitis in that a slightly older age group (40–70 years) tends to be affected and about 60% of cases are in the arm or leg. Head or neck lesions are certainly no more common and may even be more rare than those of nodular fasciitis.

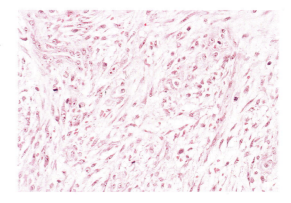

Figure 13.9 Nodular fasciitis. Higher power showing plump fibroblasts and occasional mitoses in a somewhat mucoid stroma

The usual history is of a firm subcutaneous or submucosal lesion that has developed within a few weeks and is painless. In the mouth, it may ulcerate.

Microscopy

The mass is poorly circumscribed, and may extend into underlying muscle. The connective tissue forming the mass has no discernible pattern, and consists of immature fibroblasts, including bizarre hyperchromatic giant forms with a highly malignant appearance. There are fine reticulin fibres, but little or no mature collagen apparent, and the stroma is predominantly mucoid. As the lesion matures, it becomes less abundantly cellular, giant nuclei are fewer or absent and there is more collagen. Maturation can be rapid and may develop between the time of an initial biopsy and definitive excision.

Differential diagnosis

The rarity of fasciites in the oral or perioral regions makes diagnosis difficult and the main source of confusion is with poorly differentiated sarcomas. The pathologist, therefore, needs to have the possibility of fasciitis in mind and, under such circumstances, the clinicopathological features described above should make the diagnosis possible.

Management

The essential consideration is that fasciites are benign. They have limited growth potential, less tendency to recur and extend than fibromatoses, and may even resolve spontaneously.

The treatment of choice is limited excision. This should also provide the pathologist with the junction between the lesion and surrounding tissue. Since the rapid growth of fasciitis is likely to lead to early treatment (especially in the mouth where even minute lumps cause symptoms), fasciites will usually be small and readily excised.

It is particularly important that the surgeon should not be misled by the rapid growth of these lesions into over-hasty, mutilating operations.

Fibrosarcoma

Fibrosarcoma is particularly rare in the mouth, but can occasionally be a consequence of irradiation of the region. In a series of 29 fibrosarcomas of the head and neck region, seen over a period of 32 years, Mark *et al*. (1991) noted only one each in the tongue and cheek, respectively. Four involved the mandible, one of which also involved the mastoid, tongue and hard palate. Eversole *et al*. (1973) were able to find 20 cases of fibrosarcomas of the oral soft tissues reported between 1921 and 1951.

Clinically, the peak age incidence of oral fibrosarcomas is probably between 35 and 55 years. They form initially smooth, sometimes lobulated, firm swellings, the surface of which may later ulcerate.

Microscopically, the malignant fibroblasts can be well differentiated, and form close-packed, spindle-shaped cells with large but uniform nuclei, in long interlacing bundles streaming through the mass and producing small amounts of collagen (Figures 13.10 and 13.11). At the other extreme, the fibroblast nuclei can be pleomorphic, vary in size and show frequent mitoses, and little intercellular matrix is produced.

Management

Only a minority even of poorly differentiated fibrosarcomas metastasize, but radical excision at the earliest possible stage is essential. This may be

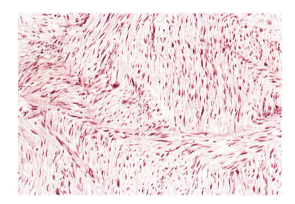

Figure 13.10   Fibrosarcoma. The characteristic fasciculated pattern is shown

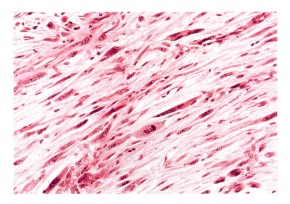

Figure 13.11 Fibrosarcoma. A moderately well-differentiated tumour with irregular elongated spindle-shaped cells, pleomorphism and mitoses

very difficult in the head and neck region and may explain the poorer prognosis for tumours in this site. Well-differentiated tumours appear to have a far better prognosis than poorly differentiated ones, but no clinical feature such as age of onset or duration of symptoms appears to affect the issue. Mark *et al.* (1991) suggest that radiotherapy should be used for patients with positive surgical margins and may be helpful in controlling high-grade tumours. There is, as yet, no firm evidence for the value of chemotherapy as ancillary treatment to radical excision, though it has frequently been used.

Because of the rarity of these tumours, reported 5-year survival rates vary widely and range from 83% for well-differentiated and 36% to zero for poorly-differentiated fibrosarcomas from all parts of the body. Of the 20 cases reviewed by Eversole *et al.* (1973), 12 were known to be alive and well for periods between 8 months and 18 years. Death is mainly from local recurrence and spread.

Fibrohistiocytic tumours and fibrous histiocytoma

The term fibrohistiocytic tumour is used by Enzinger and Weiss (1995) for a variety of tumours and tumour-like lesions which can be benign, malignant or intermediate in behaviour. Within this broad category are the xanthomas and xanthogranulomas which can be difficult to distinguish from sarcomas but are benign or even self-limiting. These tumours predominantly affect the skin or skeletal muscles and are rare in the mouth, where fewer than a dozen cases have probably been reported. The single most characteristic microscopic feature of these tumours is a storiform (knotted or tangled) pattern to the spindle cells, but the appearances are very variable with xanthomatous or myxoid areas, or many giant cells. Ultrastructural and tissue culture studies have largely supported the belief that these tumours arise from a tissue histiocyte which has fibroblastic properties and gives rise to both histiocyte-like and fibroblastic cells histologically.

Fibrous histiocytoma

From the few reports of fibrous histiocytomas arising in oral or perioral tissues, it is impossible to make generalizations about the clinical features.

Adults are affected and in the case of the most common type (in the lower extremity), the peak age is in the seventh decade. The tumour can develop in the soft tissues or bone where it produces a nondescript swelling or an area of radiolucency.

Grossly the tumour typically forms a multi-lobulated fleshy mass.

Microscopically, the most common features are short bundles of spindle-shaped cells forming storiform, matted or cartwheel patterns (Figure 13.12).

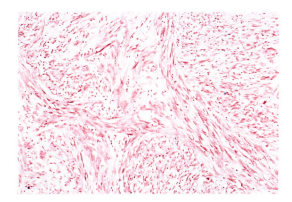

Figure 13.12 Fibrous histiocytoma. Spindle-shaped cells in the characteristic tangled or storiform pattern are shown

However, fibrosarcoma-like patterns may also be seen as well as giant cells and pleomorphic areas with plumper histiocyte-like cells and variable numbers of mitoses.

Giant cell variant of malignant fibrous histiocytoma

This tumour which has also been termed *malignant giant cell tumour of soft tissues*, consists of histiocytes, fibroblasts and osteoclast-like cells (Figure 13.13). As a consequence it may closely resemble a giant cell tumour of bone, apart from the lack of osteoid or osseous tissue. As this variant is considerably less common than the storiform type of malignant fibrous histiocytoma, little is known about its behaviour but there is nothing to suggest that it is any more benign.

Malignant fibrous histiocytoma is actively invasive and spreads particularly along tissue planes and unlike other sarcomas has a tendency to involve lymph nodes.

Management
Treatment of fibrous histiocytoma is by radical excision, including the regional lymph nodes, as the malignant variants metastasize in over 40% of cases and may do so even if microscopic features indicative of malignancy are minimal. There is some evidence that postoperative radiotherapy improves the prognosis.

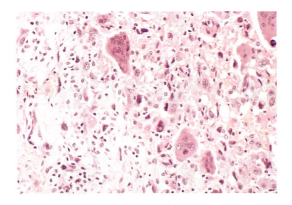

Figure 13.13 Malignant fibrous histiocytoma – giant cell variant. Mononuclear histiocyte-like cells and many osteoclast-like giant cells can be seen

Tumours of neural tissue

Traumatic neuroma

Traumatic neuromas are rare in the mouth and usually result from accidental operative damage. They are often asymptomatic and found only as small nodules in the tissues. Occasionally, they give rise to neuralgic pain, particularly if irritated, for example by a denture.

Microscopically, traumatic neuromas consist of tangled bundles of nerve fascicles separated by fibrous tissue.

Surgical excision with cryosurgery of the nerve stump is curative. When there is neuralgic pain, carbamazepine may be helpful.

Neurilemmomas (schwannomas)

Schwann cells are neuroectodermal cells which ensheath the axons. Individual peripheral nerves, which consist of a group of axons, are surrounded by a sheath of concentric layers of perineural (Schwann) cells and also collagen fibres. The epineurium ensheathes a group of nerve fascicles in a larger peripheral nerve and consists only of fibrous connective tissue.

In the mouth, neurilemmomas form small painless nodules, particularly in the tongue.

Microscopically, neurilemmomas consist of two types of tissue. Antoni A tissue, which usually predominates, forms a closely interwoven pattern of elongated spindle-shaped cells, the nuclei of which are often palisaded or regimented to produce a distinctive picture (Figure 13.14). Reticulin fibres are also abundant. Type B tissue is loose with relatively scanty, scattered and pleomorphic nuclei. Some of these may be so large and hyperchromatic as to suggest malignancy. Positive reactivity for S-100 protein tends to be considerably stronger in neurilemmomas than in neurofibromas.

Neurilemmomas should be completely excised and should not then recur.

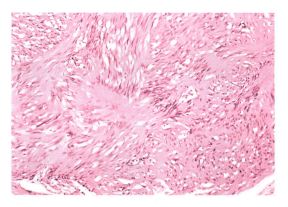

Figure 13.14 Neurilemmoma with Schwann cells showing the characteristic palisading

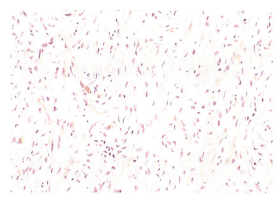

Figure 13.16 Neurofibroma. The neural elements stain brown with S-100 antibody

Neurofibroma

Solitary neurofibromas are uncommon and, when they are found, the patient should be investigated for neurofibromatosis. Clinically, neurofibromas form painless smooth nodules.

Microscopically, neurofibromas consist of elongated, bent or sinuous nuclei separated by abundant, fine and equally sinuous collagen fibres (Figures 13.15 and 13.16). Reticulin fibres by contrast are scanty. Mast cells and lymphocytes are considerably more frequently found among the fibres than in neurilemmomas (Johnson *et al.*, 1989), but reactivity for S-100 protein is patchy and variable. Occasionally, a neurofibroma develops in the inferior dental nerve and is seen radio-

graphically as a fusiform expansion of the inferior dental canal.

Complete excision should be curative.

Plexiform neurofibroma

Plexiform neuromas are exceedingly rare in the mouth. They consist of poorly organized mixtures of nerve fibrils usually unmyelinated and tangled, but sometimes also normal or hypertrophied nerve fibres (Figure 13.17). There is diffuse proliferation of spindle cells of neural origin, myxoid areas and, often, fat. Mast cells, as in many other fibro-proliferative disorders, are conspicuous and appear to contribute to the overgrowth of neural fibrous

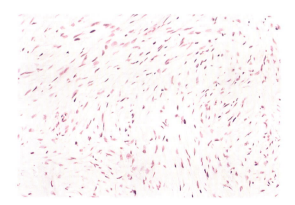

Figure 13.15 Neurofibroma

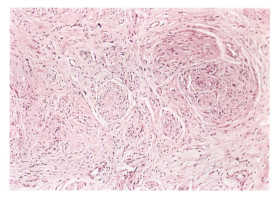

Figure 13.17 Neurofibroma: plexiform type

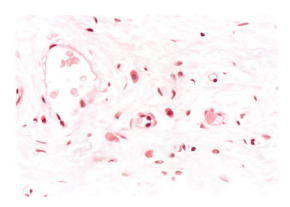

Figure 13.18   Neurofibroma showing mast cells

tissue (Figure 13.18). Compact bundles of cells apparently originating from the peri- or epineurium proliferate into the surrounding tissues. Excision should be curative, but plexiform neurofibromas are frequently a sign of von Recklinghausen's disease or multiple endocrine neoplasia syndrome.

Neurofibromatosis (von Recklinghausen's disease)

Neurofibromatosis is one of the phacomatoses ('neurodermatoses') which are genetically determined hamartomatous or neoplastic diseases of the skin and nervous system. There are two genetically and phenotypically distinct forms of neurofibromatosis, namely peripheral and central. The peripheral type (NF I) accounts for over 90% of cases; the central type (NF II), characterized by bilateral acoustic neuromas, accounts for the remainder. Neurofibromatosis (type I) is one of the most common autosomal dominant disorders, and the prevalence of the disease may approach 1 in 3000 of the population.

Clinically, the characteristic features of peripheral neurofibromatosis are multiple coffee-coloured (café-au-lait) macules which typically start to appear within the first year of life, cutaneous and sometimes skeletal neurofibromas and Lisch nodules (brownish, dome-shaped hamartomas of the iris). The severity of the disease ranges from inconspicuous to grossly disfiguring tumorous

deformities. The skin tumours start to develop at or near puberty, frequently cause itching while actively growing and in severe cases can form in hundreds or even thousands.

The café-au-lait spots resemble freckles but appear in sites shielded from sunlight, such as the axillae. In the absence of obvious neurofibromas, the diagnosis of the disease depends on finding multiple café-au-lait spots and Lisch nodules.

Neurofibromas affect the head and neck region in over 25% of cases, but involve the mouth or jaws in only approximately 5% of cases.

Microscopically, the tumours are typically plexiform neurofibromas which are strongly suggestive, if not diagnostic, of von Recklinghausen's disease or multiple endocrine neoplasia syndrome which may be associated.

Neurofibromas (Figure 13.19) are even more common than plexiform neuromas, but are not distinguishable from those unassociated with von Recklinghausen's disease. Neurilemmomas may sometimes also be found.

Bones can be involved as a result of tumours growing from nerve fibres and forming subperiosteal or more central, cyst-like areas of radiolucency. Localized expansion of the inferior dental canal may, therefore, be seen. Bone destruction may also result from formation of fibroma-like masses containing giant cells.

The café-au-lait spots show melanin hyperpigmentation of both keratinocytes and melanocytes, usually with scattered abnormally large melanin granules (giant melanosomes).

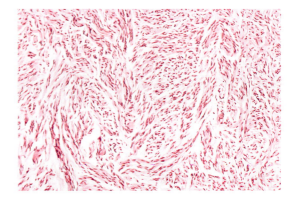

Figure 13.19   Neurofibroma. A cellular example shows interlacing elongated cells with dark, bent nuclei from a patient with neurofibromatosis

Management

Isolated tumours can be excised for functional or cosmetic reasons and recurrence is unusual. However, sarcomatous change develops in up to 10% of these neurofibromas. Other serious complications include disfigurement, mental handicap or other neurological disease such as epilepsy or paraplegia due to spinal neurofibromas. Skeletal abnormalities and central nervous system tumours, particularly gliomas of the optic nerves or chiasma, may also develop. Acoustic neuromas, contrary to earlier descriptions, are rarely associated.

Mucosal neuromas in endocrine adenoma syndromes

Oral mucosal neuromas, particularly along the lateral borders of the tongue, are a feature of multiple endocrine adenoma syndrome type III (Williams and Pollock syndrome) in which they are associated with medullary carcinoma of the thyroid and phaeochromocytoma.

Neuromas in this syndrome resemble the plexiform or traumatic types, but may be more fibrotic if traumatized.

The recognition of one of these unusual tumours in the mouth is an indication for investigation for endocrine adenoma syndrome, which they may antecede.

Malignant schwannomas and neurofibrosarcomas

Malignant tumours of nerve sheath origin may be malignant schwannomas or neurofibrosarcomas. However, there is no universally agreed terminology and it is probably justifiable to include them both in the single category of neurogenic sarcoma as there is no clear evidence that histological minutiae affect the prognosis.

Malignant schwannomas

These consist of plump spindle-shaped cells arranged in bundles which may be whorled or be interlacing. A matrix of looser fibroblastic cells or of a more mucinous nature may be apparent. In well-differentiated tumours, Antoni type A tissue may be recognizable, but in all types excessive cellularity, nuclear hyperchromatism and mitoses are typical features. One characteristic appearance is that of an area of necrosis surrounded by elongated cells with a palisaded arrangement. Care must be taken not to confuse so-called ancient neurilemmoma which can show foci of atypia. Staining for S-100 protein is frequently positive.

Neurofibrosarcomas

These tumours tend to resemble other fibrosarcomas so closely that their neural origin may not be recognizable unless they can be seen to be in continuity with neural tissue or a typical area of neurofibroma (Figures 13.20 and 13.21). They are usually composed of interlacing bundles of spindle-shaped cells (but looser and shorter than those of fibrosarcomas and with bent nuclei), either densely aggregated or more loosely arranged in a mucinous or myxoid matrix. The malignant nature of the tumour may be obvious from the cellularity and nuclear changes, but in

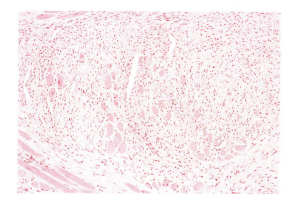

Figure 13.20 Neurofibrosarcoma. The behaviour of this tumour, invading muscle, illustrates its malignant character more dramatically than the microscopic appearances

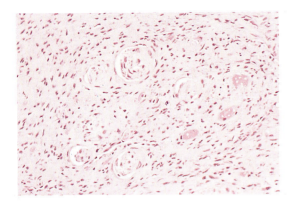

Figure 13.21 Neurofibrosarcoma showing some nuclear pleomorphism and small neural elements (neurites)

other cases mitoses may be scanty and the cells lack any significant nuclear abnormalities. However, at the periphery particularly, invasion or tissue destruction may be seen.

Management

Radical excision is the treatment of choice. However the recurrence rate is high as the tumour may infiltrate along the nerve sheath or spread via the bloodstream, and the value of radiotherapy is controversial. Spread to lymph nodes, by contrast, is uncommon. Neville *et al.* (1991) reported 3 patients with oral neurofibrosarcomas: all died from their disease. DiCerbo *et al.* (1992) reported a case of malignant schwannoma of the palate in a patient who survived 7 years after excision before being lost to follow-up.

Cervical paraganglionomas (chemodectomas, 'glomus tumours')

Paraganglionomas arise from neuroendocrine cells associated with autonomic ganglia. Paraganglionomas in the head and neck include (in order of frequency) carotid body (chemodectoma), jugulotympanic (glomus jugulare and glomus tympanicum), intravagal (glomus vagale), laryngeal, nasal and orbital tumours. True glomus tumours (glomangiomas) are described later among the blood vessel tumours.

Ten per cent are multiple and, in 8%, other neural crest tumours are associated. Normally these tumours are benign, but up to 6% may be frankly malignant and capable of metastasizing.

Overall, these tumours comprise only 0.01% of head and neck tumours. However, they are important in the differential diagnosis of masses in the head and neck. Glomus jugulare tumours may masquerade as deep or, rarely, as superficial lobe parotid tumours. Carotid body tumours may mimic deep lobe parotid tumours, branchial cysts or cervical lymphadenopathy, while Lustman and Ulmansky (1990) have reported a paraganglionoma causing a rubbery exophytic lump on the tongue.

Microscopically, paraganglionomas are characterized by the grouping of the cells in clusters or nests which are often sharply demarcated. The tumour cells typically have rounded nuclei and prominent cytoplasm which ranges from conspicuously granular to clear, sometimes with well-defined cell membranes. Neurosecretory granules, which are argyrophilic, can usually be identified by Grimelius staining, but if this fails electron microscopy may be necessary.

The correlation between the histological features and malignancy is poor. Central necrosis of the cell nests, mitotic activity and invasion of vascular spaces are features or malignancy, but can also sometimes be seen in benign paraganglionomas. However, only about 5% of carotid paraganglionomas are malignant, while malignancy in jugulotympanic paraganglionomas is virtually unknown.

Management

CT and angiography are the investigations of choice. These tumours are vascular and angiograms show their location, pattern, vascular supply and extent. Carotid body tumours lie between the internal and external carotid arteries, and spread them apart, whereas glomus jugulare tumours usually displace them forwards. As pressure on these tumours causes turbulence in the carotid blood flow, the non-invasive Doppler ultrasound (MAVIS – Mobile Arterio-Venous Imaging System) imaging technique can be used to aid diagnosis.

Treatment is by surgical excision; nevertheless, as these are slow-growing tumours and only a minority are malignant, some authors have advocated avoidance of active intervention. However, many such tumours can be peeled off the carotid adventitia with judicious tying off of feeder vessels; others require resection and reconstruction of the carotid vessels using a Javid shunt to maintain cerebral circulation. In some tumours, the vascular component is so abundant as to cause troublesome bleeding at operation. Incomplete excision is followed by recurrence. Radiotherapy has also been advocated, but the majority of these tumours appear to be relatively radioresistant.

Tumours of fatty tissue

Lipoma

Lipomas occasionally form within the mouth, particularly from the buccal fat pad or, rarely, within major salivary glands. They form soft fluctuant swellings with a distinctive creamy colour when submucosal. In approximately 5% of patients, lipomas are multiple. The tendency to develop multiple lesions is sometimes inherited as a simple autosomal dominant trait.

Microscopically, lipomas consist of mature fat cells enclosed within fine areolar tissue and surrounded by a fibrous capsule. Many of these tumours contain fibroblasts intermingled with the fat cells and are known as fibrolipomas.

Excision is curative.

Liposarcoma

Liposarcomas are rare tumours, particularly in the mouth. They show a wide variety of appearances, but well-differentiated liposarcomas can be recognized microscopically by obvious fat formation, foamy fat containing lipoblasts and signet-ring cells (vacuolated lipoblasts) (Figures 13.22 and 13.23). Characteristic, irregularly shaped giant cells within foamy cytoplasm may also be present.

Liposarcomas are considerably more cellular than lipomas and may be so cellular as to make their

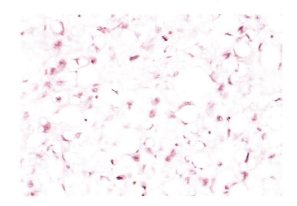

Figure 13.22 Liposarcoma. Low-power view shows a moderately cellular tumour. The pleomorphic cells contain lipid to form signet-ring cells (lipoblasts)

lipoblastic origin less obvious. When fat is present, it usually resembles embryonal adipose tissue and consists of fat cells in myxoid tissue. Liposarcomas which consist entirely of embryonal adipose tissue resemble myxomas.

Management
Radical excision is the treatment of choice, but the margins are frequently difficult to define at operation. Radiotherapy may be useful post-operatively or for palliation, particularly of the myxoid variant if surgery fails. Recurrence is common and is largely related to the degree of differentiation.

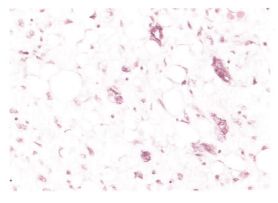

Figure 13.23 Liposarcoma. High power shows extreme nuclear pleomorphism

Diseases of muscle

Muscle pathology is a specialized field and few muscle diseases significantly affect the oral tissues. The recognition of muscle diseases in oral specimens is also made more difficult by the normal variations in size of muscle bundles in this part of the body. Artefacts resulting from surgical damage, or preparation of the specimen, further complicate the problems of diagnosis.

Muscle degeneration and regeneration

Muscle degeneration and regeneration are most likely to be seen as a result of trauma or involvement of muscle in infections or malignant tumours.

Muscle degeneration is characterized by hyaline change with loss of cross striations, vacuolation and, ultimately, necrosis. Infiltration by inflammatory cells and phagocytosis are early consequences.

Regeneration frequently follows muscle damage and is characterized by basophilia of the fibres, indistinct striations, increased number and size of nuclei sometimes with prominent nucleoli (sarcolemmal giant cells), and formation of variably sized but often small fibres (Figure 13.24).

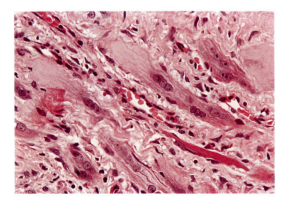

Figure 13.24 Muscle damage and regeneration. Striking sarcolemmal giant cells can be seen

Inflammatory myopathies: polymyositis and dermatomyositis

These types of myositis are traditionally grouped with the connective tissue diseases and may be immunologically mediated. Adults are mainly affected: women twice as often as men. Muscle pain and weakness, particularly of the proximal limb muscles, are the main features. Involvement of the flexors and dysphagia may be prominent but the facial and eye muscles are typically spared. Various types of rashes and, sometimes, Sjögren's syndrome, may be associated.

Microscopically, the chief finding is concurrent muscle degeneration and regeneration, associated with infiltration by mononuclear cells and phagocytosis of damaged muscle by histiocytes. Though autoantibodies to extractable nuclear antigen and rheumatoid factor may be associated, there is no specific immunological diagnostic test. Diagnosis, therefore, depends on the clinical, electromyographic and biopsy findings, and raised plasma creatinine phosphokinase (CPK) levels.

Proliferative myositis

This uncommon pseudo-sarcomatous disorder, which may be related to proliferative fasciitis, occasionally affects the masticatory muscles to produce a firm, rapidly growing tumour-like swelling. The head and neck region overall is the site of 33% of cases, but Fujiwara *et al.* (1987), in describing the immunohistochemical findings in an oral specimen, could find only one other earlier case. Adults over 45 are chiefly affected.

Microscopically, proliferative myositis consists of a loose arrangement of highly pleomorphic cells and has an infiltrative growth pattern. Giant cells resembling ganglion cells, or rhabdomyoblasts with basophilic or amphophilic cytoplasm, and sometimes two nuclei with conspicuous nucleoli, are prominent (Figure 13.25). These giant cells are separated by loose, oedematous, proliferating fibroblasts; inflammatory cells are scanty or absent. Remnants of degenerating muscle fibres may be seen, particularly near the periphery. Fujawara *et al.* (1987) found that the ganglion-like cells did not stain for desmin or myoglobin and

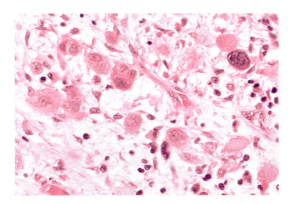

Figure 13.25   Proliferative myositis. Cytologically alarming, large basophilic cells, some with multiple, hyperchromatic nuclei, are shown

suggested that they were of myofibroblastic or macrophage origin.

Hardly surprisingly, a diagnosis of malignancy and particularly of rhabdomyosarcoma was initially made in 14 of the 33 cases reviewed by Enzinger and Dulcey (1967). Nevertheless, proliferative myositis is completely benign, as shown by its tendency to spontaneous regression.

Biopsy is essential to establish the diagnosis, but no further surgical intervention may then be necessary. At most, limited local reduction of the masses may be required for cosmetic reasons.

Myositis ossificans

This rare, benign proliferative process can be confused histologically with osteosarcoma. Solitary myositis ossificans (traumatic or ossifying myositis) may follow chronic trauma or an isolated blow to a muscle, but in at least 50% of cases there is no history of injury. Experimentally, trauma to muscle does not reproduce the pathological features of this condition.

Clinically, the masseter or temporalis muscle, usually in a teenager or young adult, can be affected and a localized, painful nodule develops within the affected muscle. A faint, delicate pattern of ossification typically starts to appear after about 3 weeks and may rarely cause ankylosis (Chapter 7).

Microscopically, there is typically initial reactive fibroblastic proliferation and organization of any haematoma present. In the developed lesion, there is usually characteristic zoning with a border of irregular trabeculae of cellular osteoid and woven bone surrounding a highly vascular central mass of proliferating, immature fibroblasts which are typically pleomorphic and have prominent mitoses. The picture is readily mistaken for sarcomatous change, but the process is benign and self-limiting. Sarcomatous change that has occasionally been reported in ossifying myositis does not seem to have been fully authenticated.

Treatment is by wide surgical excision of the ossifying mass. Recurrences are very common, but systemic bisphosphonates may help to prevent them.

Extraskeletal osteosarcoma and chondrosarcoma

These rare tumours are mentioned only to emphasize the fact that, though pseudo-sarcomatous diseases have been described above, it is also possible for true osteosarcomas or chondrosarcomas to develop in soft tissues. Care must, therefore, be taken not to dismiss osteosarcoma-like or chondrosarcoma-like changes as benign merely because they are within soft tissues. In the case of fibrous histiocytoma also, Enzinger and Weiss (1995) suggest that all gradations may exist from typical soft tissue fibrous histiocytomas to those with small foci of osteoid and typical osteosarcomas.

Granular cell tumour ('myoblastoma')

This oddity, once thought to be a degenerative disease of muscle, appears from its ultrastructural features and, more recently, from reports of positive staining with neuron-specific enolase and for the presence of S-100 ('brain specific') protein, to originate from Schwann cells or their precursor cells. Other ultrastructural reports have suggested an origin from undifferentiated mesenchymal cells and, in any case, S-100 protein is not specific for neural cells. Stewart *et al.* (1988) found that skeletal muscle stained weakly and that 50% of rhabdomyomas also stained positively for S-100 protein. They also found that 70% of granular cell tumours were invested by muscle and only 5% by nerve.

Clinically, the tongue is the most frequent site though overall, granular cell tumours are uncommon. Adults aged between 30 and 60 years are chiefly affected and the tumours often form small circumscribed lumps or firm areas just under the surface. Occasionally, the lesion is large and prominent, or resembles a carcinoma clinically. Rarely, they may develop in the midline of the tongue and then be mistaken for median rhomboid glossitis.

Microscopically, the appearance is difficult to reconcile with a neural origin, as the large granular cells frequently merge with muscle fibres (Figure 13.26). The granules, which are eosinophilic and PAS positive, may be so coarse as to make the cells conspicuous or so fine as to make them difficult to see. The cell membranes are typically well-defined. Frequently the overlying epithelium undergoes pseudo-epitheliomatous hyperplasia which may be mistaken for a carcinoma and be treated as such (Figure 13.27) (Ogus and Bennett, 1978–79).

Granular cell tumours respond to local excision but can recur if excision is inadequate. Multiple primary lesions have also been reported.

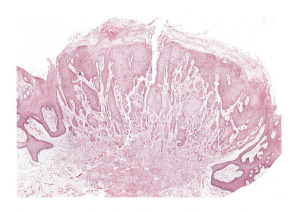

Figure 13.27   Granular cell tumour. There is striking pseudoepitheliomatous hyperplasia of the overlying epithelium

Congenital granular cell epulis

This rare entity is found on the alveolar ridge of the newborn and forms a soft rounded swelling a few millimetres across, or may be so large as to protrude from the mouth. The upper jaw is most often affected and at least 80% of affected infants are female.

Microscopically, the mass consists of closely packed granular cells with prominent cell membranes and among which is a delicate network of capillaries. These cells are S-100 negative, but stain positively for myogenous markers such as myosin and actin and are probably of mesenchymal origin. Rarely, small odontogenic rests may be present (Figure 13.28). Unlike granular cell myoblastoma, the overlying epithelium is thin and flat and the granular cells are invested by muscle fibres.

Management
Treatment is by excision, but the congenital epulis does not apparently recur, even if excision is incomplete, or may even regress spontaneously. This suggests that it is a hamartoma.

Rhabdomyoma

Cardiac rhabdomyomas, which are usually associated with one of the phacomatoses, are relatively

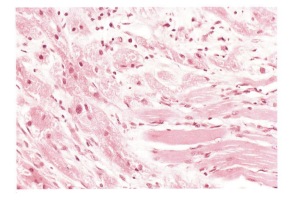

Figure 13.26   Granular cell tumour. Granular cells appear to merge with the surrounding muscle fibres

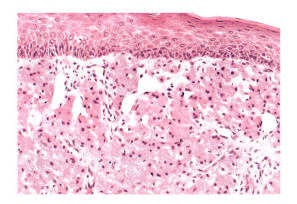

Figure 13.28 Congenital epulis. The flat layer of epithelium overlies a mass of pink, granular cells

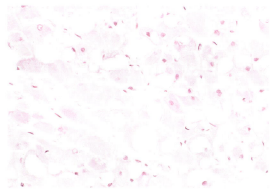

Figure 13.29 Rhabdomyoma. The vacuolated cells give the tumour a fatty appearance

common but the extracardiac rhabdomyoma is one of the rarest of all tumours. Ferlito and Frugona (1975), from a review of the world literature, estimated that there had been only about 50 reports of extracardiac rhabdomyomas. Corio and Lewis (1970) were able to identify 13 more cases from the Armed Forces Institute of Pathology files, but were able to find reports of only 16 cases of oral rhabdomyomas.

Clinically, oral rhabdomyomas affect men at least twice as frequently as women, with a peak age between 50 and 60 years. The tumour typically forms a slow-growing, painless swelling.

Microscopically, rhabdomyomas are well circumscribed or encapsulated and consist of large cells which may contain such large vacuoles as to appear fatty and sometimes cause the granular eosinophilic cytoplasm to have a spidery outline (Figure 13.29). The cell membranes are sharply defined. In haematoxylin and eosin stained sections, cross-striations can, with careful examination, be found but are more readily demonstrable using PTAH (Figure 13.30). PAS staining shows glycogen in the cytoplasm and in the peripheral vacuoles.

Diagnosis depends on showing cross-striations and absence of any features of malignancy.

Rhabdomyosarcoma

Though overall rare, rhabdomyosarcomas are among the most common sarcomas found in the mouth and second only to AIDS-related Kaposi's sarcoma.

These tumours form rapidly growing, soft swellings which (apart from the botryoid type which is unlikely to be seen in the mouth) are nondescript in character. In the series of 49 oro- and nasopharyngeal rhabdomyosarcomas of Dito and Batsakis (1962) there were 30 in the palate or tongue and 31 in the nasopharynx. Of these patients, 79% were aged under 12 years.

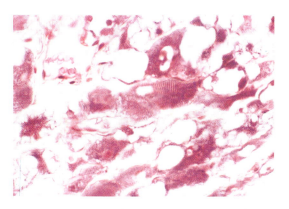

Figure 13.30 Rhabdomyoma. The cells contain large vacuoles and striation is made conspicuous by PTAH staining

Management
At operation, the tumour may shell out readily and recurrence is uncommon.

Microscopically, rhabdomyosarcomas are categorized as (a) embryonal, (b) alveolar, and (c) pleomorphic types, depending upon the predominant pattern. The embryonal type is the most common and accounts for about 75% of all cases. It is particularly common in the head and neck area and most examples are seen in children under the age of 12 years. Alveolar rhabdomyosarcoma tends to affect a somewhat older age group and is more frequent in the soft tissues of the extremities. Pleomorphic rhabdomyosarcoma is rare and most often forms in the large muscles of the extremities in adults aged over 45 years, but many authorities believe that many tumours formerly thought to be adult pleomorphic rhabdomyosarcomas should be recategorized as malignant fibrous histiocytomas.

Embryonal rhabdomyosarcoma consists of sheets of ovoid or spindle cells which may be tightly packed or interspersed in a loose myxoid stroma. Some of the round and spindle cells have eosinophilic cytoplasm which may stream out to form racquet- or strap-shaped cells. Cross-striations may be seen, but their presence is not essential for diagnosis. Glycogen is also present in the better differentiated cells, but is usually dissolved out in processing to leave multivacuolate, spider-web cells. Some embryonal rhabdomyosarcomas are highly pleomorphic and contain foci of varying size of larger bizarre cells.

Alveolar rhabdomyosarcoma tends to affect a somewhat older age group; it is considerably less common than the embryonal type and is only occasionally seen in the mouth. It consists of ill-defined nests of ovoid or round cells around central alveolar spaces (Figure 13.31). The individual alveoli are separated by fibrous septa. Multinucleated tumour giant cells are often also present.

Pleomorphic rhabdomyosarcoma, which most often affects adults over the age of 45 years, consists of round, pleomorphic cells of variable size and with varying amounts of cytoplasm which may be eosinophilic (Figure 13.32). Some may be racquet- or tadpole-shaped (Figure 13.33), but rarely show cross-striations. Many tumours previously thought to be adult pleomorphic rhabdomyosarcomas are probably malignant fibrous histiocytomas.

Diagnosis of rhabdomyosarcoma can be difficult and depends primarily on the identification of neoplastic rhabdomyoblasts, though cells with well-marked cross-striations are present in only

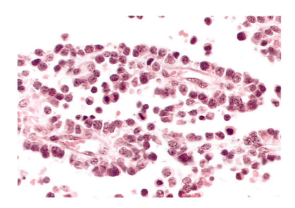

Figure 13.31 Alveolar rhabdomyosarcoma. Viable neoplastic cells can be seen adhering to the fibrous septa while degenerating cells are floating away

20–60% of cases and mainly in the embryonal type. Myoglobin is the most specific marker, but is usually negative in poorly differentiated tumours. Immunostaining for desmin, vimentin and myosin are widely used and when positive serve to distinguish poorly differentiated rhabdomyosarcomas from other small round cell tumours such as Ewing's sarcoma. However, Rangdaeng and Truong (1991) found that up to 17% of non-myogenic tumours stained with muscle-specific actin or desmin or both.

Management and prognosis

The prognosis is poor with local recurrence or distant metastases in many cases. Lymph nodes, often at a distance, may be involved in up to 50% of

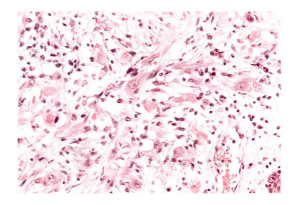

Figure 13.32   Pleomorphic rhabdomyosarcoma

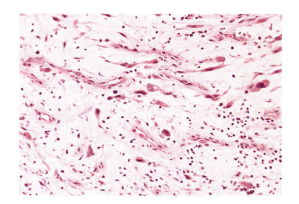

Figure 13.33   Rhabdomyosarcoma showing typical strap- and tadpole-shaped cells

cases, but favoured sites of metastases are the bones or lungs.

It appears that combination therapy has greatly improved the prognosis. For this purpose, radical surgery should be followed by intermittent multi-drug chemotherapy.

Tumours and hamartomas of blood and lymphatic vessels

Leiomyoma and angioleiomyoma

Leiomyomas are rare in the mouth and arise from muscle cells in the walls of blood vessels. They are termed angioleiomyomas or leiomyomas according to whether or not their vascular origin is apparent. The tongue is the most common site and lesions form slowly growing nondescript swellings which are usually painless. Angioleiomyomas may have a bluish colour due to the prominent vascular component.

Microscopically, leiomyomas consist of interlacing bundles of spindle-shaped cells. The nuclei are often blunt-ended and myofibrils can be demonstrated by PTAH staining. Differentiation from other spindle cell tumours such as neurofibromas may be difficult and depend on electron microscopy to demonstrate myofibrils. Immunocytochemistry may be helpful, but neurogenous tumours may also stain positively for desmin, actin and vimentin. Angioleiomyomas consist of thick-walled blood vessels and bundles of smooth muscle so that their nature is more obvious (Figure 13.34).

Treatment

Leiomyomas and angioleiomyomas are benign and respond to conservative excision.

Leiomyosarcomas

Leiomyosarcomas are exceptionally rare in the mouth. Poon *et al.* (1987) could find only 24 documented cases in the preceding 75 years. Clinically, they form initially painless, nondescript smooth swellings.

Microscopically, leiomyosarcomas are spindle cell tumours with elongated, weakly eosinophilic cells with blunt-ended nuclei like leiomyomas, but show cellular pleomorphism and mitotic activity. Differentiation from other malignant spindle cell tumours is frequently difficult unless myofibrils can be demonstrated by electron microscopy or other means. Positive staining for muscle-specific actin

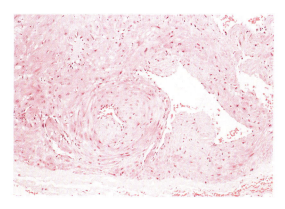

Figure 13.34   Leiomyoma – vascular type (angioleiomyoma). Recognizable smooth muscle fibres surround small and large vascular channels

and desmin is helpful, but some leiomyosarcomas fail to stain.

Treatment is surgical excision, but there is an exceedingly poor prognosis.

Haemangiomas

Most haemangiomas are hamartomas of blood vessels. They are either congenital, capillary type (vascular naevi) or cavernous and may then increase in size with age.

Haemangiomas form flat or prominent, soft purplish lesions which characteristically blanch under pressure and may bleed profusely if traumatized. Extensive, usually capillary-type, haemangiomas are a cause of macroglossia. Haemangiomas (usually cavernous or mixed type) can also rarely form intraosseous tumours (Chapter 5).

Microscopically, capillary haemangiomas consist of a dense mass of capillaries or imperforate rosettes of endothelium (Figure 13.35). Cavernous haemangiomas consist of dilated, blood-filled vascular spaces with endothelial linings and are frequently poorly circumscribed (Figure 13.36).

Intramuscular haemangiomas are a rare variant and, in the perioral region, are most likely to form in the masseter muscles as a slow-growing sometimes painful mass. The overlying skin may become purplish red and warm to the touch. Angiography is necessary to confirm the diagnosis.

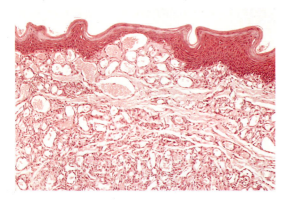

Figure 13.35 Capillary haemangioma. This submucosal tumour consists of capillaries and imperforate rosettes of endothelium

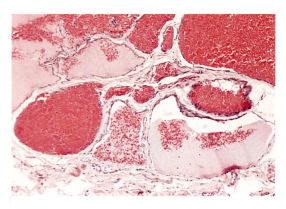

Figure 13.36 Cavernous haemangioma. Large blood-filled spaces are lined by a single layer of endothelial cells

Treatment

Superficial haemangiomas should be recognizable clinically and treatment should usually be avoided. Early onset haemangiomas may regress spontaneously, but regression is unlikely in adults. Even prominent cavernous haemangiomas, despite the possibility of being bitten, may cause little or no trouble, but if there has been significant or recurrent bleeding then an attempt should be made to eradicate them using selective embolization. For large tumours, preoperative angiography is essential to determine their extent and if possible to identify feeder vessels.

Small, predominantly capillary lesions respond well either to cryotherapy or injection of sclerosing agents such as sodium tetradecyl sulphate, which gives better cosmetic results than surgical excision in such sites as the lips. Alternatively, laser surgery can be used.

Extensive, mixed capillary/cavernous haemangiomas are more common in the masseteric region of the cheek. Following angiography and control of the feeder vessels, such lesions, which are often diffuse, should be removed surgically as completely as possible. The margins are then infiltrated with sclerosant, and full-thickness compression sutures (tied over cotton rolls externally to protect the skin) are placed for 5 days.

Extensive, especially cavernous, lesions can be excised after preoperative angiography and ligation of all feeder vessels. Alternatively, intra-tumoral ligation can be combined with injection of sclerosant solutions (Popescu, 1985). This less radical approach is suitable for diffuse cavernous lesions where surgical ablation would result in gross cosmetic deficit.

It is not usually possible to excise large haemangiomas of the tongue completely as this may require total glossectomy and excision of a large part of the floor of the mouth. Considerable morbidity or disability would thus result. A better alternative is to partially debulk the haemangioma to allow normal tongue function to be retained. Following angiography, tapes are placed around major feeder vessels and a soft intestinal clamp is fixed across the tongue at the line of resection. The excess tissue can then be excised and the resection margin oversown with non-resorbable sutures. Healing should be uncomplicated and further surgery can be undertaken if the haemangioma enlarges in later years.

Sturge–Weber syndrome and mucocutaneous angiomatosis

Vascular naevi of the skin may be isolated abnormalities or part of a syndrome such as the Sturge–Weber syndrome. The latter comprises angiomatosis within the distribution of the trigeminal nerve and of the leptomeninges of the same side, leading to epilepsy or hemiparesis and, usually, mental defect. A more limited form consists only of a diffuse vascular naevus of the face and of the underlying oral tissues including the gingivae. This type may have sharply defined lower and midline boundaries. When the gingivae are involved, the swollen tissue can cause false pocketing and inflammation or, rarely, local trauma can induce the formation of a rapidly growing, sarcoma-like mass.

These naevi are developmental anomalies and usually consist of grossly dilated vessels. There may be a genetic component in their aetiology, as suggested by several syndromes of which they are a feature. Similar lesions can also be induced by the drug thalidomide given during pregnancy or be a feature of the fetal alcohol syndrome.

Isolated naevi are rarely of clinical significance unless they are visible and disfiguring. Ugly angiomas of the face can be treated by means of skin grafting, liquid nitrogen cryotherapy or laser-induced fibrosis.

Glomus tumours (glomangiomas)

True glomus tumours arise from specialized arteriovenous shunts involved in body temperature regulation. Though glomus tumours may, to some degree, resemble paraganglionomas microscopically, glomangioma is a preferable term. They are rare oral tumours, but Geraghty *et al.* (1992) reported a case and reviewed 14 previous examples.

Microscopically, the cell of origin appears to be a modified smooth muscle cell, and the tumours typically consist of small dark cells with punched-out nuclei and little cytoplasm, surrounding dilated vascular channels lined by endothelium.

Treatment
Simple excision is usually effective and recurrence is rare.

Lymphangiomas

Lymphangiomas are more uncommon than haemangiomas but, like them, may be superficial or deep and capillary or cavernous.

Superficial lymphangiomas are pale or pink, translucent and may have a finely nodular surface. They may blacken when traumatized as a consequence of bleeding into the lymphatic spaces. Deep lymphangiomas particularly affect the tongue and are·another rare cause of macroglossia, or can affect the lip causing macrocheilia.

A rare variant is the lymphangioma of the alveolar ridge of neonates.

Microscopically, lymphangiomas differ little from their haemangiomatous counterparts and consist of capillary or cavernous lymphatic channels but which appear empty or filled with eosinophilic colloidal material (Figure 13.37). However, capillary lymphangiomas frequently cannot be distinguished from haemangiomas if there has been pre- or perioperative bleeding into the capillary spaces. Cystic hygroma is a term given to cavernous haemangiomas with unusually large, cyst-like lymphatic spaces; it is most common in the neck.

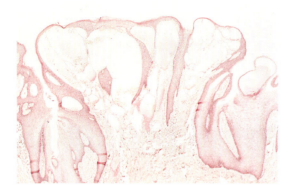

Figure 13.37 Lymphangioma showing dilated superficial lymph channels producing a lobulated swelling

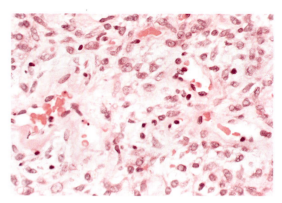

Figure 13.38 Haemangiopericytoma. A cellular area shows round and spindle-shaped cells and small vascular channels

Treatment

Lymphangiomas need only to be treated if frequently traumatized with resulting inflammation and increased swelling. However, lymphangiomatous macroglossia may interfere with swallowing, cause drooling and, when traumatized, enlarge and may become infected. Excision is then necessary. Small lesions can be completely resected. Limited resection, sufficient to restore normal function, can be carried out on large lesions and there is a good chance that the lesion will remain static after growth is complete. Large lymphangiomas in the neck may require such extensive dissection that complete removal may not be possible.

Haemangiopericytoma

Haemangiopericytoma is a rare tumour and its most common site is the skin or subcutaneous tissues. The mouth is only occasionally involved. Lesions usually form solitary, firm nodules.

Microscopically, haemangiopericytomas consist of small closely packed cells with ill-defined cytoplasm and darkly staining nuclei (Figure 13.38). Interspersed among them are slit-like or sinusoidal vascular spaces (Figure 13.39). Occasionally, the pericytes may have a palisaded configuration or may show interstitial mucoid degeneration. It may be noted that other tumours such as mesenchymal chondrosarcomas or synovial sarcomas may have extensive haemangiopericytoma-like areas.

Rare, more obviously malignant, haemangiopericytomas are more cellular, show cellular pleomorphism and mitotic activity, and sometimes areas of haemorrhage or necrosis.

Management

The behaviour of haemangiopericytomas is variable; most are entirely benign but some are infiltrative and can metastasize. One of the main problems in dealing with this tumour is, therefore, the difficulty of predicting its behaviour from the histological features.

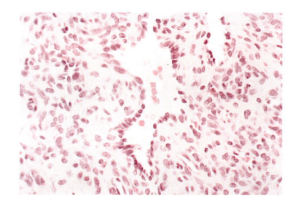

Figure 13.39 Haemangiopericytoma. Gaping thin-walled vascular spaces are surrounded by plump tumour cells

Adequate excision is the treatment of choice, as these tumours are not radiosensitive. Success has been claimed for chemotherapy of more malignant variants.

Haemangioendothelioma

In infants, there may be proliferation of the endothelial lining of capillary haemangiomas so that the endothelial cells appear rounded and the lesion consists of thin capillary channels and solid cords of cells. Such lesions are sometimes called benign haemangioendotheliomas.

A rare tumour, particularly in the mouth, is termed an epithelioid haemangioma. It may form a bluish swelling which may ulcerate. It is frequently centred on a blood vessel and characterized by rounded vacuolated cells with eosinophilic cytoplasm. These cells may be arranged in cords or small nests and surrounded by reticulin, while their matrix may have a hyaline or cartilage-like appearance. Paradoxically, vascular channels are inconspicuous.

Epithelioid haemangioendotheliomas, despite a bland cellular appearance, are regarded as being of borderline malignancy. Wide excision is the treatment of choice.

Kaposi's sarcoma

Classical (sporadic) Kaposi's sarcoma was described in 1872 in Central Europe among elderly persons of Mediterranean or Jewish origin. It is predominantly cutaneous, mainly affects the lower extremities and visceral lesions are rarely clinically apparent. Head and neck involvement is exceedingly rare. Kaposi's sarcoma with broadly similar characteristics is considerably more common in Africa, particularly in Zaire, where it formed about 12% of all malignant tumours in the pre-AIDS era. This form of Kaposi's sarcoma has both an indolent course and a good response to chemotherapy.

Clinically, AIDS-related Kaposi's sarcoma frequently involves the head and neck. The site may be oropharyngeal, cutaneous or in the cervical lymph nodes. Within the mouth, the palate is the most commonly affected site and the tumour typically produces a flat or nodular purplish lesion. It can have a similar site distribution in immunosuppressed patients, but is a relatively rare complication of such 'treatment in the West. Clinically, the differential diagnosis is from oral purpura and bacillary angiomatosis from which it can be distinguished by microscopy.

Microscopy

Kaposi's sarcoma originates in endothelial cells, as shown by the presence of the factor VIII marker. It produces florid angiomatoid proliferation with some resemblance to granulation tissue. Recognition of the tumour may, therefore, be difficult, particularly in the early stages.

In the earliest ('presarcomatous') stage of development, there is angiomatous proliferation with formation of irregular slit-like vascular spaces and perivascular cuffing by lymphocytes and plasma cells. In the intermediate stage, the angiomatoid changes are more widespread with irregular vascular spaces, together with perivascular proliferation of spindle-shaped and angular cells. Finally, the picture becomes increasingly dominated by proliferation of the interstitial spindle-shaped and angular cells and mitoses may be prominent (Figures 13.40 and 13.41). There is typically also extravasation of erythrocytes and deposition of haemosiderin, and there may be central necrosis.

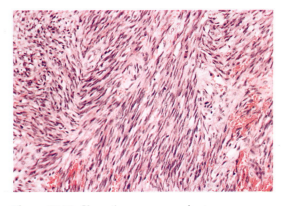

Figure 13.40 Kaposi's sarcoma – early stage. Inflammation and dilated vascular channels with areas of interstitial haemorrhage and angioblastic and spindle cell proliferation are shown

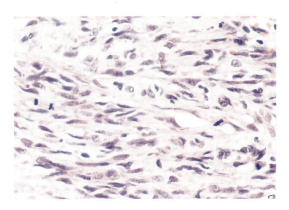

Figure 13.41   Kaposi's sarcoma. Later stage showing mainly spindle cells, some in mitosis, and smaller vascular spaces

Management

In 'classical' (sporadic) Kaposi's sarcoma, radiotherapy is the accepted treatment for localized disease, while combined chemotherapy is used for disseminated disease.

In the case of epidemic (AIDS-associated) Kaposi's sarcoma, a great variety of treatment regimens such as single agent, combined chemotherapy or zidovudine with alpha interferon and radiotherapy have been tried. The prognosis of the tumour itself as a result of such treatment is often good in the short term, and death is usually from the associated opportunistic infections secondary to the immunodeficiency. Symptomatic lesions within the mouth are best treated with two or three fractions of radiotherapy, to which they rapidly respond.

Bacillary epithelioid angiomatosis

Bacillary angiomatosis is a rare vasculoproliferative disease which can be seen in AIDS and in other immunodeficient patients. It can be mistaken for Kaposi's sarcoma clinically and sometimes histologically, as described by Glick and Cleveland (1993) who were able to demonstrate the causative bacteria in an oral lesion which had caused alveolar bone loss. The distinction from Kaposi's sarcoma must be made because of the therapeutic and prognostic implications.

Microscopy

The vasoproliferation can somewhat simulate that of Kaposi's sarcoma, but characteristic features of bacillary angiomatosis include the plump, epithelioid appearance of the endothelial cells which line well-formed vascular channels, and an inflammatory infiltrate, largely of neutrophils: factor VIII staining may be negative. When seen, the definitive finding is that of granular amphophilic aggregates of the causative bacilli which show positive Warthin–Starry staining.

The response to antimicrobials such as erythromycin or doxycycline is usually good.

Synovial sarcoma

Synovial sarcoma falls into none of the preceding categories. Paradoxically it affects tissues adjacent to or unrelated to joints, rather than joints themselves. The extremities, particularly the lower extremity, are most commonly involved: about 8% are in the head and neck region.

Clinically, synovial sarcoma frequently forms an insidiously growing, deep soft tissue mass which may eventually become painful and, if related to a joint, limits movement.

Microscopically, synovial sarcoma is characteristically biphasic, with both spindle cell and epithelial elements (Figure 13.42). The spindle cells are fibroblast-like while the epithelial cells, which stain positively with epithelial cell markers, are typically tall and columnar.

The spindle cells usually form the bulk of the tumour and are usually uniform, with plump nuclei and indistinct cytoplasm. They may form well-orientated streams of cells resembling a well-differentiated fibrosarcoma.

The epithelial cells can form a variety of arrangements such as whorls or solid cords, or they may confer a gland-like appearance to the area. Sometimes they may line clefts or cyst-like spaces and thus may resemble normal synovium. Occasionally, epithelial elements are so scanty and difficult to find that the tumour is termed 'monophasic'.

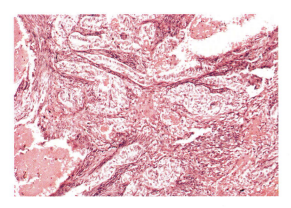

Figure 13.42 Synovial sarcoma. This biphasic tumour shows rounded, pale epithelial cells interspersed with fibrosarcoma-like spindle cells

Varying degrees of calcification or even ossification develop in about 40% of these tumours and is an important radiological feature.

Management

The prognosis of synovial sarcoma is related to the degree of differentiation rather than to the relative amounts of the two cellular components, but despite its slow growth, the tumour has a poor prognosis. The reported 5-year survival rate varies between 25% and 50%. Wide excision is necessary and radiotherapy may be beneficial, but since recurrences after limited resection may be delayed for a decade or more, it is difficult to assess cure rates. Metastases are most frequently to the lungs, but sometimes to lymph nodes or occasionally to the bone marrow.

References

Barnes, L. (1985) Tumors and tumor-like lesions of the soft tissues. In *Surgical Pathology of the Head and Neck* (ed. Barnes, L.), Marcel Dekker, New York, pp. 725–880

Chung, E.B. and Enzinger, F.M. (1981) Infantile myofibromatosis. *Cancer*, **48**, 1807–1818

Corio, R.L. and Lewis, D.M. (1970) Intraoral rhabdomyomas. *Oral Surgery*, **48**, 525–537

DiCerbo, M., Sciubba, J.J., Sordill, W.C. *et al.* (1992) Malignant schwannoma of the palate: a case report and review of the literature. *Journal of Oral and Maxillofacial Surgery*, **50**, 1217–1221

Dito, W.R. and Batsakis, J.G. (1962) Rhabdomyosarcoma of the head and neck. An appraisal of the biologic behaviour in 170 cases. *Archives of Surgery*, **84**, 112–118

Enzinger, F.M. and Dulcey, F. (1967) Proliferative myositis. Report of thirty-three cases. *Cancer*, **20**, 2213–2233

Enzinger, F.M. and Weiss, S.W. (1995) *Soft Tissue Tumors*, 3rd edn, C.V. Mosby, St. Louis

Eversole, L.R., Schwartz, D. and Sabes, W.R. (1973) Central and peripheral fibrogenic and neurogenic sarcoma of the oral regions. *Oral Surgery, Oral Medicine and Oral Pathology*, **36**, 49–62

Ferlito, A. and Frugona, P. (1975) Rhabdomyoma purum of the larynx. *Journal of Laryngology and Otology*, **89**, 1131–1141

Fujiwara, K., Watanabe, T., Katsuki, T. *et al.* (1987) Proliferative myositis of the buccinator muscle: a case with immunohistochemical and electron microscopic analysis. *Oral Surgery, Oral Medicine and Oral Pathology*, **63**, 597–601

Geraghty, J.M., Thomas, R.W.N., Robertson, J.M. *et al.* (1992) Glomus tumour of the palate: case report and review of the literature. *British Journal of Oral and Maxillofacial Surgery*, **30**, 398–400

Glick, M. and Cleveland, D.B. (1993) Oral mucosal bacillary epithelioid angiomatosis in a patient with AIDS associated with rapid alveolar bone loss: case report. *Journal of Oral Pathology and Medicine*, **22**, 235–239

Johnson, M.D., Kamso-Pratt, J., Federspiel, C.F. *et al.* (1989) Mast cell and lymphoreticular infiltrates in neurofibromas. Comparison with nerve sheath tumors. *Archives of Pathology and Laboratory Medicine*, **113**, 1263–1270

Lustman, J. and Ulmansky, M. (1990) Paraganglioma of the tongue. *Journal of Oral and Maxillofacial Surgery*, **48**, 1317–1319

Mark, R.J., Sercarz, J.A., Tran, L. *et al.* (1991) Fibrosarcoma of the head and neck. *Archives of Otolaryngology and Head and Neck Surgery*, **117**, 396–401

Neville, B.W., Hann, J., Narang, R. *et al.* (1991) Oral neurofibrosarcoma associated with neurofibromatosis type I. *Oral Surgery, Oral Medicine and Oral Pathology*, **72**, 456–461

Ogus, H.D. and Bennett, M.H. (1978–79) Carcinoma of the dorsum of the tongue: a rarity or misdiagnosis. *British Journal of Oral Surgery*, **16**, 115–124

Poon, C.K., Kwan, P.C., Yin, N.T. *et al.* (1987) Leiomyosarcoma of gingiva. Report of a case and review of the literature. *Journal of Oral and Maxillofacial Surgery*, **45**, 888–894

Popescu, V. (1985) Intra-tumoral ligation in the management of orofacial cavernous haemangiomas. *Journal of Maxillofacial Surgery*, **13**, 99–107

Rangdaeng, S. and Truong, L.D. (1991) Comparative immunohistochemical staining for desmin and muscle-specific actin. A study of 576 cases. *American Journal of Clinical Pathology*, **96**, 32–45

Siniluoto, T.M.J., Luotenen, J.P., Tikkakoski, T.A. *et al.* (1993) Value of pre-operative embolization in surgery for nasopharyngeal angiofibroma. *Journal of Laryngology and Otology,* **107,** 514–521

Speight, P.M., Dayan, D. and Fletcher, C.D.M. (1991) Adult and infantile myofibromatosis: a report of three cases affecting the oral cavity. *Journal of Oral Pathology and Medicine,* **20,** 380–384

Stewart, C.M., Watson, R.E., Eversole, L.R. *et al.* (1988) Oral granular cell tumors: a clinicopathologic and immunocytochemical study. *Oral Surgery, Oral Medicine and Oral Pathology,* **65,** 427–435

Vally, I.M. and Altini, M. (1990) Fibromatoses of the oral and paraoral soft tissues and jaws. *Oral Surgery, Oral Medicine and Oral Pathology,* **69,** 191–198

Weprin, L.S. and Siemers, P.T. (1991) Spontaneous regression of juvenile nasopharyngeal angiofibroma. *Archives of Otolaryngology and Head and Neck Surgery,* **117,** 796–799

14

Lymphoreticular and granulomatous diseases

Lymphoreticular diseases are diverse clinically and pathogenetically but can share a variety of features. In particular, immunity depends on normal function of the lymphoreticular system, so that lymphoreticular diseases frequently lead to immunodeficiencies. Conversely, lymphomas are a recognized complication of AIDS and other immunodeficiencies.

Lymphoreticular tumours – lymphomas

The main examples of solid lymphoid tumours are the lymphomas. Leukaemias, by contrast, typically do not form solid tumours but affect the bone marrow and blood. However, lymphocytic lymphomas may have features of both diseases. Myeloma and Langerhans cell histiocytosis also arise from lymphoreticular cells, but particularly affect bones and are discussed in Chapter 5.

Lymphomas are solid tumours of any type of lymphocyte; they are all malignant. They comprise Hodgkin's disease and non-Hodgkin's lymphoma. Their aetiology is unknown, but lymphomas are more frequent in the following:

- rheumatoid arthritis, Sjögren's syndrome and benign lymphoepithelial lesion
- immunosuppressive treatment, particularly for organ transplantation, and cytotoxic chemotherapy

- AIDS
- irradiation.

Exposure to asbestos has been reported to be associated with an increased incidence of oral lymphomas, but this has not been widely confirmed.

Lymphomas, particularly Hodgkin's disease, are rare tumours in the mouths of otherwise healthy persons, though they relatively frequently involve the cervical lymph nodes. The majority of oropharyngeal lymphomas develop in Waldeyer's ring, but are usually in the tonsils. Salivary glands, particularly the parotids which have a lymphoid component, can occasionally also be affected. By contrast, lymphomas in AIDS can account for 2% of oral neoplasms.

Clinical features

Adults are predominantly affected and lymphomas within the mouth form nondescript, usually soft, painless swellings, which may become ulcerated by trauma. The regional lymph nodes are not necessarily involved at first and diagnosis depends on the microscopic findings and related investigations.

Nasopharyngeal lymphoma is a rare cause of midfacial destructive disease, and can cause swelling and ulceration of the palate as the presenting feature, as discussed later.

Microscopically, lymphomas consist of B or, less often, T lymphocytes which, according to their stage of differentiation, give rise to different types of tumour, but morphological differences between these cells are frequently very slight. This is, therefore, a particularly difficult area of light microscopy and there are many classifications, of which the Working Formulation (Table 14.1) and a

Table 14.1   Working Formulation for non-Hodgkin's lymphomas

Behaviour	Histology
I. Low grade	Small lymphocytic Follicular, small cleaved cell Follicular, mixed small cleaved and large cell
II. Intermediate grade	Follicular, large cell Diffuse, small cleaved cell Diffuse, mixed small and large cell Diffuse, large cell
III. High grade	Large cell, immunoblastic Lymphoblastic Diffuse, small non-cleaved cell

simplified histological classification (Table 14.2) are given. The Working Formulation relates histology with behaviour but does not include T cell lymphomas. The simplified histological classification shows the main currently recognized types of non-Hodgkin lymphomas. However, precise categorization is best left to specialists.

Non-Hodgkin lymphomas appear as solid sheets of lymphocytes which may be predominantly small or large. Invasion or destruction of adjacent tissues may be seen and helps to confirm the malignant nature of these tumours. They may be diffuse or have a follicular pattern (Figures 14.1–14.5). Most (but not all) follicular lymphomas are low grade and have a better prognosis.

An additional problem in the mouth is that, if traumatized, superimposed inflammatory changes can cause a lymphoma to resemble a reactive lesion microscopically.

Table 14.2   Simplified histological classification of non-Hodgkin lymphomas

1. Lymphocytic
2. Follicle centre cell
3. Immunoblastic
4. Burkitt-type lymphoma
5. MALT cell lymphoma
6. T cell lymphomas

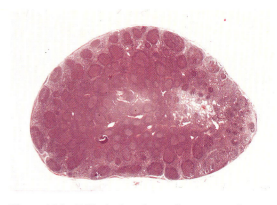

Figure 14.1   Follicular lymphoma. Low-power view shows multiple abnormal follicles

Investigation

In addition to the cytological features, which are used to decide the grade of a tumour, a useful test is the detection of a change from polyclonality (production of both lambda and kappa immunoglobulin light chains) of benign lymphoepithelial or reactive lesions to monoclonal production, usually, of kappa light chains by the neoplastic cells. Immunophenotyping is used to establish the lineage of the tumour cells as a guide to treatment.

Management

Clearly, a critical factor is whether the tumour is primary or is the initial manifestation of disseminated disease. In addition to biopsy, therefore,

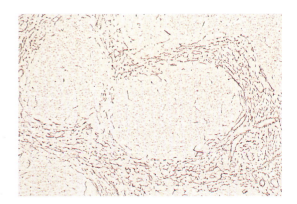

Figure 14.2   Follicular lymphoma. The follicles are clearly delineated by reticulin staining

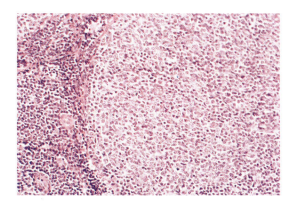

Figure 14.3 Follicular lymphoma: high-power view

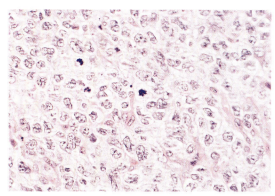

Figure 14.5 Diffuse, large cell, poorly differentiated lymphoma

staging investigation is necessary to determine the extent of spread of the tumour. Preliminary examination consists of physical examination, blood picture, chest radiographs, bone marrow biopsy and CT scanning to detect affected nodes in the abdomen.

The few cases with disease localized to a single node or extranodal site (stage I) and those with limited spread (stage II) are usually treated by irradiation. However, the majority of patients with oral or perioral lymphomas have disseminated disease (stage III or IV) and treatment is by combination chemotherapy. Oral disease, such as ulceration and infection, are common complications of such treatment. The overall 5-year survival rate for non-Hodgkin lymphomas is about 30%.

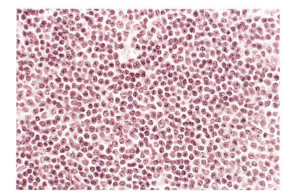

Figure 14.4 Well-differentiated diffuse lymphocytic lymphoma

Burkitt's lymphoma

This type of lymphoma, endemic in East Africa, has its onset in childhood, and has aroused interest by its association with the Epstein–Barr virus (EBV).

Clinically, Burkitt's lymphoma is peculiar in its onset at an average age of 7 years, and its predominantly extranodal distribution, with jaw involvement as the single most common initial site. Spread to the surrounding oral soft tissues and parotid glands and involvement of non-lymphoid abdominal viscera are common.

Over 95% of cases respond completely to single dose chemotherapy and though there is a high relapse rate, especially in those with widespread disease, the overall survival rate is approximately 50%. Also unlike other lymphomas, there is little or no response to radiotherapy.

Microscopically, Burkitt's lymphoma is a small cell lymphoma containing scattered histiocytes which, characteristically, give the otherwise dark sheets of cells a so-called starry-sky appearance (Figure 14.6).

A histologically similar tumour is rarely encountered in children in the West, but differs in that gut-associated lymphoid tissue is predominantly affected and it is rarely associated with the EBV genome or high EBV antibody titres. Lymphoma resembling Burkitt's lymphoma microscopically can also be a complication of immunosuppressive treatment and of AIDS and, in about 50% of the latter, is associated with EBV.

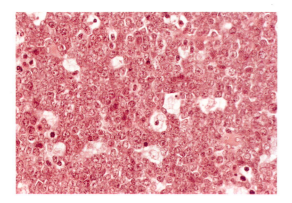

Figure 14.6 Burkitt's lymphoma. The classical starry-sky appearance due to scattered macrophages with pale vacuolated cytoplasm is shown

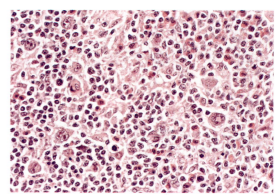

Figure 14.8 Hodgkin's disease: mixed cellularity type with Reed–Sternberg cells, lymphocytes, plasma cells and eosinophils

Hodgkin's disease

Hodgkin's disease frequently involves the cervical lymph nodes (where it may be mistaken for a submandibular salivary gland tumour) but only exceptionally rarely affects the mouth and is not clinically distinguishable from a non-Hodgkin's lymphoma.

Microscopically, Hodgkin's disease typically shows a mixed and pleomorphic picture of large, pale Hodgkin's cells as well as lymphocytes, eosinophils and fibroblasts (Figures 14.7–14.11). Moreover, the cellular picture varies widely, as indicated in the classification (Table 14.3).

Hodgkin's cells are histiocyte-like and have large nucleoli or have paired (mirror-image) nuclei (Reed–Sternberg giant cells); diagnosis depends largely on recognizing these cells. However, these cells are frequently difficult to find and, as with non-Hodgkin's lymphoma, any superimposed inflammation adds to the difficulties.

Hodgkin's disease may not readily be distinguished from non-Hodgkin's lymphomas by the microscopic features. However, it is important to make the distinction, as the chance of permanent cure of some types of Hodgkin's disease is now high as a result of irradiation of localized disease or combined chemotherapy. The overall 5-year survival rate may be 80%.

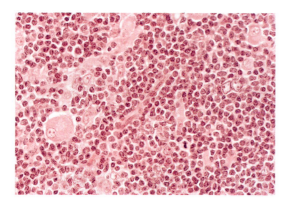

Figure 14.7 Hodgkin's disease: lymphocyte-predominant type with sheets of small lymphocytes and scattered large, pale Hodgkin's cells

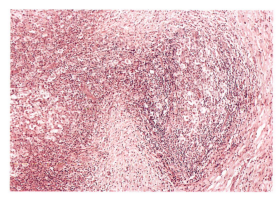

Figure 14.9 Hodgkin's disease: nodular sclerosis type with fibrous bands separating the neoplastic cells, many of which are pale

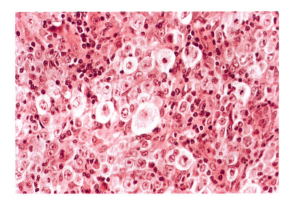

Figure 14.10   Hodgkin's disease: nodular sclerosing type showing the characteristic pale 'lacunar' cells

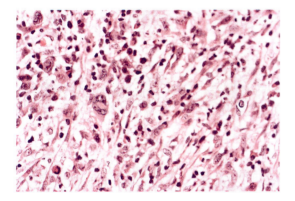

Figure 14.11   Hodgkin's disease: lymphocyte-depleted type showing gross cellular pleomorphism and diffuse fibrosis

Table 14.3   Rye classification of Hodgkin's lymphoma

- Nodular sclerosis
- Lymphocyte-predominant
- Mixed cellularity
- Lymphocyte-depleted

Causes and management of enlarged cervical lymph nodes

Dental and periodontal infections are by far the most common causes of cervical lymphadenopathy, but there is a great variety of possible causes including life-threatening diseases and, as mentioned earlier, enlargement of the cervical lymph nodes is a well-recognized early manifestation of lymphomas.

In most cases the cause of cervical lymphadenopathy is readily apparent. However, in the case of metastases without an obvious primary tumour it is essential to exclude the rare, occult and often minute, nasopharyngeal carcinoma. Second, in conditions where lymph nodes show proliferative activity it is essential to confirm or exclude a lymphoma and, if present, to start treatment as soon as possible. At the same time, it is also important to exclude non-malignant lymphoproliferative disorders to avoid serious overtreatment. Finally, increasing numbers of cases of lymphadenopathy due to HIV disease must be expected and in such patients lymph node biopsy should usually be avoided to lessen the risk of transmission of infection. Several of the diseases listed in Table 14.4 have been discussed earlier and will not be considered further here.

Indications for lymph node biopsy

These can be summarized as follows (Stansfeld and d'Ardenne, 1992):

For diagnosis of persistent unexplained lymphadenopathy   Infective causes can usually be readily eliminated, but persistently enlarged cervical nodes are often a cause for anxiety. Hard or rubbery nodes in older persons are especially likely to be due to neoplasms. Soft, slightly enlarged nodes in children are frequently of no serious significance.

To make or help in the diagnosis of lymphadenopathy associated with systemic disease   Biopsy is only justified if all other investigations have failed. One purpose of lymph node biopsy in such cases is to exclude lymphoma; however, the microscopic findings may reveal an infection such as tuberculosis or a connective tissue disease such as lupus erythematosus, of which cervical lymphadenopathy is very occasionally the presenting feature.

Table 14.4　Important causes of cervical lymphadenopathy

I. INFECTIONS
  1. *Bacterial*
    (a) Dental, tonsils, face or scalp
    (b) Tuberculosis
    (c) Syphilis
    (d) Cat scratch disease
    (e) Lyme disease

  2. *Viral*
    (a) Herpetic stomatitis
    (b) Infectious mononucleosis
    (c) HIV infection

  3. *Parasitic*
    Toxoplasmosis

  4. *Possibly infective*
    Mucocutaneous lymph node syndrome
    (Kawasaki's disease)

II. NEOPLASMS
  1. *Primary*
    (a) Hodgkin's disease
    (b) Non-Hodgkin's lymphoma
    (c) Leukaemia, especially lymphocytic

  2. *Secondary*
    (a) Carcinoma – oral, salivary gland or
        nasopharyngeal
    (b) Malignant melanoma
    (c) Ewing's sarcoma
    (d) Other mesenchymal tumours

III. MISCELLANEOUS
    (a) Sarcoidosis
    (b) Sinus histiocytosis
    (c) Angiofollicular hyperplasia
    (d) Drug reactions
    (e) Connective tissue diseases

To confirm an already suspected diagnosis　Removal or aspiration cytology of enlarged cervical nodes is mandatory in any patient with a carcinoma, treated or untreated, even when it seems that there is some other cause such as dental infection.

Similarly, in a patient with a known immunologically-mediated disease such as Sjögren's syndrome, enlargement of cervical lymph nodes may be due to infection secondary to the dry mouth, but may be due to lymphoma – a recognized hazard of this disease.

To assess the extent of spread of malignant disease　Block dissection of clinically affected nodes is frequently an essential part of the surgical treatment of carcinoma of the mouth, but removal of lymph nodes can also be part of a staging procedure for lymphoma to determine the choice of treatment.

To monitor the progress of lymphomas　Since the aim of treatment is curative, particularly in the case of Hodgkin's disease, further lymph node examinations may be required if nodes remain enlarged or enlarge during an apparent remission.

In such cases, the node may show persistence of the original tumour, the development of a different tumour (possibly as a consequence of cytotoxic chemotherapy) or an opportunistic infection secondary to immunosuppression by the tumour, or its treatment, or both.

Surgical considerations

Removal of cervical lymph nodes is not to be undertaken lightly. Though accessible, they are in close proximity to vital structures. Skill is also needed to remove enlarged and diseased nodes without traumatizing them. Pulling on a node, squeezing or crushing with forceps can damage or tear the capsule or damage the architecture. From the pathologist's viewpoint, cervical lymph nodes are a preferred group as they are least likely to show scarring or fatty involution.

Generally speaking, the choice of node to be removed for diagnostic purposes is the largest or, better, a group of enlarged nodes if several are involved. Removal of the most accessible node may be easier, but may necessitate another operation if it provides insufficient information.

Surgical management of an excised lymph node
In view of the number of investigations that may have to be applied to lymph nodes, particularly to confirm the diagnosis of lymphoma and to assign it to a precise category, it is important to excise lymph nodes with great care to avoid trauma and to treat the node in a systematic fashion, to enable the widest range of investigations to be carried out. Investigations should include:

- light microscopy
- touch (imprint) preparations and cytochemistry
- fresh frozen material for immunocytochemistry
- special fixation for other immunocytochemistry or electron microscopy and, sometimes,
- fresh material for culture.

Discussion with the pathologist is desirable to confirm which of these investigations are required in the light of the clinical picture and other findings.

Avoidance of physical trauma is essential, as lymphoma and lymphocytic leukaemia cells are fragile and when damaged can appear as mere basophilic smears (nuclear streaking) (Figures 14.12 and 14.13). This is seen particularly in small biopsies of intra-oral lymphomas, but is less likely when nodes are excised intact; the problem then may be to ensure complete fixation throughout the specimen.

Pathologists frequently prefer to cut up fresh lymph nodes themselves, but if this is not feasible, a lymph node may be cut across its long axis to provide immediate access of fixative to the full cross-section for light microscopy. The main specimen for light microscopy can be fixed in buffered formalin unless the pathologist prefers a mercury-based or other fixative such as Methacarn.

Touch preparations The unfixed fresh-cut surface of the node can be touched on to a glass microscope slide and allowed to settle under its own weight. Undue pressure should be avoided

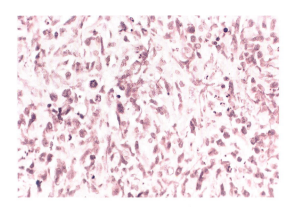

Figure 14.13 Lymphoma: adequately preserved tissue from the same tumour as in Figure 14.12 has shown it to be a poorly differentiated lymphoma

and the specimen must *not* be smeared. The touch preparation should immediately be fixed and stained with haematoxylin and eosin when rapid diagnosis is required. Other touch specimens can be used for special stains and for immunocytochemistry.

Straight frozen sections are generally considered undesirable because of changes during freezing, the risk of using up too much material or damaging the specimen in the operating theatre. At worst the diagnosis may remain in doubt and inadequate or unsatisfactory material may be left for light microscopy and other important investigations.

Immunocytochemistry A thin (1 mm if possible) section should be taken from the unfixed specimen and placed in Methacarn or other preferred fixative for immunocytochemistry, particularly if a lymphoma is suspected, and B or T lymphocyte phenotyping is required, although nowadays many markers will react with paraffin-embedded, formalin-fixed material.

Plastic-embedded specimens and electron microscopy Part of a 1 mm cross-section of the fresh node should be fixed in glutaraldehyde for electron microscopy if required, or alternatively 'semi-thin' (1 μm) sections can be cut for light microscopy and show good nuclear detail.

Part of a slice should be sent fresh for culture if a mycosis or bacterial infection is suspected.

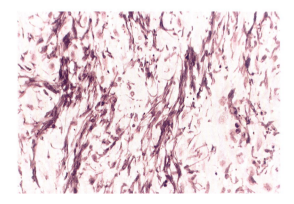

Figure 14.12 Lymphoma: mishandling of the specimen has caused nuclear streaking and made diagnosis impossible

Tuberculous cervical lymphadenopathy

Tuberculous infection of the cervical lymph nodes is a primary infection, and accounts for less than 10% of tuberculosis in Britain. *Mycobacterium tuberculosis* (human) accounts for over 90% of the isolates, and most of the patients are adults, mainly immigrants of Asian or Afro-Caribbean origin in this area. Non-tuberculous ('atypical') mycobacteria, particularly *M. avium intracellulare* or *scrofulaceum* are now the major cause of cervical mycobacterial lymphadenitis in immunocompetent children. As discussed earlier (Chapter 2), the incidence of mycobacterial infections is growing and multiply resistant strains are emerging.

The site of entry of the infection is probably the tonsil in most cases, but entry through the oral mucosa with formation of a minute painless ulcer has been described in children.

Clinically, tuberculous involvement of cervical lymph nodes gives rise to firm swelling, usually of a group of nodes which typically become matted. Later an abscess or sinus may form, or there may be progressive fibrosis and eventual calcification. The clinical picture is therefore variable, and the diagnosis is usually only made after excision of a node. If a tuberculous ('cold') abscess and sinus form, excision should be carried out and incision is contraindicated.

Diagnosis depends on finding granulomas (Figure 14.14) in which mycobacteria should be demonstrable by Ziehl–Nielsen staining or by immunofluorescence using auramine-rhodamine.

However, infection by non-tuberculous mycobacteria even in immunocompetent children is likely to give rise to poorly defined or irregular granulomas without palisading, or ill-defined aggregates of epithelioid histiocytes. Caseation may not be seen, but there may be areas of necrosis with numerous neutrophils, Ziehl–Nielsen staining is also negative, as described by Pinder and Colville (1992). Culture of the mycobacteria is required, but the tuberculin skin test should be positive unless the patient is severely immunodeficient.

In addition to any surgery, a course of isoniazid should be given.

Syphilis

The cervical lymph nodes are enlarged, soft and rubbery when the primary chancre is in the mouth or on the lip. They are also involved in the widespread lymphadenopathy characteristic of the secondary stage.

Diagnosis is by finding *Treponema pallidum* in a direct smear from the oral lesion in the primary stage, and thereafter by the serological findings, as discussed earlier (Chapter 8). Lymph node biopsy is not indicated.

Only a few hundred cases of syphilis are detected annually in England, but even when it was more frequent oral lesions were rarely seen and some perhaps go unrecognized.

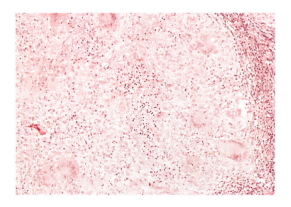

Figure 14.14 Tuberculosis. Epithelioid granulomas and multinucleated giant cells are typical

Cat scratch disease

This infection is very common in the USA and, though rare in Britain, is increasingly frequently found. The history is usually but not invariably of a scratch by a cat, followed by the appearance of a papule which may suppurate, at the site of inoculation. There is mild fever, malaise and regional lymphadenitis, which develops – weeks after exposure. The lymph nodes soften and typically suppurate. Conjunctivitis may be associated: encephalitis is a rare complication.

Microscopically, there is destruction of the architecture of the lymph nodes, necrosis and lymphocytic infiltration with formation of histiocytic granulomas and central suppuration.

These appearances can readily be mistaken for one of the deep mycoses. However, it may be possible to demonstrate the causative organism, *Afipia felis* (a small Gram-negative bacillus) by use of a silver (Warthin–Starry) stain at the site of inoculation or in the lymph nodes. Even if this fails, the clinical picture is characteristic and the diagnosis can be confirmed by a skin (Rose–Hanger) test using a sterilized extract of cat scratch disease pus.

The disease is typically mild and self-limiting but may lead to suppuration and sinus formation. The response to antibacterials is variable and difficult to evaluate in view of spontaneous resolution in many cases. However, Collipp (1992) has reported that treatment with sulphamethoxazole led to prompt healing without suppuration in 71 children, whereas 30 patients given other antimicrobials had more prolonged disease and, in 7 of them, suppuration that required drainage.

Lyme disease

Lyme disease is caused by a spirochaete, *Borrelia burgdorferi*, which is transmitted by insects, particularly by deer ticks. The disease is worldwide.

Clinically, the chief manifestations are a rash, enlarged regional lymph nodes, fever and often other systemic symptoms. The rash (erythema chronicum migrans) is characteristic and spreads outwards from the site of the insect bite. The main chronic effect is arthritis, particularly of the knees. The onset may be within weeks or more than a year after acquisition of the infection. Involvement of the temporomandibular joint is rare.

Neurological complications develop in about 15% of patients. They are typically heralded by neck pain and stiffness, and include facial palsy or other cranial nerve lesions.

Diagnosis is by the clinical picture and confirmed serologically or sometimes by demonstration of the spirochaete by means of silver stains in a skin biopsy.

The spirochaete is sensitive to penicillin or tetracycline which should be given as early as possible. However, joint pain may recur or destructive arthritis may develop later.

Infectious mononucleosis

Infection by the Epstein–Barr virus causes a self-limiting lymphoproliferative disorder characterized by polyclonal activation of B lymphocytes. In children, especially, there is generalized lymphadenopathy, typically with conspicuous enlargement of the cervical nodes, sore throat and fever. In adolescents, lymphadenopathy may be less conspicuous and there is a vague illness with fever. In the anginose form of the disease, there is a sore throat, palatal petechiae, tonsillar exudate and pharyngeal oedema which may be severe. The clinical features are distinctive in most cases, but rarely there is more persistent lymphadenopathy which may mimic a lymphoma. Confusion may be compounded if a lymph node is taken for biopsy, as the appearances can also be mistaken for those of a lymphoma.

Syndromes clinically similar to infectious mononucleosis can also result from toxoplasmal, cytomegalovirus or HIV infection.

Microscopically, the lymph node architecture is severely distorted or even destroyed and replaced by gross follicular hyperplasia with irregular germinal centres containing transforming lymphocytes which may show mitoses. Many histiocytes and large immunoblastic cells, which may resemble Reed–Sternberg cells, are associated. Lymphocytes may infiltrate the pericapsular tissues.

The diagnosis can be made on the microscopy of this lymphoma-like picture by a specialist, but is more likely to be made by a peripheral blood picture showing the atypical (monocyte-like) lymphocytes, a heterophil antibody (Paul–Bunnell) test and, if necessary, demonstration of a raised titre of EBV antibodies.

Patients are prone to characteristic macular rashes on the trunk when given ampicillin or amoxycillin, but are not necessarily allergic to penicillin.

Acquired immune deficiency syndrome

Lymphadenopathy is one of the most frequent manifestations of HIV infection, as discussed later in this chapter. Soon after infection there may be a transient glandular fever-like illness or later there may be generalized and persistent lymphadenopathy. Current estimates suggest that over 50% of patients with lymphadenopathy as the sole manifestation of HIV infection will develop full-blown AIDS within less than 4 years.

Lymph node biopsy is not recommended for diagnosis. The microscopic appearances are described later, as are clinical features which may suggest the diagnosis.

Toxoplasmosis

Toxoplasma gondii is a common intestinal parasite of many domestic animals, particularly cats. It is a low-grade pathogen but can affect previously healthy persons, particularly young women. Infection can be acquired by ingestion of oocytes and four main types of disease can result:

1. Acute toxoplasmosis in normal children or adults can cause a disease very similar to infectious mononucleosis, with cervical lymphadenopathy as the most common feature. Parotid swelling has also been described. Atypical lymphocytes are present in the blood, but there is no heterophil antibody production. Usually the infection is self-limiting.
2. In immunodeficient patients, such as those with AIDS, toxoplasmosis causes disseminated disease and, particularly, encephalitis.
3. In pregnant women, toxoplasmosis is an important cause of fetal abnormalities.
4. Toxoplasmal chorioretinitis with impairment or loss of sight is usually a result of congenital infection, but can also occasionally result from severe infections in previously healthy adults.

The microscopic appearances are not in themselves diagnostic. However, follicular hyperplasia, sinus histiocytosis and scattered foci (rather than granulomas) of pale histiocytes standing out conspicuously against a dense background of lymphocytes, is strongly suggestive (Figures 14.15 and 14.16). Merozoites are rarely seen.

The diagnosis is confirmed serologically by a high or rising titre of antibodies or by several other immunological methods.

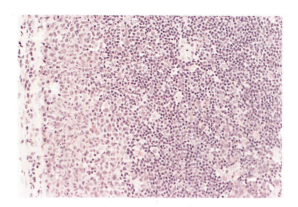

Figure 14.15   Toxoplasmosis. Sinus histiocytosis has produced a picture simulating a lymphoma

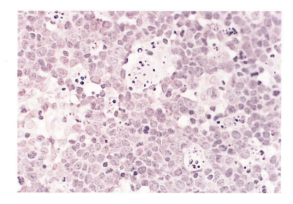

Figure 14.16   Toxoplasmosis. Large, pale-staining histiocytes contain angular, haematoxyphilic fragments

Treatment
This is required only for severe infections and is with pyrimethamine and a sulphonamide.

Mucocutaneous lymph node syndrome (Kawasaki's disease)

Kawasaki's disease is endemic in Japan and there have been outbreaks in Hawaii and the USA. In Britain, it causes approximately 100 deaths per annum.

The distribution of cases suggests that the disease may be an infection, but no agent has been identified with certainty.

Children aged under 5 years are mostly affected. Typical features are a generalized, often morbilliform rash and erythematous stomatitis. Swelling and cracking of the lips and pharyngitis quickly follow and the palms and soles become red, swollen and indurated. A unilateral mass of cervical lymph nodes is characteristic, abdominal symptoms are common and change of mood ('extreme misery') is typical. Approximately 20% of patients develop heart disease. The overall mortality is 1–3% as a result of heart failure secondary to coronary artery disease or dysrhythmias secondary to myocardial ischaemia.

The diagnosis may sometimes be made early by lymph node biopsy showing microscopic vasculitis, associated with fibrinous thrombi in small vessels and patchy necrosis. Arteritis resembling polyarteritis nodosa has its main effects on the coronary arteries. However, the diagnosis is more likely to be made from the clinical and, particularly, the electrocardiographic findings.

There is no specific treatment, but aspirin, despite the possible risk of Reye's syndrome, should be given to reduce vascular damage and thrombotic phenomena. Intravenous gamma globulin has also been advocated.

Sinus histiocytosis

Sinus histiocytosis is typically seen in nodes draining carcinomas, but is a rare cause of cervical lymphadenopathy. It is characterized by prominent distended lymphoid sinusoids. The sinuses are filled with histiocytes and the endothelial cells are often grossly hypertrophied. The condition is benign.

Sinus histiocytosis with massive lymphadenopathy (Rosai–Dorfman disease)

This disease is also rare, but particularly affects Blacks. As the name implies, lymphadenopathy can

be gross. Salivary glands and other sites are occasionally involved. Fever and neutrophil leucocytosis may be associated, but most cases resolve spontaneously.

Microscopically, the lymph node sinuses are filled with very large histiocytes, some of which have engulfed lymphocytes, and there is a reactive plasmacytosis.

Giant (angiofollicular) lymph node hyperplasia (Castleman's disease)

This rare condition usually affects the thorax, but can occasionally cause a cervical mass resembling a lymphoma. Its cause is unknown, but it can be a complication of HIV infection.

Microscopically, the salient features are gross hyperplasia of lymphoid follicles, with the lymphocytes forming tight concentric layers round blood vessels with swollen endothelial cells which frequently proliferate (Figure 14.17). The interfollicular tissue is highly vascular. Several variants of this picture have been described and in the rare plasma cell type there may be monoclonal immunoglobulin production and other abnormalities.

Though the condition is benign, the mass may be so large that resection may be justified. This not merely confirms the diagnosis, but is usually

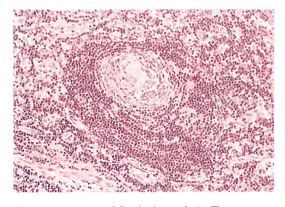

Figure 14.17 Angiofollicular hyperplasia. The thickened, hyalinized vessels and lymphoid hyperplasia can be seen

curative. Otherwise a short course of high-dosage corticosteroids or a single other immunosuppressive drug is effective, but combination cytotoxic chemotherapy should be avoided and the condition is not radiosensitive.

Lymphomatous change is a rare but recognized complication and malignant blood vessel tumours are another. In AIDS, giant lymph node hyperplasia may be associated with Kaposi's sarcoma.

Angiolymphoid hyperplasia with eosinophils (epithelioid haemangioma, Kimura's disease and related diseases)

Kimura's disease is rare in the West but common in China, Japan and Singapore. It is characterized by mucosal or cutaneous nodules which can be mistaken clinically for lymph nodes. However, these nodules, when in the mouth, are more likely to resemble pyogenic granulomas. Involvement of the parotid and submandibular glands and of the cervical lymph nodes has been described in Oriental patients.

Microscopically, there is proliferation of lymphoid tissue and blood vessels leading to formation of thick-walled capillaries (Figures 14.18 and 14.19). Eosinophils are conspicuous in the stroma and may form dense foci with central necrosis. In addition to

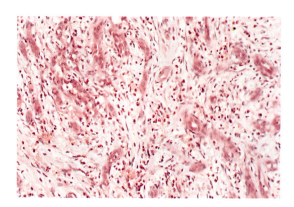

Figure 14.19 Angiolymphoid hyperplasia with eosinophils. High-power view of central area shows thick-walled capillaries with prominent endothelial cells, and eosinophils in the interstitial tissue

peripheral blood eosinophilia, serum IgE levels are frequently raised.

Excision is curative but may have to be repeated.

In the West, lesions with a somewhat similar histological picture may be seen, but peripheral eosinophilia is absent. Lymphoid hyperplasia is less prominent, but vascular proliferation may be conspicuous. These lesions should usually be categorized as epithelioid haemangiomas.

Phenytoin and other drug-associated lymphadenopathies

Of the many possible side effects of phenytoin, lymphadenopathy may rarely develop within a few weeks or months, but more frequently after long-term treatment. Lymphadenopathy caused by phenytoin (unlike that caused by many other drugs) is not generally associated with serum sickness-like symptoms of fever, rashes and joint pains. The importance of phenytoin-associated lymphadenopathy is that the microscopic changes can mimic a lymphoma.

Cervical lymph nodes are frequently first affected, but lymphadenopathy usually becomes widespread. The microscopic appearances are varied, but the nodal architecture can be completely obliterated by a pleomorphic picture with proliferation of large immunoblast-like cells which may

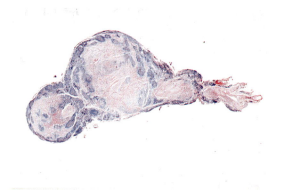

Figure 14.18 Angiolymphoid hyperplasia with eosinophils. Low-power view shows a lobulated mass with a rim of lymphocytes surrounding a central area of vascular and smooth muscle proliferation

be binucleate or multinucleate, and appearances which can closely mimic Hodgkin's disease. There also appears to be a slight risk of lymphoma if the condition is allowed to progress.

The diagnosis is likely to be made from the history of treatment with phenytoin, or suggested from the finding of associated gingival hyperplasia. If the latter is absent and the patient fails to disclose the necessary information about drug treatment so that lymph node biopsy is carried out, an expert opinion is needed to distinguish these changes from lymphoma.

Substitution of phenytoin with another anticonvulsant such as carbamazepine should allow the lymphadenopathy to subside and confirm the diagnosis.

Other drugs which can cause lymphadenopathy include penicillin (rarely), phenylbutazone (virtually obsolete) and some other non-steroidal anti-inflammatory drugs, and some antimalarials. As mentioned earlier, lymphadenopathy with these drugs is frequently associated with serum sickness-like features.

Immunodeficiency diseases

In immune deficiency states the activity of one or more components of the immune system is defective. The main consequence is that, in the more severe types, the ability to combat infections is so impaired that they are the chief cause of death. This is shown strikingly in the acquired immune deficiency syndrome (AIDS), which is both transmissible and exceptionally severe.

Immune deficiencies can be primary or acquired (Table 14.5) and can affect B or T lymphocytes, or both. However, the role of T lymphocytes in regulating B lymphocyte activity often means that a T cell defect affects antibody production. Alternatively, there can be failures of production of individual antibodies such as IgA or of complement components.

Clinically, any patient who develops recurrent infections, particularly if the infections .respond poorly to treatment or are caused by otherwise harmless microbes (opportunistic infections), must be suspected of being immunodeficient.

Table 14.5   Important causes of immunodeficiency

PRIMARY (GENETIC)

T or B lymphocyte defects (Swiss-type agammaglobulinaemia, Di George's syndrome, etc.)

IgA deficiency

Complement component deficiencies

SECONDARY (ACQUIRED)

Infections – HIV, other severe viral or bacterial infections, malaria, etc.

Drug induced – immunosuppressive and anticancer treatment

Malnutrition (worldwide a major cause of immunodeficiency)

Cancer (particularly of lymphoreticular cells)

Diabetes mellitus

The severe primary immunodeficiencies are rare and, unless a marrow transplant can be given, are usually fatal in childhood. The main causes of *severe* immunodeficiency in the developed world are HIV infection and immunosuppressive treatment for organ transplantation or other purposes. Many cancer patients are also severely immunodeficient as a result both of the neoplasm and of the cytotoxic drugs used for its treatment.

Oral manifestations of immunodeficiencies

The main effect, as mentioned earlier, is the abnormal susceptibility to infections, particularly candidosis or viral infections such as herpes. Similar but generally less severe infectious complications to those seen in AIDS are to be expected and are usually the chief cause of death. Deficiency of complement components, particularly C3, also increases susceptibility to infection but is rare.

Acquired immune deficiency syndrome (AIDS)

The acquired immune deficiency syndrome is epidemic in parts of the USA and Africa. It is worldwide in distribution and several millions have been infected. It is almost useless to quote statistics because of the rate at which the disease is spreading. However, by 1992, more than 7000 cases and over 4000 deaths from this cause had been reported in Britain, despite the fact that the infection rate is the lowest in Europe. In the USA, cases of AIDS exceeded 100 000 during 1989, but this figure had doubled by 1992. In addition, many times these numbers of persons in all parts of the world have acquired the infection and may be able to transmit it, but have not yet had any clinical effects.

AIDS is transmissible to health care personnel, particularly surgeons, dental surgeons and nurses, via needles or other sharp instruments. However, the risk of acquiring the infection by this means is considerably smaller than that of hepatitis B.

Aetiology

AIDS is caused by a retrovirus, the human immunodeficiency virus (HIV), mainly HIV 1. HIV 2 is as yet only widely prevalent in West Africa. AIDS in the absence of HIV infection is currently a source of controversy.

The chief mode of transmission is by male homosexual activity which accounts for over 70% of cases in Britain. Heterosexual transmission is far less common in the Western world than in Africa. Once infected, pregnant women can transmit the infection to the fetus. Transmission by blood or blood products has caused intravenous drug abusers to be at risk. Many haemophiliacs have acquired the disease from infected blood products but heat treatment of clotting factor concentrates should have eliminated this risk.

The incubation period of AIDS is highly variable and may be related to the infecting dose of virus. In the case of male homosexuals, the incubation period is on average approximately 5 years, but study of sera stored before the disease was recognized shows that it can be as long as 14 years. Testing of apparently healthy infected persons also shows deterioration of immune function long before the disease becomes clinically apparent and it is still not clear whether all those who develop prodromal signs, such as generalized lymphadenopathy, will develop the full, lethal syndrome.

Immunology

The human immunodeficiency virus directly infects lymphocytes and other cells which carry the CD4 marker. In particular, the virus depresses the number of T helper (CD4) cells and reverses the ratio of helper to suppressor lymphocytes. Macrophages and monocytes can engulf the virus and some monocytes also express the CD4 receptor to which the virus binds. These cells probably have a major role in the propagation and pathogenesis of the infection.

Antibody is produced in response to the virus but is not protective and there is no evidence as yet that the virus is ever eliminated from the body. Antibodies to HIV indicate only that infection has been acquired and all seropositive persons must be assumed to be capable of transmitting the virus. Though the detection of these antibodies is often misnamed, by the press, 'the AIDS test', it is of little value in predicting the development of full-blown disease. The immune responses and serological consequences of HIV are not as yet clear, but it has become apparent that, rarely, antibodies to HIV may not appear for periods of up to 3 years after infection. In others, antibodies may disappear from the blood late in the disease. Antibody detection is not therefore 100% reliable, but has been a useful means of detecting the majority of HIV-infected persons, particularly among blood donors.

Detection viral antigens, such as p24, in the blood provide a more direct and reliable indicator of infection. Moreover, minute amounts of the virus in the form of provirus DNA in lymphocytes can be detected by using the polymerase chain reaction. The presence or absence of viral antigens can, therefore, be correlated with the serological findings and can, for example, be used when the history and clinical features are at variance with the serological findings.

The main effect of depletion of T helper cells is deepening depression of cell-mediated immunity. This can be demonstrated by such means as declining responses of lymphocytes to antigens *in vitro*, and impaired or absent delayed hypersensitivity responses, long before any clinical signs of the disease appear. Apparently paradoxically, there is also polyclonal B lymphocyte activation resulting in hypergammaglobulinaemia and autoantibody production. The main effect of the immunodeficiency and chief cause of death is infection by a wide variety of microbes, particularly opportunistics.

In addition to its effects on the immune system, the human immunodeficiency virus also attacks the central nervous system, cells of which carry receptors for the virus.

Clinical aspects

The possible courses of events after infection by HIV are shown in Figure 14.20 but, as mentioned earlier, it is still uncertain whether any symptomless carriers of the virus will ultimately remain healthy.

As can be seen from Figure 14.20, the earliest clinical manifestation of infection can be a transient illness resembling glandular fever, associated with antibody production. Thereafter, in progressive cases, markers of declining cell-mediated immunity eventually become detectable and later various clinical syndromes, previously termed AIDS-related complex (ARC), may develop. The classification of HIV infection by stages has been developed by the Center for Disease Control (CDC) but a new, combined WHO/CDC clinical classification has been proposed to include specific diseases and immunological findings. Generalized lymphadenopathy syndrome (GLS), in which there is widespread persistent enlargement of lymph nodes, is a typical early sign of developing disease. However, the course of AIDS is highly variable and none of the prodromal symptoms appears to be obligatory.

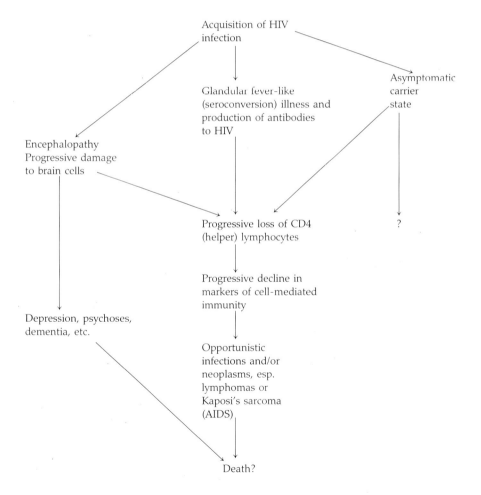

Figure 14.20   Some typical consequences of acquisition of HIV infection

The first clinical sign may therefore be *Pneumocystis carinii* pneumonia or Kaposi's sarcoma.

The full syndrome of AIDS is characterized by multiple infections by bacteria, fungi, parasites and viruses (Table 14.6). Many of these infections, such as *P. carinii* pneumonia, are opportunistic and virtually unknown in normal persons.

Though infections are the main cause of death, there is also a greatly increased incidence of tumours, particularly Kaposi's sarcoma and lymphomas which frequently affect the oral or perioral tissues. In normal persons these tumours are not merely uncommon or rare but are particularly rare in the oral tissues.

The second major manifestation of AIDS is, in addition to opportunistic infections or tumours involving the central nervous system, neuropsychiatric disease which can range from psychi-atric disturbance resembling depression, to dementia and death. These neurological disorders may be associated with, but can develop in the absence of, immunodeficiency.

A third but lesser manifestation of AIDS in some patients is autoimmune disease, particularly thrombocytopenic purpura or, less frequently, a disease resembling lupus erythematosus.

Once AIDS has developed, the outcome is invariably fatal usually within 2–3 years, though the course of the disease may be modified to some degree by drugs such as zidovudine and vigorous treatment of the infections.

The terminal stages of AIDS can be horrifying. A young patient may be emaciated with persistent diarrhoea, suffering a multiplicity of infections, covered with skin lesions, breathless from *P. carinii* pneumonia, frequently with a malignant tumour, and sometimes also blind and demented.

Table 14.6   Important opportunistic infections in AIDS

VIRAL
Herpes simplex
Varicella zoster
Cytomegalovirus
JC virus

BACTERIAL
Campylobacter spp.
Legionellosis
Pseudomonas aeruginosa
Staphylococcus aureus
Streptococcus pneumoniae
Haemophilus influenzae
Mycobacterium tuberculosis
M. avium-intracellulare
Other non-tuberculous mycobacterioses
Shigellosis

MYCOSES
Aspergillosis
Candidosis
Coccidioidomycosis
Cryptococcosis
Histoplasmosis
Mucormycosis

PARASITIC AND OTHER
Cryptosporidiosis
Giardiasis
Isosporosis
Microsporidiosis
Pneumocystis carinii

Orofacial manifestations of AIDS

More than 75% of patients with AIDS have orofacial manifestations, and thrush is a common early sign of the immunodeficiency. Orofacial manifestations of AIDS are listed in Table 14.7 and discussed in more detail below.

Prediction of progression of AIDS

The current estimate is that at least 60% of HIV seropositive individuals will develop the disease, but increasing evidence of silent infections with greatly delayed antibody production and retrospective studies of 'pre-AIDS' stored sera may cause such estimates to appear modest.

Haematological markers, indicative of progression to AIDS, include the presence of viral antigens in the serum, high beta 2 microglobulin levels and failure of or greatly depressed antigen-induced interferon gamma production. Fewer than 0.2×10^9 CD4 (T helper) lymphocytes per litre or a total lymphocyte count of less than 1×10^9 per litre represent advanced disease.

Clinical indicators of a poor prognosis are oral thrush or herpes zoster or other persistent or recurrent infections, hairy leukoplakia, unexplained constitutional symptoms, cutaneous anergy and

Table 14.7 Oral disease in HIV infection

INFECTIONS
Fungal
  Thrush and other forms of candidosis
  Mucosal lesions of deep mycoses
  (cryptococcosis, histoplasmosis, etc.)

Viral
  Herpes simplex
  Herpes zoster or varicella
  Oral hairy leucoplakia (EBV-associated)

Bacterial
  Mycobacterium tuberculosis and non-tuberculous
  ('atypical') mycobacterioses
  Klebsiella pneumoniae
  Escherichia coli
  E. cloacae

TUMOURS
Lymphomas
Kaposi's sarcoma

SALIVARY GLANDS
Swelling (cystic, proliferative or neoplastic)
Xerostomia

NEUROLOGICAL
Facial palsy
Trigeminal neuropathy

OTHERS
Purpura
Pigmentation
Major aphthae
Necrotizing gingivitis
Accelerated periodontitis
Delayed wound healing

lymphadenopathy. Between approximately 20% and 70% of such patients can be expected to develop full-blown disease within a period of less than 5 years.

The possibility of transmission of HIV infection during oral surgery is a source of anxiety. Oral infections and other features of AIDS or its prodromes may enable patients to be recognized. A young adult male who develops thrush for no apparent reason is likely to have AIDS, but if he has oral Kaposi's sarcoma it is virtually pathognomonic. However, there are many more patients who are infective but without overt signs to suggest the possibility. At the time of writing there may be 20 000 or more antibody-positive, potentially

infective persons in Britain and the number rises each month.

All patients must now, therefore, be regarded as potentially infective and treated with full aseptic precautions as for hepatitis B. The only small crumbs of comfort are that HIV is considerably less easily transmitted than hepatitis B.

Most health care workers who have developed AIDS have not acquired it as a result of their occupation. However, a few nurses have become infected as a result of needle-stick injuries and accidentally injecting themselves with a significant amount of infected blood. By contrast, many other needle-stick injuries have apparently failed to transmit the infection.

As to the risk to dental and general surgeons, at least two of the latter in the Western world are known to have died from the disease, acquired at operation. By contrast, only one dental surgeon is known to have acquired the disease as a consequence of his occupation. He was working in New York (by far the highest incidence area in the Western world), did not practise a high standard of infection control and had had many needle-stick injuries. No other dental surgeons, even in high incidence areas, are known to have acquired the disease occupationally.

Nevertheless, as mentioned earlier, all patients must be regarded and treated as potentially infective. Though the risk of acquiring AIDS during dental treatment may be very small, the consequences of doing so are so appalling as to be avoided by all means possible. Currently, the chance of acquisition of hepatitis B is considerably greater, because of its greater prevalence and ease of transmission, but is avoidable by immunization.

Oral lesions in AIDS

In a review of 2235 HIV-positive homosexual or bisexual men in San Francisco, Feigal *et al.* (1991) found that the most frequent oral lesions were hairy leucoplakia (18.7%), thrush (6.6%) or erythematous candidosis (2.1%), Kaposi's sarcoma (1.6%) and oral ulcers (2%). However, the frequency of such lesions varies in other groups. Kaposi's sarcoma, for example, is particularly common in homosexual men.

Candidosis   Oral thrush may be seen in over 70% of patients at some stage. It is indicative of declining immunity, and other infections may be associated or are likely to follow. Thrush may be concurrent with oral herpes to produce a confusing clinical picture.

In approximately 50% of patients with HIV-associated thrush, AIDS is likely to develop within 5 years.

Most of the other types of candidosis, such as angular stomatitis, generalized mucosal erythema or hyperplastic candidosis, have also been reported in AIDS patients.

Viral infections   Herpetic stomatitis is less common than might be expected. Severe orofacial zoster may be indicative of a poor prognosis.

Cytomegalovirus can be found in some oral ulcers and the possible role of the Epstein–Barr virus in hairy leucoplakia is discussed below.

Papillomaviruses have been isolated from proliferative lesions, such as verruca vulgaris, condyloma acuminatum and focal epithelial hyperplasia in patients with AIDS.

Bacterial infections   A variety of infections by bacteria which rarely affect the oral tissues, such as *Klebsiella pneumoniae*, *Enterobacter cloacae* and *Escherichia coli*, have been reported.

In the later stages there may be oral lesions secondary to systemic infections, particularly myco-bacterial ulcers.

Deep mycoses   Histoplasmosis or cryptococcosis can give rise to proliferative or ulcerative lesions. Histoplasmosis can also destroy the adrenal glands and occasionally cause Addison's disease with oral hyperpigmentation.

Hairy leucoplakia   This lesion, characteristic of HIV infection, is so called because hair-like filaments of keratin may extend from the surface, but more commonly the whitish surface has a vertically corrugated surface. The plaque is soft, usually painless and is most frequently seen along the lateral borders of the tongue. It has been discussed more fully in Chapter 9.

The chief importance of hairy leucoplakia is as an index of prognosis. Over 80% of patients with this lesion are likely to develop full-blown AIDS within 3 years. However, hairy leucoplakia can also rarely be seen in immunodeficient patients such as those receiving renal transplants and does not appear to be unique to HIV infection.

Surgical excision of hairy leucoplakia is not indicated.

Tumours   Nearly 50% of patients with AIDS have a malignant tumour at the time of presentation. By far the most frequent are Kaposi's sarcoma and non-Hodgkin lymphomas. Unlike non-AIDS patients these tumours are particularly frequent in the head and neck region.

The aetiology of AIDS-associated tumours is unknown, though it is suspected that they may be viral and secondary to the immunodeficiency.

Kaposi's sarcoma   This tumour is particularly common in male homosexuals with AIDS, but uncommon in intravenous drug abusers and rare in haemophiliacs who have acquired the infection from contaminated blood products.

Clinically, a common oral site is the hard palate where the tumour forms a purple area or, later, a nodule which bleeds readily. Kaposi's sarcoma in the mouth, particularly in a young male who is not receiving immunosuppressive treatment, is virtually pathognomonic of AIDS. Kaposi's sarcoma has been discussed more fully in Chapter 13.

Non-Hodgkin lymphomas   AIDS-related lymphomas can develop in intra-oral sites, in salivary glands or in cervical lymph nodes. Typical sites within the mouth are the palate or alveolar ridge, where the tumours form soft painless swellings which do not ulcerate unless traumatized.

Microscopically, these tumours frequently resemble Burkitt's lymphoma and are of intermediate or, more frequently, high-grade malignancy as discussed earlier.

Lymphadenopathy

Enlargement of lymph nodes is particularly characteristic of AIDS and its prodromes, especially the early glandular fever-like syndrome and the later generalized lymphadenopathy syndrome (GLS). Cervical lymphadenopathy is probably the most common head and neck manifestation of HIV infection.

Microscopically, typical findings are smaller numbers of T-helper cells in the paracortical region associated with greater numbers of T-suppressor cells there and in the follicles. Follicles may initially be hyperplastic but later undergo involution. The lymph nodes become virtually or entirely functionless.

Enlargement of the cervical lymph nodes may also be due to lymphomas.

Autoimmune disease

The most common autoimmune phenomenon in AIDS is thrombocytopenic purpura. This can give rise to purple patches in the mouth and may be mistaken for Kaposi's sarcoma. As with other types of purpura, prolonged bleeding may follow surgery.

Other autoimmune diseases reported in AIDS are lupus erythematosus, but salivary gland disease resembling Sjögren's syndrome does not seem to have a similar basis.

Gingivitis and periodontitis

HIV-related periodontal disease includes necrotizing gingivitis and accelerated periodontitis.

Salivary gland disease

The main effects, which are described in more detail in Chapter 11, include:

● parotitis, possibly due to Epstein–Barr virus or cytomegalovirus, appears to affect children with AIDS particularly
● a Sjögren-like syndrome with xerostomia in adults, though autoantibodies characteristic of this disease are lacking
● parotid swellings due to benign lymphoepithelial lesion, which are frequently cystic, bilateral and identifiable by CT scanning.

Parotid swelling due to Kaposi's sarcoma has also been reported but it is rare in the salivary glands.

Recognition of parotid cysts or microscopic diagnosis of Sjögren-like changes, particularly in a young adult male, are important indicators of HIV infection of which the surgeon should be aware when dealing with a tumour-like lesion of salivary glands.

Neurological complications

Orofacial effects include facial palsy and trigeminal neuropathy.

Miscellaneous oral lesions

● Mucosal ulcers – these include major aphthae and can be a troublesome feature which can interfere with eating and accelerate deterioration of health
● Necrotizing oral ulceration of an ill-defined nature has also been reported and aphthae-like lesions are common oral signs of HIV infection
● Oral hyperpigmentation – in a few cases, pigmentation may be secondary to Addison's disease due to fungal destruction of the adrenals; alternatively, it appears to be a complication of treatment with zidovudine or to be due to an unknown mechanism.

No doubt, with the passage of time, yet other orofacial manifestations of AIDS will be reported. AIDS-related arthritis, for example, was only firmly identified approximately 7 years after the disease was first characterized.

Surgical considerations in AIDS and its prodromes

With the growing prevalence of HIV infection and the severity of its consequences, it is overwhelmingly important to the oral surgeon to recognize the oral and perioral manifestations. Though surgical intervention is rarely indicated for AIDS-related lesions, oral surgery may be necessary for treatment of concomitant disease. Prevention of cross-infection, as discussed earlier, and awareness of the patient's low resistance to secondary infection are then major considerations. However, it does not appear that patients with HIV infection are particularly prone to infective complications from dental procedures such as extractions. Occasionally, biopsy of a lesion, particularly if it proves to be a Kaposi's sarcoma, may suggest hitherto unsuspected HIV infection.

Primary IgA deficiency

IgA deficiency is common in that it affects approximately 1 in 700 of the population. The chief effects are:

- recurrent respiratory infections (especially if IgG_2 is also lacking)
- atopic disease (frequently)
- connective tissue disease (uncommonly).

Despite the fact that IgA is the only antibody secreted in the saliva in significant amounts, IgA deficiency may not be associated with any increase in frequency of oral infections. This may in part be due to secretion of other immunoglobulins in the saliva when IgA is absent. However, Porter and Scully (1993) have reported that in 39 of these children aphthae-like ulcers were present in 61%, thrush in 25%, recurrent herpes labialis in 25%, and only 9% had no orofacial lesions.

Hereditary angio-oedema

Hereditary angio-oedema causes localized areas of oedema resembling allergic angio-oedema, but results from a genetically determined deficiency of C1 esterase inhibitor. Deficiency of this enzyme results in prolonged complement activation and release of kinin-like substances, typically in response to minor trauma including oral surgery. Oedema typically affects the oral and perioral regions, where it can endanger the airway.

Significant clinical manifestations frequently do not appear until later childhood or adolescence and the abdomen or extremities are other sites which may be affected. Abdominal pain, nausea or a rash may herald an attack. In the absence of treatment, the mortality may be as high as 30%.

The most effective treatment is with the androgenic steroids, such as stanozolol, which should be given daily, usually 2.5–10 mg for an adult.

Allergic angio-oedema

Allergic angio-oedema is typically an IgE-mediated reaction and can be precipitated by drugs such as penicillin or antisera. Acute oedematous swelling frequently affects the face and neck region and can endanger the airway. Such reactions should be managed as for anaphylactic emergencies with adrenaline plus intravenous antihistamines or corticosteroids. Mild cases may respond to oral antihistamines.

Granulomatous diseases

The term granuloma is traditionally used *clinically* for lesions characterized by proliferation of granulation tissue as in apical granulomas or, in a more specialized sense, for 'midline granulomas', as described below. *Histologically*, the term granuloma refers only to conditions where there is formation of tuberculosis-like follicles microscopically. These consist of rounded collections of large, pale histiocytes ('epithelioid cells'), sometimes surrounded by lymphocytes and often containing giant cells. The causes of this type of reaction are heterogeneous: it is usually a manifestation of cell-mediated immunity, but the immunological abnormalities associated with these diseases are very varied. The more important examples are shown in Table 14.8. Many of them can affect the cervical lymph nodes (as described above) or the mouth.

Midline granuloma syndrome (lethal midline granuloma, midfacial destructive disease, etc.)

Midline granulomas are granulomas mainly in the sense of the clinical appearance of granulomatous destruction of tissues, particularly of the nasal cavity, but sometimes extending into the mouth.

Table 14.8   Important examples of granulomatous diseases

INFECTIONS
Tuberculosis and non-tuberculous mycobacterioses
Leprosy
Syphilis
Deep mycoses, particularly histoplasmosis,
cryptococcosis, blastomycosis and coccidioidomycosis
Cat scratch disease
Toxoplasmosis

REACTIVE
Foreign body reactions
Secondary to carcinoma or radiotherapy

UNKNOWN CAUSES
Wegener's granulomatosis
Sarcoidosis
Crohn's disease
Orofacial granulomatosis

Proliferation, ulceration and crusting of the nasal or paranasal tissues typically leads to destruction (occasionally gross) of the midfacial tissues. Later, other organs are involved and the outcome is typically fatal. One cause of this previously mysterious syndrome has now been identified as being a lymphoma, but since it is not clinically distinguishable from Wegener's granulomatosis it is also discussed here.

Specific infections such as tuberculosis, leprosy or the deep mycoses may rarely produce a somewhat similar clinical picture but only the idiopathic types are discussed here. These comprise two main diseases, namely:

● Wegener's granulomatosis – a form of necrotizing vasculitis
● peripheral T cell lymphomas.

Wegener's granulomatosis

Wegener's granulomatosis, in its fully developed form, typically comprises the triad of granulomatous inflammation of the nasal region and pulmonary and lung involvement.

Wegener's granulomatosis is frequently (but unjustifiably) classified with the connective tissue

diseases, but there are no immunological abnormalities linking it with those diseases. Neutrophil anticytoplasmic antibodies have been detected in Wegener's granulomatosis, but are not specific to it.

Clinically, men seem to be more frequently affected and the peak age incidence is between 40 and 55 years.

Early features of Wegener's granulomatosis typically consist of granulomatous inflammation and variable degrees of destruction of the nasal cavity. Later, destruction of the nasal septum can lead to a saddle-nose deformity. Wegener's granulomatosis can also give rise to oral ulcers or to a distinctive type of oral lesion, namely a proliferative gingivitis with a granular surface and deep red in colour. It has been described as 'strawberry gums' and can involve a few or many teeth. It can form the earliest clinical manifestation of the disease and, after confirmation by biopsy, can allow treatment to be started at an early stage. Approximately 10% of patients with Wegener's granulomatosis have oral lesions.

Microscopically, there is widespread inflammation with a mixed cellular picture and, frequently, numerous eosinophils. However, an essential feature is a necrotizing vasculitis of small arteries, associated with giant cells (Figure 14.21). The giant cells are not necessarily directly involved in the vasculitis and may as frequently be found in the adjacent tissues. They are typically compact with four or five nuclei and an irregular outline, but may resemble Langhans giant cells. Granulomas, though characteristic of this disease, are inconspicuous, usually difficult to find and rarely seen in

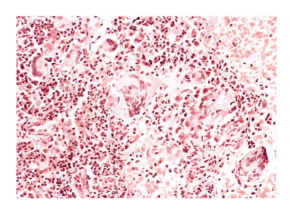

Figure 14.21   Wegener's granulomatosis. Multinucleate giant cells can be seen in the dense acute-on-chronic inflammatory infiltrate

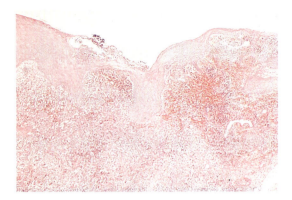

Figure 14.22   Wegener's granulomatosis. A gingival biopsy shows epithelial hyperplasia and inflammation

oral biopsies, as are foci of necrosis and micro-abscesses (Devaney *et al.*, 1990). Biopsies of gingival lesions typically show only the giant cells and are unlikely to show vasculitis, since arteries of sufficient size are unlikely to be included. In addition, gingival tissues show superficial proliferation throwing the epithelium up into folds which produce the granulomatous appearance seen clinically (Figure 14.22).

Diagnosis and management

Later manifestations are typically pulmonary cavitation, and renal disease which is likely to be fatal. Joint pains are common and rashes are sometimes a feature. The diagnosis must be confirmed by biopsy at the earliest possible moment and detection of neutrophil anticytoplasmic antibodies. Examination of the nasopharynx, chest radiographs, renal function tests and, if appropriate, lung biopsy should also be carried out. Haematuria is likely to indicate glomerulonephritis and a poor prognosis.

Early treatment with cytotoxic drugs such as cyclophosphamide or azathioprine may be successful. Arrest of the disease with cotrimoxazole has been reported on several occasions but remains a controversial treatment (Hoffman *et al.*, 1992).

Peripheral T cell lymphomas

Some of these tumours, when in the nasopharyngeal region, can cause midfacial destruction.

The cellular picture is pleomorphic and a variety of terms had been given to these lesions until the introduction of T cell markers confirmed their nature. Confusion has arisen particularly because of the tendency in these lymphomas for the tumour cells to surround or destroy blood vessels and so closely mimic true vasculitis.

Clinically, these tumours, by their involvement of the nasal passages, are not reliably distinguishable, in their earlier stages, from Wegener's granulomatosis. The age and sex distribution seems also to be similar.

Early features are nasal obstruction and sero-sanguinous discharge from or crusting of the nostrils. In advanced cases, massive destruction of the centre of the face and secondary infection may develop.

Oral lesions, unlike those of Wegener's granulomatosis, typically consist of palatal swelling, which is boggy in character, and ulceration. The latter may consist of no more than a small central crater or result from extensive palatal necrosis. Bone destruction can lead to loosening of upper teeth. Involvement of regional lymph nodes is unusual until the tumour disseminates.

Microscopically, the cellular picture is pleomorphic, with many large or immunoblast-like cells and relatively few small lymphocytes. A striking feature is the angiocentric distribution of the tumour cells and angiodestruction which mimics vasculitis (Figures 14.23 and 14.24). Epithelium may also be invaded and extensive areas of necrosis may be seen. Unlike Wegener's granulomatosis, giant cells are absent and granulocytes few unless infection is superimposed. However, in

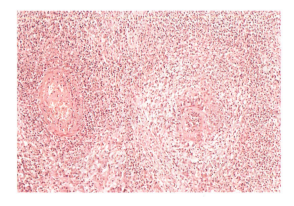

Figure 14.23   Peripheral T cell lymphoma showing angiocentric distribution

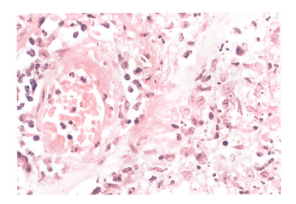

Figure 14.24 Peripheral T cell lymphoma. Angiodestruction by the pleomorphic lymphomatous infiltrate

biopsies from the mouth the picture is frequently obscured by necrosis, superimposed inflammation and consequently a much more mixed cell population.

Diagnosis and management
Adequate biopsy is essential. In the case of palatal involvement the biopsy should extend deeply and be repeated if necessary to obtain material uncontaminated by superimposed inflammation or necrosis.

Some of these tumours have a slow and remittent course, but eventually disseminate. The main principles of treatment are radiotherapy, usually with combination chemotherapy.

Midline granuloma syndromes – summary

Wegener's granulomatosis and nasopharyngeal T cell lymphomas can present indistinguishable nasopharyngeal disease, comprising ulceration, discharge, granulation and crusting. Wegener's granulomatosis can cause destruction of the nasal septum, but T cell lymphomas can ultimately cause more severe midfacial destruction. Extension into the mouth of a T cell lymphoma is most likely to be via the palate which appears ulcerated as a result of perforation. Wegener's granulomatosis, by contrast, can cause a proliferative gingivitis (strawberry

gums) or mucosal ulceration: either may be the presenting feature.

Microscopically, the essential lesion of Wegener's granulomatosis is a necrotizing arteritis with giant cells. T cell lymphomas present a pleomorphic cellular picture, but can show angiocentric and angiodestructive infiltrations which mimic arteritis. Identification of T cells by immunocytochemistry is required. Spread of Wegener's granulomatosis is particularly to the lungs and kidneys. Late-stage nasopharyngeal lymphoma disseminates in a generally similar way to other lymphomas.

Tuberculosis

This infection has been discussed earlier in this chapter and in Chapter 8.

Deep mycoses

Granuloma formation is typical of mycoses such as histoplasmosis, as discussed in Chapter 2.

Sarcoidosis

Sarcoidosis is a chronic disease of unknown cause, in which non-caseating epithelioid cell granulomas form, particularly in the lungs, lymph nodes (especially the hilar nodes), liver, skin (frequently of the face), eyes, bones, nerves and salivary glands.

Oral lesions are uncommon, but the most frequently affected sites are the gingivae, lips, palate and buccal mucosa, usually with painless swelling, or solitary or multiple soft nodules. In over 50% of patients with bilateral hilar lymphadenopathy, biopsy of the minor labial salivary glands shows typical granulomas. Clinically evident involvement of the major salivary glands is uncommon, but can cause tumour-like swelling or so-called Mikulicz's syndrome (Chapter 11).

Microscopically, the essential features of sarcoidosis are non-caseating epithelioid-cell granulomas, sometimes compact and numerous, surrounded by lymphocytes and containing variable numbers of multinucleated giant cells (Figure 14.25).

Many minor abnormalities of immune responses but, in particular, limited depression of cell-mediated immunity (as shown by anergy to some antigens such as tuberculin) and frequently hypergammaglobulinaemia are detectable. Paradoxically, patients are not unusually susceptible to infection, and frequently also treatment with immunosuppressive drugs, namely corticosteroids, is effective.

Diagnosis

This depends on the combined clinical and laboratory findings and, in particular, evidence of pulmonary involvement, biopsy of affected tissue and a positive Kveim test. Granuloma formation in labial salivary glands may obviate the need for pulmonary biopsy and thus facilitate diagnosis.

Treatment

Treatment with systemic corticosteroids is effective but justified only to control pulmonary fibrosis, eye or cerebral lesions or hypercalcaemia.

Crohn's disease

Crohn's disease is of unknown aetiology. It most frequently affects the ileocaecal region causing thickening and/or ulceration. Effects include abdominal pain, variable constipation or diarrhoea and sometimes obstruction and malabsorption.

Many other sites may become involved either before or after gut involvement. Orofacial involvement is relatively frequent and may occasionally also precede abdominal changes. The main effects are diffuse soft or tense swelling of the lips, or mucosal thickening. A cobblestone-like thickening of the buccal mucosa, with fissuring and hyperplastic folds, is characteristic. The gingiva may be erythematous, diffusely enlarged and granular. A minority of patients have painful ragged, linear or aphtha-like oral ulcers. Some patients have glossitis due to iron, folate or vitamin B_{12} deficiency that can result from malabsorption. Abdominal symptoms such as colicky pain, and alternating constipation and diarrhoea, if associated with the characteristic oral changes, are strongly suggestive of Crohn's disease.

Microscopically, oral lesions typically show dilated lymphatics, focal aggregations of lymphocytes and irregular, perivascular mononuclear cell infiltrates

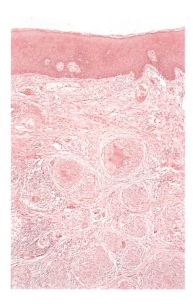

Figure 14.25   Sarcoidosis. Discrete, non-caseating epithelioid granulomas can be seen

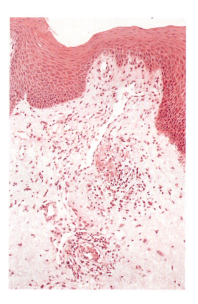

Figure 14.26   Crohn's disease. There is oedema of the superficial corium, lymphangiectasia and loosely-formed epithelioid granulomas

and, in particular, loose, non-caseating granulomas, with or without multinucleate giant cells in the corium, but often few in number (Figure 14.26). The overlying oral epithelium may be normal or ulcerated.

The oral symptoms may resolve when intestinal Crohn's disease is under control, or may respond to oral sulphasalazine or to intralesional injections of triamcinolone. No special precautions are necessary for oral surgery unless the patient is having systemic corticosteroids or is anaemic due to malabsorption.

Melkersson–Rosenthal syndrome and cheilitis granulomatosa

Melkersson–Rosenthal syndrome, in its rare complete form, comprises facial palsy, facial swelling and fissured tongue. The aetiology is unknown.

Zimmer *et al.* (1992) have described 42 patients and reviewed the findings in 220 reported cases. Labial swelling was most common (84% of cases). Initially recurrent, it tends to become persistent due to progressive fibrosis. Facial swelling is less common. The buccal mucosa may have a cobblestone pattern indistinguishable from that in Crohn's disease. Facial palsy, which can be the first sign, develops in up to 36% of cases. It is typically recurrent over many years, is usually unilateral, and can be partial or complete. Permanent weakness of the facial muscles may follow. The tongue is fissured in 50–60% of cases, but has no other special features.

Microscopy
Typical epithelioid granulomas may be close set, contain many large Langhans-type giant cells and be surrounded by lymphocytes. Fibrosis is seen in long-standing cases. The appearance cannot be distinguished microscopically from sarcoidosis and other granulomatous diseases, and like sarcoidosis the serum angiotensin-converting enzyme level may be raised.

Treatment
Persistent lip swelling sometimes responds to intralesional injection of corticosteroids, but relief is usually only temporary. After some years, the lip swelling becomes permanent, in which case surgical reduction may be indicated. Dramatic effectiveness has been claimed for methotrexate (Leicht *et al.*, 1989), but enthusiasm for treatment with cytotoxic drugs may not be widespread.

Isolated swelling of the lips, with similar microscopical appearances, is termed *cheilitis granulomatosa (Miescher's syndrome)*, but may be an incomplete form of Melkersson–Rosenthal syndrome.

Foreign body reactions

Granulomas in response to implantation of foreign bodies are usually readily recognizable because of the clinical circumstances, most frequently implantation of amalgam or extrusion of root canal filling material. Such material is usually visible microscopically either directly or by polarized light. Amalgam frequently, however, causes no reaction in the tissues.

In starch granulomas (from glove powder), the granules should be recognizable by polarized light, but may cause confusion because they can induce caseation. Beryllium and zirconium (once used in dentifrices) can cause widespread and severe foreign body reactions.

Food implanted into the tissues can sometimes cause a florid reaction with giant cells, while leguminous matter can produce a particularly characteristic reaction (pulse granuloma – Chapter 2). A granulomatous reaction can also develop in relation to endogenous material such as keratin (as in ruptured epidermal cysts) or sequestra.

Granulomatous reactions secondary to radiotherapy or chemotherapy

After treatment (usually radiotherapy) of oral carcinoma, regional lymph nodes may become enlarged and firm, as if due to tumour spread. Removal of such a node sometimes shows only a granulomatous (sarcoid-like) reaction, probably as a response to reaction products from treatment of the tumour.

The finding is of no clinical significance apart from the need to reassure the patient.

Granulomatous reactions of unknown cause

The diagnosis of granulomatous reactions in oral tissues frequently depends on ancillary investigations, as suggested earlier. However, once the major causes have been eliminated, a significant proportion of oral granulomatous reactions are of unknown cause. In some, the patient may develop Crohn's disease or sarcoidosis some time later. Many others, however, remain healthy. In some of them the granulomatous reaction appears to result from common food additives such as cinnamon or tartrazine. Such causes can only be confirmed by an exclusion diet which, if faithfully maintained, may sometimes greatly lessen the swellings.

The term *orofacial granulomatosis* has been introduced for this otherwise healthy group. However, this term must not be confused with midline (midfacial) granulomas which are potentially lethal diseases, as discussed above, in view of their utterly different effects and outcomes.

Otherwise, it is essential to maintain regular follow-up to ensure that systemic disease such as Crohn's disease or sarcoidosis is not missed before it reaches an advanced stage. Symptomatic treatment can be given as for granulomatous cheilitis.

Differential diagnosis of oral granulomatous lesions

It is frequently impossible to identify the cause of a granulomatous disease from an oral biopsy alone, but various clinicopathological features are helpful and suggest appropriate systemic and laboratory investigations (Tables 14.9 and 14.10).

Table 14.9   Major features of important granulomatous diseases

Disease	Oral mucosal lesions	Cervical lymph nodes	Salivary glands	Systemic or other lesions
Tuberculosis	Ulceration, usually tongue	−	Rarely	Pulmonary cavitation (reactivation)
Tertiary syphilis (granulomas exceptionally rare)	Leucoplakia (premalignant or malignant)	−	Historically mainly	CVS or CNS disease
Deep mycoses	Ulcers and/or tumour-like lesions	Rarely	Rarely	Usually disseminated disease
Cat scratch disease	−	++	Rarely	Conjunctivitis, fever Encephalitis
Sarcoidosis	Typically gingival swelling	+++	++ esp. minor glands	Lungs; facial palsy; Xerostomia
Crohn's disease	Cobblestone mucosal swellings; ulcers	+	−	Ileitis, fistulas, malabsorption*
Melkersson–Rosenthal syndrome	Lip swelling, fissured tongue	−	Minor glands	Facial palsy
Cheilitis granulomatosa	Lip swelling	−	Minor glands	−
'Orofacial granulomatosis'	Lip or gingival swelling	−	−	−
Wegener's granulomatosis	Gingival swelling; mucosal	−	Rarely	Nose, lung and renal disease
Foreign body reactions	Minor swelling or pigmentation	−	Mainly with tumours†	−

* Malabsorption due to ileal disease can cause anaemias and consequent oral lesions.
† Particularly in Warthin's tumour and occasionally in mucoepidermoid carcinomas.

Table 14.10 Oral features of important granulomatous disease and confirmatory findings

Disease	Oral features of granulomas	Confirmatory tests
Tuberculosis	Numerous epithelioid follicles, Langhans giant cells, caseation, dense peripheral lymphocytic infiltrate	Sputum culture, chest radiograph (bacteria rarely found in oral granulomas)
Sarcoidosis	Many, compact epithelioid follicles, no caseation, peripheral lymphocytic infiltrate	Chest film, labial gland biopsy, blood picture serum ACE and calcium levels, Kveim test
Crohn's disease	Isolated, loose, poorly formed follicles, often deeply situated; occasional giant cells, scanty inflammatory cells	History of bowel dysfunction or pain, abdominal radiographs (if appropriate); blood picture
Deep mycoses	Organisms typically difficult to find if granulomas prominent; sometimes central necrosis in granulomas; dense inflammatory infiltrate; special stains may show many yeast forms or hyphae	Culture of any unfixed material; immune function (?HIV+); patient from endemic area?
Cat scratch disease	Multiple epithelioid granulomas with central suppuration, in lymph nodes; dense surrounding infiltrate; bacteria may be demonstrable with Warthin–Starry stain	Papule or pustule at inoculation site, conjunctivitis? Rose–Hanger skin test
Tertiary syphilis	Plasma cells prominent but granulomas rarely seen; inflammation may be non-specific	Both specific and non specific serological tests positive if untreated
Wegener's granulomatosis	Dense mixed inflammatory infiltrate, granulomas ill-defined and hard to find; arteritis; giant cells randomly distributed	Raised titre of anti-neutrophil cytoplasmic antibodies

References

Collipp, P.J. (1992) Cat-scratch disease: therapy with trimethoprim-sulphmethoxazole. *American Journal of Diseases of Children*, **146**, 397–399

Devaney, K.O., Travis, W.D., Hoffman, G. *et al.* (1990) Interpretation of head and neck biopsies in Wegener's granulomatosis. A pathologic study of 126 biopsies in 70 patients. *American Journal of Surgical Pathology*, **14**, 555–564

Feigal, D.W., Katz, M.H., Greenspan, D. *et al.* (1991) The prevalence of oral lesions in HIV-infected homosexual and bisexual men: three San Francisco epidemiological cohorts. *AIDS*, **5**, 519–525

Hoffman, G.S., Kerr, G.S., Leavitt, R.Y. *et al.* (1992) Wegener granulomatosis: an analysis of 158 patients. *Annals of Internal Medicine*, **116**, 488–498

Leicht, S., Youngberg, G. and Modica, L. (1989) Melkersson–Rosenthal syndrome: elevations in serum angiotensin converting enzyme and results of treatment with methotrexate. *Southern Medical Journal*, **82**, 74–76

Pinder, S.E. and Colville, A. (1992) Mycobacterial cervical lymphadenitis in children: can histological assessment help differentiate infections caused by nontuberculous mycobacteria from *Mycobacterium tuberculosis?* *Histopathology*, **22**, 59–64

Porter, S.R. and Scully, C. (1993) Orofacial manifestations in primary immunodeficiencies involving IgA deficiency. *Journal of Oral Pathology and Medicine*, **22**, 117–119

Stansfeld, A.G. and d'Ardenne, A.J. (eds) (1992) *Lymph-node Biopsy and Interpretation*, 2nd edn, Churchill Livingstone, Edinburgh

Zimmer, W.M., Rogers, R.S., Reeve, C.M. *et al.* (1992) Orofacial manifestations of Melkersson–Rosenthal syndrome. A study of 42 patients and review of 220 cases from the literature. *Oral Surgery, Oral Medicine and Oral Pathology*, **74**, 610–619

Index

Numbers in italics refer to pages with illustrations

Abscess,
  in actinomycosis, 30
  apical, 36
  brain, 36
  buccal, 28
  in glossitis, 162
  lung, 26
  palatal, 29
  parotid, *218*, 219
  soft tissue, 28, 29
  submasseteric, 29, 122
  tuberculous, 296
Acanthosis, 192
  syphilitic, 170
Acanthosis nigricans, 156
Acquired immune deficiency
    syndrome (AIDS), 297–298,
    301–308
  Addison's disease in, 186
  aetiology, 302
  aphthous stomatitis in, 145
  autoimmune disease in, 304, 307
  bacillary epitheloid angiomatosis,
    286
  bacteriaemias in, 36
  clinical aspects, 303
  condyloma acuminatum in, 192
  cryptococcosis in, 34
  cytomegalovirus infection in, 140
  deep mycoses in, 30
  herpes zoster in, 138
  immunity in, 302
  infections in, 306
  Kaposi's sarcoma in, 285
  lymph glands in, 306
  lymphomas in, 289
  neurological complications, 307
  opportunistic infections in, 304
  orofacial manifestations, 304, 305
  pigmentation in, 187
  prediction of progression, 304
  purpura and, 181
  stomatitis, 138
  surgery in, 307
  terminal stages, 304
  tuberculosis and, 140
  tumours in, 306
  ulcers and, 143

AIDS-related complex, 303
Actinic radiation,
  cancer and, 195
Actinomyces israelii, 29
Actinomycosis, 29
  features of, 29
  osteomyelitis in, 21
  sulphur granules, 30, *30*
Addison's disease, 173, 186
Adenoameloblastoma, 64
Adenocarcinomas, 193
Adenoid cystic carcinoma, *9*
Adenoid squamous carcinoma, 213
Adenolymphoma, 12
Adenomas, 193
Adentomatoid odontogenic tumour,
    64, *65*
Afipia felis, 297
Age,
  cancer and, 194
Alcohol,
  cancer and, 197
Allbright's syndrome, 112
Allergic angio-oedema, 308
Allergic sialadenitis, 223
Allergic stomatitis, 158
Alveolar rhabdomyosarcoma, 280,
    280
Alveolar ridge,
  cancer of, 200
Amalgam tattoo, 185, *186*
Amelanotic melanoma, 181
Ameloblastic carcinoma, 63
Ameloblastic fibro-adenoma, 69
Ameloblastic fibroma, 68, *68, 69*
  granular cell, 69
Ameloblastic fibro-odontomas, *69*
Ameloblastic fibrosarcoma, 69, *70*
Ameloblastic sarcoma, 69
Ameloblastoma, 38, 39, 59, *60, 61,
    62, 63*
  acanthomatous, 61
  basal cell, 62
  clinical features, 59
  cysts in, 56, 60
  desmoplastic, 62
  extraosseous, 59
  follicular, 60

  granular cell, 61
  histological diagnosis, 6
  malignant, 63, *63*
  management, 62
  maxillary, 62
  odonto-, 63
  plexiform, 61
  primary extraosseous, 63
  radiography, 59
  unicystic, 59, 60, 63
Amputation neuroma, 8, *8*
Amyloidosis, 66, 96, 97, *98*
Anaemia,
  drug-induced, 169
  Fanconi's, 198
  glossitis, 160, 161
  sickle cell, 110
Anaesthesia,
  Ludwig's angina and, 26
Anaplastic carcinomas, 201
Aneurysmal bone cyst, 55–56, *55,
    56, 84*
  aspiration, 19
  with chondroblastoma, 89
Angina bullosa haemorrhagica, 181
Angiofibroma,
  nasopharyngeal (juvenile), 263,
    263
Angiofollicular hyperplasia, *299*
Angioleiomyoma, 281
Angiolymphoid hyperplasia, 300,
    300
Angio-oedema, 308
Angiosarcoma of bone, 94
Angular stomatitis, 171, 180
Antibiotic stomatitis, 180
Antrum,
  mucosal cysts of, 57, *57*
Anxiety states, 231
Aphthae, recurrent
  see under Aphthous stomatitis
Aphthous stomatitis,
  aetiology, 143
  clinical features, 143
  clinical variants, 144
  management, 144
  minor, 144
  recurrent, 137

Arachnodactyly, 110
Arthralgia, 125
Arthritis, 156
Asbestos, 289
Aspergillosis, 33, *33*
Aspergillus fumigatus, 33
Aspiration, 8–11
  fine-meedle, 8, 11
  simple, 10
Autoimmune disease, 307

B-cells, 96
  in AIDS, 301
  in Sjögren's syndrome, 227
B-cell lymphomas, 8, 95, 256
Bacillary epitheloid angiomatosis,
  286
Bacteraemias, 35
Bacterial infections,
  in AIDS, 306
  fascial space, 24
Bacteroides fragilis, 20
Basal cell adenocarcinoma, 252
Basal cell carcinoma, 50
Behçet's syndrome, 144, 145
Benign migratory glossitis, 174
Benign monoclonal gammopathy,
  98
Betel, 197
Bidi smoking, 196
Bifid uvula, 104, 110
Biopsy, 1
  artefacts in, 2
  in malignant disease, 2
  needle, 10
  technique, 2
Birbeck granules, 99
Blastomyces dermatiditis, 34, 35
Blastomycosis, 34
Blood blisters, 181
Blood vessels,
  cancer invasion of, 207
  hamartomas, 281
  tumours of, 281
Bloom's syndrome, 198
Blue naevi, 182, *183*
Bohn's nodules, 45
Bone,
  aneurysmal cyst, *see Aneurysmal
    bone cyst*
  angiosarcoma, 94
  brittle, 107
  cancer invasion of, 207
  fibro-osseous lesions, 112
  fibrosarcoma, 92
  fibrous dysplasia, 112, *113*
  genetic disease, 103
  haemangioma, 93, *93*, 94
  in hyperparathyroidism, 118
  in hypophosphatasia, 109
  leiomyosarcoma of, 94

marble disease, 108
metabolic disease, 109
Paget's disease, 22, 84, 92, 116,
    117, 118
phantom disease, 120
plasmacytoma, 97
primary lymphoma, 95
remedial surgery, 97
Stafne's cavity, 56, *56*, 217, 259
in thalassaemia, 111
Bone cysts, 54, *55*
Bone disease,
  investigation of, 14
Bone islands, 2, 23, 119
Bony overgrowths, 79
Borrelia burgdorferi, 297
Borrelia vincentii, 27
Botryoid odontogenic cysts, 46
Brain abscess, 36
Branchial arch syndrome, 105
Branchial cysts, 274
Breast cancer, 101, 118
Breslow thickness, 185
Brittle bone disease, 107, *109*
Buccal abscess, 28
Buccal mucosa,
  cancer of, 200
Bullous disease, 181
Bullous erythema multiforme, 155
  drug-induced, 160
Bullous pemphigoid, 154
Burkitt's lymphoma, 95, 291, *292*

Calcifying epithelial odontogenic
    tumour (CEOT), 65, *65*, *66*
Calcifying giant cell tumour, 89
Calcifying odontogenic cysts, 51, *51*,
    67
Cancer,
  accuracy of site identification,
    203
  actinic radiation and, 195
  aetiology of, 194
  age and, 194
  alcohol and, 197
  association with leucoplakia, 195,
    200
  candidosis and, 198
  chemotherapy, 205
  classification, 201
  clinical presentation of, 199
  definitions, 193
  dental factors in, 199
  epidemiology, 193
  genetics, 198
  grading methods, 204
  infections and, 198
  leucoplakia and, 195, 200
  local spread of, 206
  management of, 205
  metastases, 206

after initial treatment, 210
to lymph nodes, 207
trends in mortality, 210
microscopy, 201
pipe smoking and, 196
racial aspects, 195
radiotherapy, 205, 208–209
STNMP classification, 205
sex incidence, 194
site frequency, 194
size of, 204
staging, 201, 203
surgery for, 205
TNM classification, 202
tobacco use and, 196
*see also Carcinoma, Tumours, types,
    sites etc*
Cancrum oris, 27, *28*
Candida albicans, 171, 173, 191
Candidal leucoplakia,
  cancer and, 198
Candidosis, 142, 161, *163*, 170, 179,
    232
  in AIDS, 305
  cancer and, 198
  causing erythema, 180
  diagnosis, 11
Candidosis syndromes, 172, 173
Capillary haemangioma, *282*
Carcinogens, 195
Carcinoma,
  ameloblastic, 63
  anaplastic, 201
  basal cell, 213
  epidermoid, 213
  Merkel cell, 213
  multiple, primary, 211
  spindle cell, 213, *213*
  spread in mouth, 296
  squamous, *see Squamous cell
    carcinoma*
  variations, 213
  verrucous, 201, *211*, 212
Carcinoma-in-situ, 178
Carcinosarcoma,
  of salivary glands, 254
Carotid body tumours, 274
Castleman's disease, 299
Cat scratch disease, 296, 314, 315
Cavernous haemangioma, *282*, *282*
Cavernous sinus thrombosis,
    26–27
Cell mediated immunity, 160
Cell proliferations, 8
Cellulitis,
  acute, *24*
  causes, 24
  cervicofacial, 23
  sublingual, 25
  submandibular, 25
  submaxillary, 25
Cemental tumours and dysplasias,
    71, 75, *75*

Cementoblastoma, 72, *72, 73,* 82
Cemento-osseous dysplasia, 76, *76*
Cemento-ossifying fibroma, 72, *73,*
    74, 79
Central giant cell granulomas, 117
Central giant cell lesions of jaws,
    82, 83
Cervical lymphadenopathy,
    causes of, 294
    syphilitic, 296
    tuberculous, 296
Cervical lymph nodes,
    in cat scratch disease, 296
    drug-related disease, 300
    enlarged, 293
    metastases in, 207
    removal of, 294
    surgical management, 294
Cervical paraganglionomas, 274
Cervicofacial cellulitis, 23
Cheek,
    abscess of, 28
    fibrosarcoma, 268
Cheek-biting, 168
Cheilitis granulomatosa, 313, 314
Chemodectomas, 274
Chemotherapy,
    reactions to, 313
Cherubism, 83, 114, *115*
Children,
    AIDS in, 222
    arthritis in, 129
    Burkitt's lymphoma in, 291
    calcifying odontogenic cysts, 52
    eruption cysts, 45
    glossitis in, 164
    melanotic neuroectodermal
        tumour, 94, *95,* 185
    myofibromatosis, 265
    odontoameloblastoma, 63
    osteomyelitis, 21
    parotitis in HIV infection, 231
    recurrent parotitis in, 219, *220*
    salivary gland tumours, 257
Chondroblastoma, 89, *89, 90*
Chondroma, 86, *87*
Chondromyxoid fibroma, 88, *89*
Chondrosarcoma, 86, *87,* 277
    management, 87
    mesenchymal, 88, *88*
    prognosis, 87
Chorioretinitis, 298
Cinnamon-related lesions, 158
Clear cell adenoma, 244
Clear cell odontogenic carcinoma,
    66
Cleft lip, 103, 105, 106
    surgical aspects, 104
Cleft palate, 104, 105, 106
    in Marfan's syndrome, 110
    surgical aspects, 104
Cleidocranial dysplasia, 109
Clinical investigations, 1

histopathological diagnosis, 5
Codman's triangles, 82, 84
Coeliac disease, 143
Cold sores, 136, 138
Collagenase, 39
Complement, 150
Computed tomography, 12, *13*
Condensing osteitis, 21, *21*
Condylar hyperplasia, 132
Condylar neck fracture, 122
Condyloma acuminatum, 191
Congenital defects, 103
Congenital heart disease, 106
Conjunctivitis, 156
Contact hypersensitization, 158
Corticosteroids in aphthous
        stomatitis, 145
Costen's syndrome, 132
Cowden's syndrome, 191
Cranial arteritis, 129, *129, 130*
Craniofacial defects, 103
Crohn's disease, 4, 136, 143, 312,
    312, 314
    buccal abscess in, 28
Crouzon's disease, *107, 108*
Cryotherapy, 179
Cryptococcosis, 33
Cryptococcus neoformans, 33
Cyclosporin, 145
Cylindroma of salivary glands, 247
Cystic hygroma, 283
Cystic neoplasms, 56
Cyst-like lesions, 54–56
Cysts, 38–58
    see also different types and sites
    in ameloblastoma, 60
    antral, 57
    apical periodontal, *see Cysts,*
        radicular
    aspiration, 10
    bone resorbing factors, 39
    botryoid, 46
    calcifying odontogenic, 51, *51,* 67
    characteristics, 39
    in chondromyxoid fibroma, 89
    in cleidocranial dysplasia, 109
    dental lamina of newborn, 45
    dentigerous, 44, 45
    diagnosis, 10
    differential diagnosis, 39
    epithelial proliferation, 38
    eruption, 45, *45*
    follicular, *see Cysts, dentigerous*
    frequency of types, 38
    gingival, 45, *46*
    globulomaxillary, 53
    Gorlin, 67
    growth of, 39
    hydrostatic effects of fluids, 38
    lateral periodontal, 46
    mechanisms of formation, 38
    median mandibular, 53, *54*
    multiple in Gorlin-Goltz

syndrome, 50
    nasolabial, 53
    nasopalatine, 52, *53*
    neoplastic change in lining, 57
    in odontomas, 76
    origins of, 38
    paradental, 44
    primordial, 51
    radicular, 40, *41, 42,* 43, 44
        aspiration, 42
        clefts in, 42
        cyst wall, 41
        differential diagnosis, 42
        enucleation, 43
        epithelial lining, 40
        fluid, 42
        lateral, 40
        marsupialization, 43
        treatment, 42
    residual, 40
    salivary glands, 217
    sialo-odontogenic, 46, *47*
    simple bone, 54
    solitary haemorrhagic of bone,
        54
Cytomegalovirus infection, 140, 222,
    222
    in AIDS, 306

Darier's disease, 152
Deficiency states, 161
Dental factors in cancer, 199
Dental lamina cyst of newborn, 45
Dentigerous cysts, 44–45
Dentino-genesis imperfecta, 108
Denture-induced hyperplasia, 260,
    261
Denture-induced stomatitis, 180
DNA hybridization, 11
Dermatitis herpetiformis, 155
Dermatomyositis, 276
Dermoids,
    sublingual, 57, *58*
Desmoplastic fibroma, 91
Desquamative gingivitis, 147, 148,
    155
Diabetes mellitus, 146, 176
    necrotizing fasciitis and, 27
    rhinocerebral mucormycosis and,
        32
Diffuse fibrous hyperplasia, 266
Diffuse sclerosing osteomyelitis, 22,
    22
Di George's syndrome, 173
Discoid lupus erythematosus, 149,
    173
Down's syndrome, 103, 106, 190
Drugs,
    oral mucous reactions, 159
    pigmentation and, 187
Dry mouth, 160

Dyskeratosis congenita, 168, 198
Dysphagia, 125
Dysplasia, 178, 179
Dysplastic leucoplakias, 6

Ear disease,
    affecting temporomandibular
        joint, 127
Ehlers-Danlos syndromes, 134
Embryomas,
    in salivary glands, 258
Embryonal rhabdomyosarcoma, 280
Eminectomy, 134
Enamel pearls, 78
Endocarditis,
    infective, 35, 36, *36*, 106
Endocrine adenoma syndromes,
    273
Endocrine candidosis syndrome,
    173
Eosinophilic granuloma, 98
    multifocal, 99
    traumatic, 100
Eosinophilic ulcer, 100
Epidermolysis bullosa, 152
Epiphseal chondromatous giant cell
    tumours, 89
Epithelial dysplasia, 166, 178, *178*
Epithelial hyperplasia, 192
Epithelial-myoepithelial carcinoma,
    251, *251*
Epithelial tumours, 190–216
Epitheloid haemangioma, 285, 300
Epstein-Barr virus, 175, 220, 291,
    297
Epulis,
    congenital, 278, *279*
    congenital granular cell, 278
    fibrous, 260, *261*
    giant cell, 262
    neoplastic, 263
    in pregnancy, 261, 262
Eruption cysts, 45, *45*
Erythmatous candidosis, 180
Erythema chronicum migrans, 297
Erythema multiforme, *156*
Erythematous stomatitis, 299
Erythroplakia, 180
Erythroplasia, 179, 180
Ewing's sarcoma, 22, 85, 90, *91*
    metastases from, 101
Exfoliative cytology, 10
Exfoliative stomatitis, 160
Exophthalmos, 108
Exostoses, 79
Eyes in Stevens-Johnson syndrome,
    155

Facial clefts, 103–106
Facial nerve,

care of, 237
Facial palsy, 221, 313
Familial fibrous dysplasia, 114
Familial mucocutaneous candidosis,
    172
Fanconis anaemia, 198
Fascial space infections, 23
Fasciitis, 266
Fast neutron therapy, 209
Fatty tissue,
    tumours of, 275
Fever blisters, 136, 138
Fibrohistocytic tumours, 269
Fibromas, 71, 260
    cemento-ossifying, 72
    giant cell, 261, *261*
Fibromatosis, 264
    gingival, 266
Fibrosarcoma, 268, *268*, *269*
    of bone, 92
Fibrosis,
    submucous, 177
Fibrous dysplasia, 22, 83, 112, *113*
Fibrous epulis, 260, *261*
Fibrous nodules, 260, *260*
Fine-needle aspiration cytology,
    8–11
First and second branchial arch
    syndromes, 105
Floor of mouth,
    cancer of, 194, 200
Fluorescence immunocytochemistry,
    7
Focal epithelial hyperplasia, 192
Follicular cysts,
    see Dentigerous cysts
Fordyce's spots, 167
Foreign body reactions, 313, 314
Fractures,
    infection and, 18
Frey's syndrome, 238
Frictional keratosis, 168
Frontal bossing, 108
Frozen sections, 4, 5
Fusobacterium nucleatum, 27

Gardner's syndrome, 80
Garrés osteomyelitis, 22
Generalized lymphadenopathy
    syndrome, 303
Genetics,
    cancer and, 198
Geographical tongue, 162, *162*
Ghost cell carcinomas, 67
Ghost cell tumour, 67
Giant cell arteritis, 129, *129*, *130*,
    164
Giant cell epulis, 262
Giant cell fibroma, 261
Giant cell granuloma, 82, *83*, 83
Giant cell tumours, 84, 92, 119

calcifying, 89
    of chondroblastoma, 56
    Paget's disease and, 117
Giant cell variant,
    of malignant fibrous histiocytoma,
        270
Giant lymph node hyperplasia, 299
Gigantiform cementoma, 76
Gingiva,
    cancer of, 200
    in Crohn's disease, 312
    cysts of, 45, *46*
    drug-induced hyperplasia, 160
    fibromatosis, 266, *266*
    giant cell fibroma, 261
    lichen planus, 147, 148
    pigmentation, 187
Gingivitis,
    in AIDS, 307
    acute ulcerative, 137
    desquamative, 147, 148, 155
    plasma cell, 158
Glandular fever, 140, 297
Globulomaxillary cysts, 53
Glomangiomas, 283
Glomus tumours, 274, 283
Glossitis, 161
    acute, 164
    in anaemia, 160, 161
    benign migratory, 162, 174
    median rhomboid, 163, *163*
    syphilitic, 199
Goldenhar syndrome, 105
Gorlin cyst, 67
Gorlin-Goltz syndrome, 48, *49*, 50,
    51, *51*
Graft versus host disease, 146
Granular cell ameloblastic fibroma,
    69
Granular cell epulis, 278
Granular cell tumour, 277, *278*
Granuloma,
    from foreign bodies, 313
    frozen sections, 5
    giant cell 82, *83*
    familial, 172
    pulse, 23
    pyogenic, 261, *262*
Granulomatous diseases, 308
    differential diagnosis, 314
    features of, 314, 315
Granulomatous reactions, 313, 314
Grinspan syndrome, 146
Gumma of palate, 141
Gunshot wounds, 19

Haemangioendothelioma, 285
Haemangioma, 10, 181, 282
    of bone, 93, *93*, 94
    epithelioid, 300
    intrabony, *95*

Haemangioma (*cont.*)
  of jaw, 120
  types of, 93
Haemangiopericytoma, 284, *284*
Haemangiopericytoma-like
    mesenchymal chondrosarcoma,
    88
Haemophilus influenzae, 164
Hairy leucoplakia, 175
  in AIDS, 175, 305, 306
Hairy tongue, 162
Harmartoma, 191
  of blood vessels, 281
Hand-foot-and-mouth disease, 137,
    139
Hand-Schuller-Christian disease, 98,
    99
Head and neck cancer, 195
Heart disease, 106, 110
Heck's disease, 192
Heerfordt's syndrome, 220
Hemifacial microsomia, 103, 105
Hereditary angio-oedema, 308
Hereditary haemorrhagic
    telangiectasia, 181
Herpes labialis, 136, 138
Herpes simplex, 136, *137*
Herpes zoster, 16, 137
  of trigeminal area, 138
Herpes virus,
  cancer and, 198
Herpetic cross-infections, 138
Herpetic stomatitis, 136, 137
Herpetiform aphthae, 133
Histiocytoma,
  fibrous, 269, *269, 270*
  giant cell, 270
  malignant fibrous, 92
Histiocytosis X, 98
Histoplasma capsulatum, 31
Histoplasmosis, 31, *31, 32*
Hodgkin's disease, 138, 256,
    292–293, *292*
  see also Non-Hodgkin's lymphoma
  Rye classification, 293
Human immunodeficiency virus
    infection, 302
  angiofollicular hyperplasia in, 299
  aphthous stomatitis and, 144
  candidosis in, 180
  consequences of, 303
  hairy leucoplakia and, 175, *175*
  Kaposi's sarcoma and, 181
  molluscum contagiosum in, 192
  osteomyelitis in, 16
  parotid cysts in, 227
  progression of, 304
  thrush in, 171
  transmission of, 305
Human papilloma virus, 190, 191,
    192
  cancer and, 198
Hyperbaric oxygen therapy, 20

Hypercalcaemia, 118, 119
Hyperkeratosis, 166, *168*
  syphilitic, 170
Hypernephroma, 251, *252*
Hyperparathyroidism, 83, 118, *119,*
    262
Hyperplasia,
  denture-induced, 260
  diffuse fibrous, 266
  verrucous, 211
Hyperplastic candidosis, 170, 171,
    171
Hypersensitivity, 158
Hypertension, 146
Hyperventilation syndrome, 123
Hypoadrenocorticism, 186
Hypoparathyroidism, 173
Hypophosphatasia, 109
Hysterical trismus, 123

Immunocytochemistry, 7
Immunodeficiency,
  see also AIDS etc
  bacteriaemias in, 36
  causes of, 301
  cytomegalovirus infection in, 140
  herpetic cross-infection in, 138
  oral manifestations, 301
  osteomyelitis and, 16, 19
Immunodeficiency disease, 301
  see also AIDS
Immunoglobulins,
  in lupus erythematosus, 150
Immunoglobulin A deficiency, 308
Immunosuppression,
  deep mycoses in, 30
  necrotizing fasciitis and, 27
Infantile myofibromatosis, 265
Infections 16–37
  see also specific conditions
  cancer and, 198
  diagnosis, 11
  sickle cell disease and, 110
  systemic, 35
Infectious mononucleosis, 140, 297
Infective endocarditis, 35, 36, *36,*
    106
Inflammatory bowel disease, 157
Intestinal polyposis, 186
Intra-alveolar carcinoma, 64
Intraosseous salivary gland tumours,
    66
Investigations, 1–15
  biopsy, 1
  clinical, 1
  CT scans, 12, *13*
  DNA hybridization, 11
  exfoliative cytology, 10
  fine-needle aspiration cytology, 8,
    11
  frozen sections, 4

immunocytochemistry, 7
laboratory, 14
MRI scans, 12
medical assessment, 14
needle biopsy, 10
radionuclide scanning, 12
salivary gland flow measurement,
    14
sialography, 12
simple aspiration, 10
ultrasonography, 12

Joint replacements, 36
Junctional activity, 182, *182*
Kaposi's sarcoma, 181, 285, *285,*
    286, 300, 305
  in AIDS, 304, 305, 306, 307
Kawasaki's disease, 140, 298
Keratinization, 178
Keratoacanthoma, 212, *212,* 213
Keratoconjunctivitis sicca, 228, 229
Keratocysts, 38, 47–50
  aspiration, 10
  clinical features, 48
  development of, 50
  histology, 6
  orthokeratotic variant, 47, *49,* 49
  parakeratotic variant, 47, *48,* 49,
    50
  recurrence, 49
  treatment of, 50
Keratocytes, 39
Keratosis,
  frictional, 168
  of renal failure, 175
  smokers', 169, 188, *188*
  snuff-dippers', 169
  sublingual, 173, *174*
Keratosis follicularis, 152
Kimura's disease, 300
Koilocytes, 175
Koplik spots, 140

Laboratory investigations, 14
Langerhans cell histiocytosis, 98
Leiomyoma 281, *281*
Leiomyosarcoma, 94, 281
Lentigo maligna, 184
Leptotricia buccalis, 35
Lethal midline granuloma, 308
Letterer-Siwe disease, 98, 99
Leucoplakia, 166
  association with cancer, 195, 200
  hairy, 175, *175*
  idiopathic, 177
  premalignant potential, 177
  speckled, 177, 179
  syphilitic, 170, 198
Leukaemia, 106

Leucopenia,
  drug induced, 159
Lichenoid reactions, 160
Lichen planus, 146, *148*, 149, 173,
    187
  aetiology, 146
  cancer and, 199
  clinical features, 146
  drug associated, 149
  gingival, 147, 148
  malignant changes, 148
  management, 148
  prognosis, 148
  tongue, 161
Linear IgA disease, 154
Lip,
  canalicular adenomas, *244*
  cancer of, 194, 195, 198
    clay pipes and, 196
    spread of, 208
  carcinoma of, 193
  swelling, 313
  tumours, 234
Lipomas, 275
Liposarcoma, 275, *275*
Lockjaw, 122
Ludwig's angina, 23, 25–26
Lung,
  abscess, 36
  cancer, 118
  metastases in, 84, 92, 210
Lung disease,
  pigmentation and, 187
Lupus erythematosis, 136, 149–150,
    149, *150*, 173
  in AIDS, 307
Lyme disease, 297
Lymphadenopathy,
  in AIDS, 303, 306
  diagnosis of, 293
Lymphangiomas, 283, *284*
Lymphatics,
  tumours of, 281
Lymph nodes,
  see also cervical lymph nodes
  in AIDS, 297
  assessing cancer, 294
  drug-related disease, 300
  in glandular fever, 297
  hyperplasia, 299
  immunocytochemistry, 295
  indications for biopsy, 293
  metastases, 207
    management of, 29
  monitoring lymphomas, 294
  preparations, 295
  in sinus histiocytosis, 299
Lymphoepithelial carcinoma, 253
Lymphomas, 289, *295*
  in AIDS, 289
  biopsy, 3
  of bone, 95
  clinical features, 289

follicular, *290, 291*
lymphocytic, *291*
malignant, 90
management of, 290
non-Hodgkin's, 96, 290, 292,
    306
of salivary glands, 255
in Sjögren's syndrome, 230
Lymphoreticular diseases, 289
  frozen sections, 5
Lymphoreticular tumours, 289
  monoclonal antibodies, 7

Macroglossia, 283, 284
Magnetic resonance imaging, 12
Malignant disease, 1
See also Cancer, Tumours and specific
    lesions
  biopsies and, 2
  frozen sections, 4
  histopathological criteria, 6
  toluidine blue marking, 4
Malignant fibrous histiocytoma, 92
Malignant melanoma, 184, *184*
Malocclusion,
  affecting temporomandibular
    joint, 130
  in Marfan's syndrome, 110
  in thalassaemia, 112
Mandible,
  cancer invasion, 207
  sclerosis, 23
Mandibular block injections, 122
Marble bone disease, 108, *109*
Marfan's syndrome, 110, 134
Maxilla,
  cancer of, 207
Maxillary antrum,
  carcinoma of, 214
Maxillary osteomyelitis, 139
Measles, 140
Median mandibular cysts, 53
Melanoacanthoma, 183, *184*
Melanocytes, 181, *182*
Melanomas, 181
  amelanotic, 181
  Breslaw thickness, 185
  malignant, 184, *184*
  salivary glands and, 258
  secondary, 185
  terminology, 181
Melanosis, 188, *188*
Melanotic macule, 183, *183*
Melanotic naevi, 182
Melanotic neuroectodermal tumours
    of infancy, 94, *95*, 185
Meikerssohm-Rosenthal syndrome,
    217, 313, 314
Merkel cell carcinoma, 213
Mesenchymal chondrosarcoma, 88,
    88

Mesenchymal tissue,
  tumours of, 258, 260–288
Metals causing pigmentation, 187
Metastases, 100, *101*
  diagnosis, 11
  from chondrosarcoma, 87
  MRI scans, 12
  radiology, 12
Microscopy, 6
Midfacial destructive disease, 308
Midline granuloma syndrome, 308,
    311
Miescher's syndrome, 313
Mikulicz aphthous ulcer, 144
Mikulicz's disease and syndrome,
    212, 311
Mobile arterio-venous imaging
    system, 274
Molluscum contagiosus, 192
Mongolism, 103, 106, 190
Monoclonal antibodies, 7
Morphea, 125
Mucoceles of salivary glands, 226,
    226, 227
Mucocutaneous angiomatosis,
    283
Mucocutaneous candidosis, 186
  diffuse-type, 172
  familial, 172
  late onset, 173
  management of, 173
Mucocutaneous lymph node
    syndrome, 140, 298
Mucormycosis, 32
Mucosa,
  pigmented lesions, 180
  purple lesions, 180
  red lesions, 180
  white lesions, 166
Mucosal cysts of antrum, 57, *57*
Mucositis,
  plasma cell, 158
Mucous membrane,
  diseases of, 136–165
  infections of, 136
  pemphigoid, 153
  reaction to drugs, 159
Multifocal nodular oncocytic
    hyperplasia, 242
Multiple hamartoma, 191
Multiple myeloma, 96, *96*, 97
Mumps, 220, 221, *221*
Mumps virus, 221
Muscles,
  degeneration and regeneration,
    276
  diseases of, 276–281
Mycobacterium tuberculosis, 296
Mycoses, 314, 315
  in AIDS, 306
  deep, 30, 311, 314
  life-threatening, 31
Myoblastoma, 277

Myoepithelioma, 240, *241*
Myofibromatosis, 265
Myositis, 276
Myositis ossificans, 277
Myxoma, 70, *70*

Naevi,
    blue, 182, *183*
    compound, 182, *182*
    melanotic, 182
    pigmented, 181, 182
    vascular, 282
    white sponge, 166, *166, 167*
Naevoid basal cell carcinoma
        syndrome, 48
Nasolabial cysts, 53, *54*
Nasopalatine cysts, 52, *53*
Nasopharyngeal (juvenile)
        angiofibroma, 262, *263*
Nasopharyngeal lymphoma, 289
Neck,
    management of cancer of, 209
Necrotizing fasciitis, 27
Necrotizing sialometaplasia, 222,
        223
Needle biopsy, 10
Neoplastic epulides, 263
Neuralgia,
    post-herpetic, 139
Neural tissue tumours, 270
Neurilemmomas, 270, *271*
Neuroblastoma, 90
Neurofibroma, 272, *271, 272*
    plexiform, 271, *271*
Neurofibromatosis, 272
Neurofibrosarcomas, 273, *273, 274*
Neuroma,
    amputation, 8, *8*
    mucosal, 273
    traumatic, 270
Newborn,
    dental lamina cysts of, 45
Nicotinic stomatitis, 169
Nikolsky's sign, 151, 154
Nodular fasciitis, 267, *267*
Noma, 27
Non-Hodgkin's lymphoma, 96, 290,
        292
    in AIDS, 306
    classification, 290
    clinical features, 290
Non-odontogenic tumours, 79–102
North American blastomycosis, 34
Nose,
    chondroma of, 86
Nuclear hyperchromatism, 178
Nuclear pleomorphism, 178

Oculo-auriculovertebral dysplasia,
        105

Odontoameloblastoma, 63
Odontogenic fibroma, 71, *71*
Odontogenic fibromyxoma, *71*
Odontogenic ghost cell tumours, 67
Odontogenic myxoma, 70, *70*
Odeontogenic tumours, 59–78
    see also specific tumours
Odontomas, 76–78
    complex, 77, *77*
    compound, 76, *77*
    dilated, gestant and germinated,
        78
Oncogenes, 198
Oncocytic hyperplasia,
    multifocal nodular, 242
Oncocytoma, 242, *242*
Oncocytosis, 243
Oral nasal aspergillosis, 33
Oral submucous fibrosis, 123
Ossifying dysplasia, 113
Ossifying fibroma, 56, 79
    aggressive, 79, *79*
    juvenile active, 79, *79*
Osteitis,
    condensing, 21
Osteitis deformans, *see Paget's*
        disease
Osteitis fibrosis cystica, 118
Osteoblastoma, 81, 82, *82*
    malignant change in, 82
Osteochondroma, 80, *81*
    of temporomandibular joint, 132
    soft tissue, 81
Osteochondromatosis,
    multiple, 81
Osteoclastoma, 84
Osteogenesis imperfecta, 107, *109*
Osteoid,
    formation of, 85
Osteoid osteoma, 81, 82
Osteolysis, 120
Osteomas, 79–82
    cartilage-capped, 80
    compact and cancellous, 80, *80*
Osteomyelitis,
    acute, 16, *17*, 19
        causes, 16
        clinical features, 16
        management of, 18
        pathology, 18
    bacteria responsible, 18
    cellulitis complicating, 24
    chronic, 19, 20, 21
        with productive periostitis, 22
    chronic focal sclerosing, 21, *21*
    chronic specific, 21
    complications, 19
    diffuse sclerosing, 22, *22*
    Garrés, 22
    non-suppurative, 22
    in osteopetrosis, 108, 109
    radiation-associated, 19
Osteopetrosis, 22, 108, *109*

Osteoporosis,
    in hyperparathyroidism, 118
Osteoporosis circumscripta, 116
Osteoradionecrosis, 19
Osteosarcoma, 84, *85*, 86, 114
    extraskeletal, 91, 277
    juxtacortical, 85
    management, 85
    parosteal, 86, *86*
    periosteal, 86
    small cell, 85
Osteosclerosis, 23, 119
Oxophilic adenoma, 242, *242*

Pachyonychia congenita, 167, *167*
Paget's disease of bone, 22, 84, 92,
        116–118, *117*
Palate,
    abscess, 29
    cancer of, 196
    fibrosarcoma, 268
    gumma, 141
    herpetic stomatitis, 136
    malignant melanoma, 184
    in Marfan's syndrome, 110
    mucoceles, 226
    papillary cystadenocarcinoma, 248
    papillary hyperplasia, 191
    tumours, 234
Papillary hyperplasia of palate, 191
Papilloma, 190, *190*
Papillomatosis,
    florid, 190
Paracoccidioides brasiliensis, 34
Paracoccidioidomycosis, 34, *35*
Paradental cysts, 44
Parapharyngeal space, 25
Parathyroidadenoma, 118
Parosteal fasciitis, 267
Parotid gland,
    abscess, 218, *218*, 219
    adenocarcinoma, 248
    adenoid cystic carcinoma, 247
    benign tumours, 224
    calculi, 225
    carcinoma, 253
    cysts, 227, 231
    CT scan, 236
    duct adenoma, 243
    epithelial tumours in children, 257
    haemangioma, 257
    infection of, 217
    Kimura's disease of, 300
    lymphoma, 256
    malignant tumours, 224, 237
    melanoma, 185
    Milulicz's syndrome, 233
    mucoepidermoid carcinoma, 245
    in mumps, 221
    mycobacterial infection, 220
    obstruction, 224

Parotid gland (*cont.*)
oncocytoma, 242, *242*
papillary obstruction, 224
papillary trauma, 224
pleomorphic adenoma, 237, 238
sarcoidosis, *221*
sialosis, 233
in Sjögren's syndrome, 229
squamous cell carcinoma, 252
swelling, 220
tumours, 237
biopsy of, 2
fine-needle aspiration cytology, 8, 9
incidence of, 234
surgery of, 237
Warhin's tumour, 241
Parotitis, 217
in AIDS, 307
acute suppurative, *218*
in childhood AIDS, 222
chronic, 222
HIV infection in children, 231
recurrent, 219, *220*
Patterson-Kelly syndrome, 199
Pemphigoid, 153
Pemphigus vulgaris, 7, 11, 150–152, *151, 152,* 157
Periapical cemental dysplasia, 75
Periarticular tissues, 122
Perineural space,
cancer invasion of, 206
Periodontal cysts,
lateral, 46
Periodontitis,
in AIDS, 307
Periostitis,
chronic, 23
Peripheral T-cell lymphomas, 310, *310*
Pernicious anaemia, 180
Peutz-Jeghers syndrome, 186
Phantom bone disease, 120
Phenytoin related
lymphoadenopathies, 300
Phycomycosis, 32, *32*
Pierre Robin sydrome, 103, 104
Piezoelectric shock wave lithotripsy, 226
Pigmentary incontinence, 187, *187*
Pigmentation,
in AIDS, 187, 307
in Addison's disease, 186
drug-associated, 187
from amalgam, 185
lesions, 180
in lichen planus, 187
lung disease and, 187
in Peutz-Jeghers syndrome, 186
racial, 187, *187,* 196
terminology, 181
Pigmented lesions, 166, 180
management, 183

Pigmented macules, 183, *183*
Pilomatroxima, 67
Pindborg tumour, 65, *65, 66*
Pipesmokers, 196, 222
Plasma cell gingivitis and mucositis, 158
Plasmacytoma, *7, 96*
of bone, 97
soft tissue, 97
Pleomorphic adenoma, *236, 238, 238*
carcinoma in, 254, *254*
dysplasia in, 239
spread of, 239, 240, *240*
Pleomorphic rhabdomyosarcoma, 280, *280*
Plexiform neurofibroma, 271, *271*
Pneumocystis carinii, 304
Polyendocrinopathy syndrome, 173, 186
Polymerase chain reaction, 11
Polymorphous low-grade
adenocarcinoma, 249
Polymyalgia rheumatica, 129
Polymyositis, 276
Polyostotic fibrous dysplasia, 112
Polyposis coli, 80
Post-herpetic neuralgia, 139
Precancerous lesions, 193
Pregnancy,
gingival hyperplasia, 262
HIV infection in, 302
toxoplasmosis in, 298
Pregnancy epulis, 261, 262
Primary intraosseous carcinoma ex
odontogenic cysts, 57
Primordial cysts, 51
Prognathism, 110
Progonoma, 185
Progressive systemic sclerosis, 124
Proliferative fasciitis, 267
Proliferative myositis, 276, *277*
Prostaglandins, 39
Prostatic cancer, 100, 101
Pseudomembranous colitis, 20
Pseudosarcomatous fasciitis, 267
Psoriasis, 174, *174*
Pterygoid space, 25
Pulse granuloma, 23
Purpura, 181
drug-induced, 159
localized, 181
Pyoderma vegetans, 157
Pyogenic granuloma, 261, *262*
Pyostomatitis vegetans, 157

Race,
cancer and, 195
Racial pigmentation, 187, *187*
Radicular cysts, 40, *41, 42,* 43, 44
aspiration, 42

clefts in, 42
differential diagnosis, 42
enucleation, 43
epithelial lining, 40
fluid, 42
lateral, 40
marsupialization, 43
treatment, 42
Radiography, 11
Radionuclide scanning, 12
Radiotherapy, 208–209, 210
reactions to, 313
ulceration following, 11
Ramus osteotomies, 126
Ranula, 227
Raynaud's phenomenon, 125
Reed-Sternberg cells, 292, *292*
Reiter's disease, 156
Renal cell carcinoma, 252, *252*
Renal failure,
keratosis of, 175
Respiratory distress, 23, 26
Reye's syndrome, 299
Rhabdomyoma, 278
Rhabdomyosarcoma, 277, 279, *279, 281*
Rheumatoid arthritis, 228
of temporomandibular joint, 127, *127, 128,* 131
Rhinocerebral mucormycosis, 32, 33
Rosai-Dorfman disease, 299

Saliva,
flow measurement, 14
obstruction, 224
Salivary glands,
see also specific glands etc
aberrant tissue, 217
accessory glands and lobes, 217
in AIDS, 307
actinic cell carcinoma, 246, *246*
adenocarcinoma, 248
adenoid cystic carcinoma, 247, *247, 248, 249*
adenolymphoma, 241
aplasia and agenesis, 217
benign epithelial tumours, 238
benign lymphoepithelial lesions, 255
calculi, 224
canalicular adenomas, 243, 244
carcinoma of, 245–255
carcinoma-in-situ, 239
clear cell tumours, 244, 250
cystoadenolymphoma, *see
Warthin's tumour*
cysts of, 217, 227
cytomegalovirus infection, 222, *222*
developmental disorders, 217

Salivary glands (*cont.*)
  duct,
    atresia, 217
    carcinoma, 250, *250*
    papillomas, 244
    structures, 224
  embryoma, 258
  epithelial-myoepithelial
      carcinoma, 251
  epithelial tumours in children,
      257
  fistula, 217
  granulomatous infections, 220
  Hodgkin's disease, 256
  HIV associated disease, 231, *231,
      232*
  hypoplasia, 217
  infections, 217
  inflammatory disease, 217
  intraduct papilloma, 245
  inverted duct papilloma, 244
  irradiation damage, 232
  juxtaglandular tumours, 258
  lymphoma, 255, 256
  MRI scan, 236
  membranous basal cell adenoma,
      243, *243*
  metastasizing mixed tumour,
      254
  metastatic renal cell carcinoma,
      251, *252*
  metastatic tumours, 258
  minor,
    adenocarcinoma of, 248
    carcinoma of, 245, 247
    tumours of, 236, 237, 238, 256
  mucinous adenocarcinoma, 248
  mucoceles, 226, *226, 227*
  mucoepidermoid carcinoma, 245,
      245
  myoepithelioma, 240, *245*
  non-epithelial tumours, 255, 259
  non-neoplastic disease of,
      217–233
  obstruction, 224
  oncocytosis, 243
  oxyphilic adenoma, 242, *242*
  papillary cystadenoma, 244
  pleomorphic adenoma, *236,* 238,
      238, 239, 254
  polymorphous low-grade
      adenocarcinoma, 249, *249, 250*
  pseudo-mesenchymal tumours,
      264
  radionuclide scanning, 12
  ranula, 227
  rare carcinomas, 255
  sebaceous lymphadenoma and
      adenoma, 244
  sialadenoma papilliferum, 244
  spindle cell tumours, 264
  squamous cell carcinoma, 252
  terminal duct carcinoma, 249, *249,*

250
trabecular adenomas, 243, *243*
tubular adenomas, 234
tumours of, 234–259
    age, site and sex distribution,
        234
    biopsy of, 2, *3*
    CT and MRI scans, 12, 235
    chemotherapy, 238
    classification, 234, 235
    clinical features, 235
    diagnosis, 9
    distribution of, 234, 236
    fine needle aspiration, 9
    frozen sections, 5
    histological diagnosis, 6
    histopathological classification,
        235
    in infants and children, 257
    intraosseous, 66, 259
    radiotherapy, 238
    ultrasound in, 237
tumour-like lesions, 255
undifferentiated carcinomas, 253
Warthin's tumour, 235, 241, *241,
    242*
Salivary gland inclusion disease, 222
Sarcoidosis, 12, 220, *221,* 222, 311,
    312, 314, 315
Sarcoma,
  in Paget's disease, 117
Schwannomas, 270
  malignant, 273
Scleroderma, 123, 124, *125*
  localized, 125
Sclerotic bone islands, 23
Sebaceous lymphadenoma and
    adenoma, 244
Septicaemia, 19
Shingles, *see Herpes zoster*
Sialadenitis,
  acute bacterial, 217
  allergic, 223
  chronic, 219, 224
  HIV associated, 231
  obstructive, *219*
  post-irradiation, 222
  viral, 221
Sialadenoma papilliferum, 244
Sialadenosis, 233
Sialoblastoma, 258
Sialography, 12
Sialolithiasis, 224
Sialometaplasia, 222, *223*
Sialo-odontogenic cysts, 46, *27*
Sialosis, 233
Sicca syndrome, 227
  see also Sjögren's syndrome
Sickle cell disease, 110-111
Sinus histiocytosis, 299
Sjögren-like syndrome, 112
  in AIDS, 307
Sjögren's syndrome, 14, 149, 180,

218, 222, 227-230, *228, 229,
    230,* 231, 235, 255
  associated disorders, 228
  biopsy in, 228, 229
  compared with HIV salivary gland
      disease, 232
  complications, 230
  labial gland biopsy, *230*
  lymphoma in, 256
  salivary glands in, 218
Skin lesions in lichen planus, 147
Skull in Paget's disease, 116
Small dark cell tumours, 8
Smokers' keratosis, 152, 169
Smokers' melanosis, 188, *188*
Smoking,
  bidi, 196
  cigarette, 196
  necrotizing sialometaplasia and,
      222
  pipe, 196, 222
Snuff dipping, 169, 197, 211
Soft tissue,
  abscess, 28
  cancer invasion, 206
  osteochondromas, 81
  plasmacytoma, 97
South American blastomycosis, 34,
    35
Speckled leucoplakia, 177
Spindle cell carcinoma, 213, *213*
  of salivary glands, 264
Squamous cell carcinoma, 180, 193,
    201, 202, 203
  definition, 193
  epidemiology, 193
  of salivary glands, 252
Squamous cell papillomas, 190, *190*
Squamous odontogenic tumour, 67,
    68
Stafne's bone cavity, 56, *56,* 217,
    259
Staphylococcus aureus, 17, 21, 218
Staphylococcus epidermidis, 17
Stevens-Johnson syndrome, 155,
    160
Still's disease, 129
Stomach,
  carcinoma of, 157
Stomatitis,
  in AIDS, 306
  allergic, 158
  angular, 171, 180
  antibiotic, 180
  aphthous, *see Aphthous stomatitis*
  denture-induced, 180
  exfoliative, 160
  nicotinic, 169
  primary herpetic, 136
Stomatitis areata migrans, 162, 174
Stomatitis nicotina, 169, 222
Strawberry gums, 309
Strawberry tongue, 140

Sturge-Weber syndrome, 283
Sublingual cellulitis, 25
Sublingual dermoids, 57, 58
Sublingual gland,
    adenocarcinoma, 248
    mucous extravasation cyst, 227
Sublingual keratosis, 173, *174*
Submandibular cellulitis, 25
Submandibular duct stricture, 224
Submandibular gland,
    adenocarcinoma, 248
    adenoid cystic carcinoma, 247
    calculi, 225, *225*
    carcinoma, 253
    Kimura's disease, 300
    lymphoma, 256
    in mumps, 221
    papillary obstruction, 224
    pleomorphic adenoma, 238
    stricture, *224*
    tumours, 237
        incidence of, 234
        surgery of, 238
Submasseteric abscess, 29, 122
Submaxillary cellulitis, 25
Submucous fibrosis, 177
Sulphur granules, 30, *30*
Sun-ray appearance, 82, 84
Superior orbital fissure syndrome, 25
Synovial sarcoma, 132, 286, *287*
Syphilis, 140–142, *141, 142*
    cervical lymph nodes in, 296
    features, 314, 315
    glossitis, 199
    involving salivary glands, 220
    leucoplakia, 170, 198
    osteomyelitis, 21
Systemic lupus erythematosus 149, 173

T-cells, 96
    in AIDS, 301, 302, 304
    depletion of, 180
    in lichen planus, 147
    in Sjögren's syndrome, 227
T-cell lymphoma, 310, *310, 311*
Teething, 137
Telangiectases, 181
Telangiectatic erythema, 198
Temporomandibular joint,
    ankylosis of, 123, 126
    arthritis of, 126, 129
    dislocation, 133
    disorders of, 122-135
    extracapsular ankylosis, 123
    infection and inflammation, 122, 126
    internal derangement, 128

intracapsular ankylosis, 126
limitation of movement, 122
loose bodies in, 133
metastases, 132
neoplasm of, 126, 132
osteoarthritis, 128, *128*
osteochondritis dissecans, 133
osteoma and chondroma, 132
osteochondroma, 132
pseudo-ankylosis, 123
recurrent dislocation, 134
rheumatoid arthritis, 127, *127, 128*, 131
synovial chondromatosis, 133, 134, *134*
synovial sarcoma, 132
trauma, 123, 126
Temporomandibular pain
    dysfunction syndrome, 123, 129, 130–132
    aetiology, 130
    clinical features, 130
    management, 131
Terminal duct carcinoma, 249, *249*
Tetanus, 122
Tetany, 122
Thalassaemias, 111–112
Thrombocytic purpura, 181, 307
Thrush, 148, 170, *171*, 232
    AIDS and, 305, 306
    diagnosis, 11
Thyroid carcinoma, 273
Tobacco,
    cancer and, 196
    chewing, 169, 197, 211
    effects of, 169
    smokeless, 197
    see also Smoking
Toluidine blue marking, 4
Tomography, 11
Tongue,
    see also Glossitis
    black hairy, 188
    cancer of, 194
        metastases, 208
        presentation, 199
        spread of, 206
    carcinoma of, 170, 179
    carcinoma-in-situ, 179
        complaints, 160–164
        eosinophilic ulcer, 100
    fibrosarcoma, 268
    fissured, 313
    foliate papillitis, 163
    furred, 163
    geographical, 162, *162, 174*
    haemangioma, 283
    hairy, 162, 188
    herpetic stomatitis, 136
    hyperplastic candidosis, 171
    ischaemic necrosis, 164
    lichen planus, 146, 147, 161, 173
    lymphangioma, 283

malignant ulcer of, 200
neurilemmonas, 270
osteochondroma of, 81
sore, 161
strawberry, 140
    in syphilis, 141
tuberculosis of, 140
ulcers of, 161, 200
Torus mandibularis, 79, 80
Torus palatinus, 79
Toxoplasma gondii, 298
Toxoplasmosis, 220, 298
Treponema pallidum, 141, 296
Trigeminal herpes zoster, 16
Trigeminal neuralgia, 131
Trismus, 122, 201
    hysterical, 123
Trisomy 21 (Down's syndrome), 103, 106
Tuberculosis, 12, 140, *141*
    features of, 314, 315
    involving salivary glands, 220
Tuberculous osteomyelitis, 21
Tumour-like lesions, 59
Tumours,
    see also Cancer, Carcinoma etc
    benign or malignant, 6
    diagnosis, 4
    epithelial, 190
    frozen sections, 4
    lymphoreticular, 289
    mesenchymal tissue, 260–288
    neural tissue, 270
    non-odontogenic, 79–102
    odontogenic, 59–76
    seeding of cells, 9
    small dark cell, 8
Tzank cells, 151

Ulcers,
    in AIDS, 305, 307
    aphthous, 143
    in aspergillosis, 33
    in blastomycosis, 35
    eosinophilic, 100
    following radiotherapy, 11
    in hand-foot-and-mouth disease, 139
    in necrotizing sialometaplasia, 222, *223*
    non-infective, 142
    syphilitic, 141
    tongue, 161
    traumatic, 142
Ulcerative colitis, 143, 157
Ulcerative gingivitis, 137
Ultrasonics,
    for salivary gland tumours, 235
Ultrasonography, 12
Urethritis, 156

Uvula, bifid, 104, 110
Verruca vulgaris, 191
Verruciform xanthoma, 176, *176*, 192
Verrucous carcinoma, 201, 211, *211*
Verrucous hyperplasia, 211
Vincent's infection, 27
Vitamin B deficiency, 161, 180
von Recklinghausen's disease, 272

Warthins' tumour, 12, 235, 241, *241*, *242*
Warts, 191
Warty dyskeratoma, 152
Wegener's granulomatosis, 12, 309, *309*, 310, 314, 315
White sponge naevus, 166, *166*, *167*
Whitlow, herpetic, 138
Williams and Pollock syndrome, 273

Xanthogranulomas, 269
Xanthomas, 269
  verruciform, 176, *176*, 192
Xerostoma, 180
  causes of, 229
  functional causes, 230

Zygomatic bones, in thalassaemia, 112
Zygomycosis, 32